Pediatric Gastroenterology Case Studies

Pediatric Gastroenterology Case Studies

second edition

---

a compilation
of 64 clinical studies

William M. Liebman, M.D.
Director of Pediatric Gastroenterology
Children's Hospital Medical Center
Oakland and San Francisco, California

MEDICAL EXAMINATION PUBLISHING CO., INC.

Liebman, William M.
    Pediatric gastroenterology case studies.

    Bibliography: p.
    Includes index.
    1. Pediatric gastroenterology. I. Title.
[DNLM: 1. Gastrointestinal Diseases in infancy &
childhood--problems. WS 18 L716p]
RJ446. L52   1984   618.92'3309   84-1157
ISBN 0-87488-340-7

Printed in the United States of America

Contents

vi / Contents

Contents / vii

Preface

This collection of clinical studies represents a broad spectrum of characteristic problems encountered in the practice of pediatric gastroenterology. Each case consists of a brief history, a physical examination, and a list of pertinent laboratory data. A series of thought-provoking questions and fully discussed answers follows each case presentation. These questions were designed to help the clinician assess his or her knowledge of the given problem, and to stimulate further inquiry into especially interesting topics.

It is my hope that the material found within will serve as a catalyst for further study in the exciting and expanding "world" of pediatric gastroenterology.

Acknowledgments

The author wishes to express his thanks to the house staff and fellow colleagues for their diligent participation in the care of many of these cases. My thanks also to those of the secretarial staff who helped with the preparation of the manuscript.

notice

The author and the publisher of this book have made every effort to ensure that all therapeutic modalities that are recommended are in accordance with accepted standards at the time of publication.

The drugs specified within this book may not have specific approval from the Food and Drug Administration in regard to the indications and dosages that may be recommended by the author. The manufacturer's package insert is the best source of current prescribing information.

Case 1

RESPIRATORY DIFFICULTY AND
VOMITING IN A NEWBORN

HISTORY

A 3-day-old black female presented with increasing respiratory
distress since birth. There was associated intermittent cyanosis as well as the previously described progressive dyspnea. In
addition, with feedings there was recurrent vomiting, nonprojectile in nature, containing predominantly undigested formula.
There was no associated hematemesis, fever, diarrhea, melena, hematochezia, skin lesions, apparent swallowing difficulty,
and/or anorexia. The patient was the product of a full-term
pregnancy, apparently normal gestation and delivery, birth
weight 3.6 kg. The remainder of the past history, developmental history, family history, social history, and review of systems was noncontributory.

EXAMINATION

The patient was in moderate respiratory distress with no definite
cyanosis, increased respiratory rate 62 per minute, heart rate
160 per minute, normal temperature, weight 3.45 kg, length
52 cm. Examination of the chest revealed dullness to percussion and absent breath sounds in the left anterior and posterior
lung fields. The abdomen had a scaphoid appearance, with no
palpable masses, apparent tenderness, distention, and the liver,
spleen, and kidneys were not palpable. A few bowel sounds
were present with no bruits. Acrocyanosis was present but mucous membranes were still pink.

1

LABORATORY DATA

Hemoglobin:	14.2 gm%
Hematocrit:	43%
White blood cell count:	11,100/mm^3
PMN's:	58%
lymphocytes:	40%
monocytes:	1%
eosinophiles:	1%
Platelets:	250,000/mm^3
Urinalysis:	negative
Serum:	
sodium:	137 meq/L
potassium:	3.7 meq/L
chloride:	98 meq/L
bicarbonate:	18 meq/L
creatinine:	0.5 mg%
Chest X-ray:	(Fig. 1.1)
Upper GI series:	not done
Barium enema:	negative

QUESTIONS

1. The most likely diagnosis in this patient is
   A. tracheo-esophageal fistula
   B. diaphragmatic hernia
   C. duodenal ulcer
   D. hiatus hernia
   E. pyloric stenosis

2. The most common location of this condition is
   A. right foramen of Bochdalek
   B. right foramen of Morgagni
   C. left foramen of Morgagni
   D. left foramen of Bochdalek
   E. central defect

3. Common clinical features include which of the following?
   A. Dyspnea after birth
   B. Constipation
   C. Cyanosis after birth
   D. Diarrhea
   E. Feeding difficulties

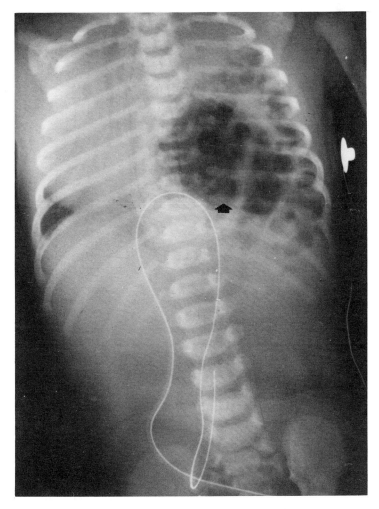

Figure 1.1   Chest film. A globular, air-filled structure is
visualized in the thoracic cavity, left side (arrow).

4.   The common physical findings include
     A. scaphoid abdomen
     B. displacement of maximal cardiac impulse
     C. absent breath sounds on the affected side
     D. visible peristaltic waves in the abdomen
     E. abdominal mass

5. Diagnosis is usually possible by which one of the following studies?
   A. Chest radiographs
   B. Electrocardiogram
   C. Barium swallow
   D. Liver-lung scan
   E. Fiberoptic upper endoscopy

6. Associated anomalies include
   A. pulmonary hypoplasia
   B. malrotation of intestine
   C. pyloric stenosis
   D. dextrocardia
   E. duodenal stenosis or atresia

7. Which of the following is the definitive treatment of this condition?
   A. Surgery
   B. Mechanical ventilation
   C. Digitalization
   D. Indomethacin
   E. Cimetidine

8. The prognosis in this condition is characterized by
   A. mortality rate of 15 to 30%
   B. mortality rate of 30 to 60%
   C. higher mortality rate in those operated upon in the immediate postnatal period or with associated anomalies
   D. decreased mortality rate in the last 10 to 20 years
   E. no change in prognosis in the last 10 to 20 years

ANSWERS AND COMMENTS

1. (B) The most likely diagnosis is diaphragmatic hernia. The presence of gas-filled bowel, i.e., stomach in this case, is demonstrated on the chest X-ray. The lung on the affected side is collapsed, and the mediastinum is displaced.

2. (D) The diaphragm is formed between the eighth and tenth weeks of gestation. (1,2) Abdominal and thoracic compartments are thereby formed. During this same stage, the gastrointestinal tract elongates into the umbilical pouch and is rotating for its return to the abdominal cavity. A disruption can lead to a diaphragmatic hernia. (1,2) A posterolateral defect in the diaphragm, the foramen of Bochdalek, is most common. More than 75 to 80% of this defect involve the left leaf of the diaphragm.

Only 1 to 2% of diaphragmatic hernias involve a retrosternal defect, the foramen of Morgagni. (1,2) The overall incidence of this anomaly is 1:4000 live births.

3. (A,C,E) The symptomatology will obviously vary according to the size and location of the defect. The most common defect, the foramen of Bochdalek, is usually large, and symptoms occur soon after birth. As gas fills the herniated bowel, dyspnea and cyanosis occur. In defects of the foramen of Morgagni, cardiorespiratory symptoms usually are milder or nonexistent, but large intestinal obstruction may be present in this defect. These symptoms principally occur with the left-sided defect, while the right-sided defect usually is associated with milder respiratory distress because the liver acts as a barrier, preventing to some extent bowel from occupying the right side of the chest. (1-9) The former defect has no sac, while the latter, an infrequent defect, usually has a membranous sac. (1-3) Feeding difficulties are present to a variable extent in all defects.

4. (A,B,C) Due to the herniated bowel occupying the chest, the abdomen will be scaphoid. Dullness to percussion and absent breath sounds will be present on the affected side. The maximal cardiac impulse site will be displaced. There will be a mediastinal shift. Peristaltic sounds over the back are not a reliable sign. (1-5,7-9)

5. (A) Roentgenographic studies will confirm the diaphragmatic hernia. Usually, contrast medium is not required because the air in the bowel will provide adequate contrast to prove the presence of intestine in the chest. Furthermore, the use of contrast medium, such as barium, may be dangerous because of possible vomiting and aspiration. However, at times, contrast studies will be necessary, usually in those patients with lesser cardiopulmonary distress. (1-5,7-9)

6. (A,B,D) The relationship of diaphragmatic hernia and survival is essentially determined by the extent of altered respiratory function. The herniated organs prevent differentiation of the lung, resulting in pulmonary hypoplasia. (1-9) This is more extensive with defects on the left side. (1-9) However, pulmonary hypoplasia is usually not present in hernias through the foramen of Morgagni. (1-9)

Midgut may be present in the chest due to a lack of normal mesenteric fixation, and thus, malrotation will be present. (1-9) Intestinal obstruction may occur due to peritoneal bands or even volvulus. (1-9)

7.   (A) Most newborns with diaphragmatic hernia are in significant respiratory distress and require immediate surgery. Oxygen must be administered; an endotracheal tube should be inserted, if necessary, after administration of a muscle relaxant. This will prevent further distention of the stomach and intestine by gas (air) forced down the esophagus. In addition, decompression of the stomach by nasogastric tube must be initiated. Ventilatory support in congenital diaphragmatic hernia is associated with a significant incidence of barotrauma, e.g., subpleural air bullae. (10) Bullous rupture can result in tension, extrapulmonary air, e.g., pneumothorax, while alveolar overdistention and rupture can result in pulmonary interstitial emphysema. These events play a role in the pathogenesis of pulmonary hypertension and cardiopulmonary decompensation. (10, 11) Surgery should be performed as soon as possible in these patients. In defects through the foramen of Bochdalek, an abdominal approach should be used in order to determine the presence of peritoneal bands or volvulus. The abdominal musculature can be stretched. If the abdominal cavity is still too small, only the skin should be initially closed. Conversely, some surgeons use the transthoracic approach in order to relieve pressure on the lung. (1-14)

For hernias of the foramen of Morgagni, surgery is recommended, although symptomatology is usually mild or nonexistent. An abdominal approach is usually used, although some surgeons use the transthoracic approach, too. (1-5,7-14)

The hypoplastic lung should be expanded carefully so as not to exceed its capacity. A catheter is left in place until the pleural space is filled completely by the fully expanded lung. However, altered aeration of the involved lobe may persist for months. Blood gas studies, previously demonstrating acidosis, low pO_2 and high pCO_2, should be followed periodically until return to normal. (1-5) Additionally, pulmonary hypertension may develop and may need medical therapy. Oral feedings may be possible on the second or third postoperative day. Gavage feedings may be preferable initially.

8.   (B, C, E) The highest mortality rate occurs in those infants with symptomatology within the first day or so of life and in those with associated malformations. (1-5, 7-14) The mortality rate continues to be high, 30 to 60%. (1-5, 7-14) Furthermore, this rate has essentially remained unchanged over the last 10 to 29 years. (1-5, 7-14) Finally, postoperatively, vasodilator responsiveness apparently has been shown to be an accurate indicator of survival chances in patients with persistent pulmonary hypertension and right to left shunts. (15)

REFERENCES

1. Raphaely, R.C. and Downes, J.J.: Congenital diaphragmatic hernia: Prediction of survival. J Pediatr Surg 8: 815, 1973.

2. Johnson, D.G., Deaner, R.M., Koop, C.E.: Diaphragmatic hernia in infancy: Factors affecting the mortality rate. Surgery 62:1082, 1967.

3. Pecora, D.U.: Ventilatory changes with Bochdalek-type diaphragmatic hernia. Am Surg 36:372, 1970.

4. Dibbins, A.W. and Wiener, E.S.: Mortality from neonatal diaphragmatic hernia. J Pediatr Surg 9:653, 1974.

5. Baran, E.M., Houston, H.E., Lynn, H.B., et al.: Foramen of Morgagni hernias in children. Surgery 62:1076, 1967.

6. DeLorimier, A.A., Tierney, D.E., Parker, H.R.: Hypoplastic lungs in fetal lambs with surgically produced congenital diaphragmatic hernia. Surgery 62:12, 1967.

7. Reale, F.R. and Esterly, J.R.: Pulmonary hypoplasia: A morphometric study of the lungs of infants with diaphragmatic hernia, anencephaly, and renal malformations. Pediatrics 51:91, 1973.

8. Allen, M.S. and Thomson, S.A.: Congenital diaphragmatic hernia in children under one year of age: A 24-year review. J Pediatr Surg 1:157, 1966.

9. Evans, C.J. and Simpson, J.A.: Fifty-seven cases of diaphragmatic hernia and eventration. Thorax 5:343, 1950.

10. Srouji, M.N., Buck, B., Downes, J.J.: Congenital diaphragmatic hernia: Deleterious effects of pulmonary interstitial emphysema and tension extrapulmonary air. J Pediatr Surg 16:45, 1981.

11. Adelman, S. and Benson, C.D.: Bochdalek hernias in infants: Factors determining mortality. J Pediatr Surg 11: 569, 1976.

12. Lister, J.: Recent advances in the surgery of the diaphragm in the newborn. Progr Pediatr Surg 2:29, 1971.

13. Chatrath, R.R., Shafie, M.E., Jones, R.S.: Rate of hypoplastic lungs after repair of congenital diaphragmatic hernia. Arch Dis Child 46:633, 1971.

14. Roy, C.C., Silverman, A., Cozzetto, E.J.: Pediatric Clinical Gastroenterology, 2nd edition. The CV Mosby Co., St. Louis, 1975, p. 99.

15. Bloss, R.S., Aranda, J.V., Beardmore, H.E.: Vasodilator response and prediction of survival in congenital diaphragmatic hernia. J Pediatr Surg 16:118, 1981.

Case 2

PERSISTENT VOMITING IN A 5-WEEK-OLD MALE

HISTORY

A 5-week-old male presented with a 2-week history of recurrent vomiting, nonbilious in nature. The vomiting would occur within 15 to 30 minutes after meals, the vomitus consisting of partially digested or digested food, and without bile. The vomiting was forceful, but the parents did not feel it was projectile. There was no associated regurgitation, fever, diarrhea, constipation, melena, hematochezia, hematemesis, jaundice, or skin lesions. The appetite was essentially unchanged and his activity level had remained relatively good. There was no similar illness in the parents, one sibling, 2 years of age, or in any individuals who had had contact with this patient. The patient was the product of a full-term pregnancy, normal gestational and delivery history, birth weight 6 lbs 7-1/2 oz. The remainder of the past history, developmental history, social history, family history, and review of systems was noncontributory.

EXAMINATION

He was a relatively alert, thin, 5-week-old white male in no apparent distress and with normal vital signs. Head circumference was 33 cm, weight 3.3 kg, length 53.5 cm. There was a possible palpable mass in the midline of the mid-upper abdomen, firm, small, and nontender. Active bowel sounds were present with no bruits. No persistaltic waves were noted. The remainder of the examination was unremarkable.

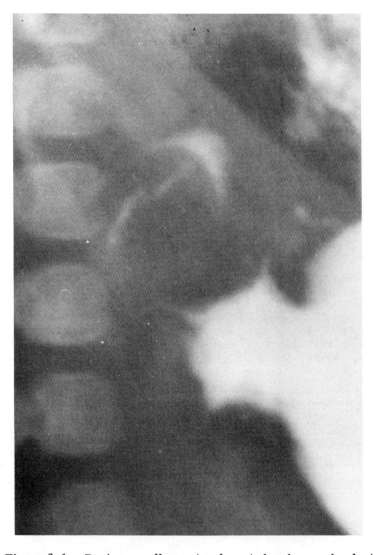

Figure 2.1   Barium swallow.   An elongated and curved pyloric
canal is shown.   The duodenal bulb is normal in shape but poorly filled.   No web or diaphragm is seen.

LABORATORY DATA

Hemoglobin:	11.9 gm%
Hematocrit:	35%
White blood cell count:	9,200/mm^3
PMN's:	45%
lymphocytes:	48%
monocytes:	5%
eosinophiles:	2%
Platelets:	225,000/mm^3
Sedimentation rate:	11 mm/hr
Serum:	
sodium:	132 meq/L
potassium:	3.8 meq/L
chloride:	92 meq/L
bicarbonate:	15 meq/L
total protein:	6.2 gm%
albumin:	4.6 gm%
SGOT:	24 units
alkaline phosphatase:	90 IU
Urinalysis:	negative
Chest X-ray:	negative
Plain films - abdomen:	gastric outline prominence
Upper GI series:	(Fig. 2.1)

QUESTIONS

1. A probable diagnosis in this child is
   A. chalasia
   B. achalasia
   C. gastric ulcer
   D. annular pancreas
   E. pyloric stenosis

2. Which of the following statements about this condition are correct?
   A. It is more common in males
   B. Its clinical presentation is predominantly in the first two weeks of life
   C. Acquired causes include trypanosomiasis (Chagas' disease)
   D. Abnormal serum gastrin levels have been frequently found
   E. Severe hypokalemia and alkalosis may result

3. Which of the following radiological findings are diagnostic
    of this condition?
    A. Double bubble pattern
    B. Railroad track sign
    C. Colon cut-off sign
    D. Shoulder sign
    E. Kantor's sign

4. Which of the following statements about treatment for this
    patient is correct?
    A. Corticosteroids are effective in reversing this condition
    B. Bougienage (dilatation) is the only effective treatment
    C. Surgery is the treatment of choice
    D. Antibiotics (broad spectrum) have been the medical
        treatment of choice
    E. There is no effective treatment for this condition

ANSWERS AND COMMENTS

1. (E) This patient has pyloric stenosis. Refer to answer 2.

2. (A,C,D,E) Pyloric stenosis is the commonest alimentary
disorder requiring surgery in the infant. The estimated incidence is 2 to 2.60 per 1,000 live births. (1-4) It usually pre-
sents at the age of 4 to 6 weeks, being characterized by vomiting, projectile in nature, associated weight loss, but voracious
appetite. Varying degrees of wasting result.
    Males are more often affected than females. In most series,
the sex ratio is 4 males to 1 female. (1-4) A genetic factor has
been suggested, and selective studies have confirmed an increased incidence in Caucasians. (1-4) An increased incidence
is also present in siblings, up to 30 times higher than anticipated. (1-4) Also, maternal relatives seem to have a higher incidence than paternal relatives. (1-5) This may relate to a
higher genetic load carried by females. (1,3) Descendants of
affected females seem to be most likely to develop hypertrophic
pyloric stenosis. (5) With regard to birth rank, despite conflicting reports, two recent studies have confirmed the predisposition of firstborn. Other implicated factors have included an increased incidence in blood groups O and B. (1-5)
    As previously mentioned, the usual presenting symptom is
vomiting, projectile and nonbilious in nature. There is associated weight loss coupled with a continued voracious appetite.
Constipation may result. The presenting signs may include abdominal distention, visible peristaltic waves traveling from the
left upper quadrant downward to the lower aspect of the right

upper quadrant, and the usual presence of an olive-sized mass in the midline of the mid-upper abdomen or in the right-upper abdomen. Evidence of dehydration is invariably present. The laboratory data include significant hypokalemia and metabolic alkalosis.

The etiology of this interesting entity has been the subject of numerous diverse studies. With pyloric ligation or even selective destruction of the myenteric plexus hypertrophic pyloric stenosis (muscle tumor) could not be reproduced. (6,7) Another focus of attention has been on a humoral factor or factors. Gastrin has been the main factor implicated in the etiology. Elevated levels of serum gastrin have been found, as well as elevated basal and peak acid outputs. (8,9) However, pyloric obstruction per se produces the previously mentioned changes, and therefore, what is cause and what is effect cannot be elucidated. More convincing, but not absolute, evidence has been the production of pyloric muscular hypertrophy in puppies by perinatal treatment with pentagastrin. (8) One explanation for the previously mentioned findings has been the common denominator of deranged gastric emptying. (8,9) Pyloromyotomy does not change mean fasting serum gastrin levels in infants. (10) Other areas of investigation have included attempted but generally unsuccessful viral and bacterial isolations. (9)

3. (B,D) The major roentgenological signs include the slow opening and elongation of the pylorus, narrowing of the pyloric canal (string sign), bending upward of the pyloric canal and indentation of the base of the duodenal bulb (shoulder sign), and layering of barium along the walls of the narrowed, elongated pyloric canal (railroad track sign). (1-5,11-14) In addition, erect survey films may demonstrate a frothy fluid level (fuzzy appearance of the air-fluid interface). (15)

4. (C) Surgery is the treatment of choice. (1-5,16-19) Use of anticholinergics, cholinergics, as well as other medical measures, are rarely if ever successful on a long-term basis. (16) Metoclopramide was not studied in this condition.

Electrolyte abnormalities must be corrected before surgical intervention. The Fredet-Ramstedt pyloromyotomy is the procedure most commonly employed and involves a splitting of the muscular layer of the pylorus, leaving the mucosa intact. (1-5, 17-19) During the first 24 to 36 hours after surgery mild vomiting may occur, but this subsides quickly. This procedure produces consistent, successful, and dramatic results.

REFERENCES

1. Dodge, J.: Infantile pyloric stenosis inheritance, psyche and soma. Irish J Med Sci 5:6, 1972.

2. Gerard, J.W., Waterhouse, J.A.H., Maurice, D.G.: Infantile pyloric stenosis. Arch Dis Child 30:493, 1955.

3. Carter, C.O. and Evans, K.A.: Inheritance of congenital pyloric stenosis. J Med Genet 6:233, 1969.

4. Laurence, K.M.: Hypertrophic pyloric stenosis. Lancet 1:224, 1963.

5. Hicks, L.M., Morgan, A., Anderson, M.R.: Pyloric Stenosis - A report of triplet females and notes on its inheritance. J Pediatr Surg 16:739, 1981.

6. Okamoto, E., Iwasaki, T., Katutani, T., Ueda, T.: Selective destruction of the myenteric plexus: Its relation to Hirschsprung's disease, achalasia of the esophagus and hypertrophic pyloric stenosis. J Pediatr Surg 2:446, 1967.

7. Mishalany, H.: Experimental study of the pathogenesis of congenital hypertrophic pyloric stenosis in puppies. J Pediatr Surg 2:212, 1967.

8. Dodge, J.A.: Neonatal pyloric hypertrophy and duodenal ulceration produced by pentagastrin. Gut 10:1055, 1969 (abstract).

9. Herweg, C., Middlekamp, J.N., Thornton, H.K., Reed, C.A.: A search into the etiology of hypertrophic pyloric stenosis. J Pediatr 61:309, 1962.

10. Wesley, J.R., Fiddian-Green, R., Roi, L.D., et al.: The effect of pyloromyotomy on serum and luminal gastrin in infants with hypertrophic pyloric stenosis. J Surg Res 20:533, 1980.

11. Jacoby, N.M.: Pyloric stenosis: Selective medical and surgical treatment. A survey of 16 years' experience. Lancet 1:119, 1962.

12. Olnick, H.M. and Weens, H.S.: Roentgen manifestations of infantile hypertrophic pyloric stenosis. J Pediatr 34: 720, 1949.

13. Caffey, J.: Pediatric X-Ray Diagnosis, 4th Edition. Year Book Medical Publishers, Inc., Chicago, 1961, p. 561.

14. Toccalino, H., Licastro, R., Quastavino, E., et al.: Hypertrophic pyloric stenosis. Clin Gastroenterol 6:279, 1977.

15. Matisonn, A.: The "frothy fluid level" in congenital hypertrophic pyloric stenosis. S Afr Med J 46:1963, 1972.

16. Day, L.R.: Medical management of pyloric stenosis. J Am Med Ass 207:948, 1969.

17. Benson, C.D. and Lloyd, J.R.: Infantile pyloric stenosis. Am J Surg 107:429, 1964.

18. Steinicke, O. and Roelsgaard, M.: Radiographic follow-up in hypertrophic pyloric stenosis after medical and surgical treatment. Acta Paediat (Uppsala) 49:4, 1960.

19. Wanscher, B. and Jensen, H.E.: Late follow-up studies after operation for congenital pyloric stenosis. Scand J Gastroenterol 6:597, 1971.

Case 3

BILIOUS VOMITING AND ABDOMINAL
WALL DEFECT IN A NEWBORN

HISTORY

A newborn white female presented with recurrent vomiting; the
vomitus contained bile-like material as well as digested foods.
In addition, there was associated abdominal protuberance and
an apparent abdominal defect. There was no associated history
of fever, hematemesis, diarrhea, constipation, jaundice, skin
lesions, or trauma. Appetite and activity remained unchanged.
Diet consisted of formula (Similac). The patient was the product
of a full-term pregnancy, normal delivery and gestational history. Birth weight was 7 lbs 2 oz. Pertinent family history
showed the mother with a history of supposed cow's milk intolerance during early childhood. The remainder of the past history, developmental history, family history, social history, and
review of systems was noncontributory.

EXAMINATION

She was alert, active, and in no distress, with normal vital
signs. Head circumference was 33 cm, length was 51 cm, and
weight 3.2 kg. The examination was unremarkable, except for
a midline abdominal defect (membrane covering) without normal
cord insertion. The anorectal examination was unremarkable.
Stool hemoccult examination was negative.

LABORATORY DATA

Hemoglobin:	14.3 gm%
Hematocrit:	44%

White blood cell count: $11,200/mm^3$
    PMN's: 48%
    lymphocytes: 43%
    monocytes: 6%
    eosinophiles: 3%
Serum:
    sodium: 141 meq/L
    potassium: 4.3 meq/L
    chloride: 104 meq/L
    bicarbonate: 22 meq/L
    calcium: 9.8 mg%
    glucose: 84 mg%
    total protein: 6.2 gm%
    albumin: 3.8 gm%
    total bilirubin: 0.8 mg%
    direct bilirubin: 0.4 mg%
    SGOT: 29 KU
    alkaline phosphatase: 110 IU
    amylase: 100 units
Urinalysis: negative
Stool:
    occult blood: negative
    reducing substances: negative
    culture: negative
    ova and parasites: negative
Chest X-ray: negative
Plain films - abdomen: (Fig. 3.1)

QUESTIONS

1. The origin of this defect is
   A. midgut (endoderm)
   B. neural tissue (ectoderm)
   C. skin (ectoderm)
   D. hindgut (endoderm)
   E. biliary tract (endoderm)

2. Which structures may be contained within this defect?
   A. Stomach
   B. Esophagus
   C. Liver
   D. Kidney(s)
   E. Spleen

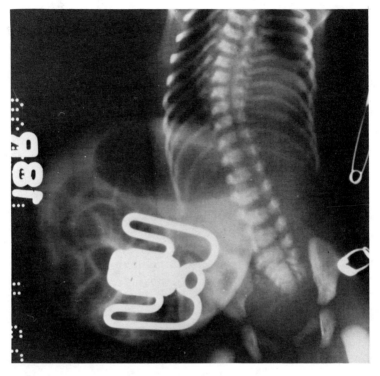

Figure 3.1   Plain film of the abdomen. Obvious large midab-domen defect extending outside body outline.

3.   This disorder has been associated with
     A. macroglossia
     B. hypocalcemia
     C. hydrocele
     D. hypoglycemia
     E. hydronephrosis

Question 4: Answer true (T) or false (F).

4.   When a large defect is present, malrotation is usually pres-ent.

5. Which one of the following complications may occur in larger defects?
   A. Duodenal ulcer
   B. Volvulus
   C. Intussusception
   D. Pancreatitis
   E. Necrotizing enterocolitis

6. After identification of this condition, which of the following constitutes appropriate treatment?
   A. At initial identification, covering of defect with moist dressings
   B. One-stage (primary) surgical repair, especially with defect less than 5 cm in diameter
   C. Primary surgical repair with any defect
   D. Staged surgical repair with any defect
   E. With large defects, staged surgical repair, using inert material covering such as silon sheets

ANSWERS AND COMMENTS

1. (A) Embryologically, the midgut lengthens, and a ventral loop connected by a stalk with the yolk sac extends into the so-called umbilical coelom. This loop allows further longitudinal growth of the small intestine. Several coiled loops form. After 10 weeks gestation these loops return to the abdominal cavity. If there is a delay in migration of these intestinal "coils" from the umbilical coelom, anomalies develop such as omphalocele, umbilical hernia. (1-4) Omphalocele occurs in approximately 1 of 6,000 live births, with a mortality nearing 50%. (1-4)

2. (C,E) With larger defects, liver, spleen, and/or parts of the gastrointestinal tract, essentially the small and large intestine may be contained within them. Omphalocele is distinguished from gastroschisis, a defect of the abdominal wall with evisceration, by the presence of a covering sac. In addition, the omphalocele does not have a normal insertion of the cord, as does gastroschisis. (1-5)

3. (A,D) The syndrome complex of omphalocele with macroglossia, advanced somatic development, adrenal cortical enlargement (hyperplasia), and neonatal hypoglycemia was first described in 1964 by Beckwith, et al. and Wiedeman. (6,7) Fifteen to thirty percent of omphaloceles are found in association with the previously described anomalies. (6-8)

4. (T) In larger defects of 5 cm in diameter or more at the base of the umbilical cord and with frequently contained structures, such as liver and spleen, malrotation is usually present. (1,2,5)

5. (B) In larger defects, malrotation is usually present, as mentioned in answer 4. In addition, due to the lack of significant attachment of this herniated intestine, volvulus may occur. (1-5)

Varying length of small intestinal atresia with resultant short bowel syndrome may also occur. Dependent upon this segmental length, nutritional consequences may be inconsequential to severe.

6. (A,B,E) Risk factors associated with mortality in infants with omphaloceles have included (1) size, (2) preoperative rupture, (3) treatment delay, (4) low birth weight, and (5) other anomalies. (3,4,12,13) Knight, et al., in particular, pointed out that assessment of the entire patient and not the size and associated mechanical problem in dealing with it is most useful in determining treatment modality.

When the omphalocele is identified, the sac should be covered with moist packs, and the abdomen wrapped. Nasogastric intubation and suction should be instituted in order to reduce and prevent an increase in size due to air accumulation in the intestine.

If the defect is 5 cm or less at the base of the cord, a primary (one-stage) repair can be contemplated. (9-15) In properly selected cases, replacement into the abdominal cavity and closure is very successful. (9-15) In larger defects, primary repair should not be attempted, or respiratory and vascular distress can result. Therefore, larger defects must be managed in a staged manner. Some authors, such as Firor (13), have mobilized skin and covered the sac, especially if it has ruptured. Others have advocated the use of prosthetic materials, such as silon sheets, for covering the defect and step-by-step reducing the contents into the abdomen. (5,9,15) Potential hazards of this approach include sepsis.

Firor (13) and a few authors have recommended a nonoperative approach (antiseptic applications) for those cases with an intact sac and a fascial defect over 2 cm in diameter, or with any part of a solid viscus in the sac. (5,9,15) Close observation is necessary. Over several weeks, complete resolution or satisfactory resolution to allow an easier surgical repair can be expected in as many as 80 to 89% of cases. (9-15) Complications have been no more frequent than with surgical approaches. (9-15)

REFERENCES

1. Mahour, G.H., Weitzman, J.J., Rosenkranz, J.H.: Omphalocele and gastroschisis. Ann Surg 177:478, 1973.

2. O'Neill, J.A. and Grosfeld, J.L.: Intestinal malfunction after antenatal exposure of viscera. Am J Surg 127:129, 1974.

3. Aitken, J.: Exomphalos. Analysis of a 10-year series of 32 cases. Arch Dis Child 38:126, 1963.

4. Knight, P.J., Sommer, A., Clatworth, H.W., Jr.: Omphalocele: A prognostic classification. J Pediatr Surg 16: 599, 1981.

5. Poh, V. and Schneiver, M.: Analysis of experience in therapy of omphalocele over the period of the last 15 years. Cesk Pediatr 21:426, 1966.

6. Beckwith, J.B., Wang, C.I., Donnell, G.N., et al.: Hyperplastic fetal visceromegaly with macroglossia, omphalocele, cytomegaly of adrenal fetal cortex, postnatal somatic gigantism, and other abnormalities. J Pediatr 65:1053 1964 (abstract).

7. Wiedeman, H.R.: Complexe malformatif familial avec hernia ombilicale et macroglossie - un "syndrome nouveau"? J Genet Hum 13:233, 1964.

8. Irving, I.M.: Exomphalos with macroglossia: A study of eleven cases. J Pediatr Surg 2:499, 1967.

9. Grob, M.: Conservative treatment of exomphalos. Arch Dis Child 38:148, 1963.

10. Kling, S.: Massive omphalocele: A method of treatment employing skin allograft. Can J Surg 10:455, 1967.

11. Schuster, S.R.: A new method for the staged repair of large omphaloceles. Surg Gynecol Obstet 125:837, 1967.

12. Simpson, T.E. and Lynn, H.B.: Omphalocele. Results of surgical treatment. Mayo Clin Proc 43:65, 1968.

13. Firor, H.V.: Omphalocele - An appraisal of therapeutic approaches. Surgery 69:208, 1971.

14. Girvan, D. P., Webster, D. M., Shandling, B.: The treatment of omphalocele and gastroschisis. Surg Gynecol Obstet 139:222, 1974.

15. Knight, P. J., Buckner, D., Vassey, L. E.: Omphalocele: Treatment options. Surgery 89:332, 1981.

Case 4

NONBILIOUS VOMITING AND ABDOMINAL
DISTENTION IN A NEWBORN

HISTORY

A newborn white male (1 day) presented with a history of vomiting which was initially nonbilious. There had been no passage
of meconium from the anorectal area. The patient was the product of a term pregnancy, apparently normal gestation, and the
delivery was stated not to be difficult. The remainder of the
past history, developmental history, family history, social history, and review of systems was noncontributory.

EXAMINATION

He had obvious abdominal distention and was in moderate distress, heart rate 180 per minute, respiration 50 per minute,
rectal temperature 37.8°C, head circumference 33.25 cm,
length 39 cm, birth weight 2.7 kg. The remainder of the examination was unremarkable except for obvious distention of the
abdomen.

LABORATORY DATA

Hemoglobin:	14.0 gm%
Hematocrit:	43%
White blood cell count:	$17,400/mm^3$
PMN's:	65%
lymphocytes:	31%
monocytes:	2%
eosinophiles:	2%
Urinalysis:	negative

Serum:
　　sodium:　　　　　　　　　　　134 meq/L
　　potassium:　　　　　　　　　　4.0 meq/L
　　chloride:　　　　　　　　　　　95 meq/L
　　bicarbonate:　　　　　　　　　19 meq/L
　　creatinine:　　　　　　　　　　0.6 mg%
　　SGOT:　　　　　　　　　　　　31 KU
　　total bilirubin:　　　　　　　　0.9 mg%
　　direct bilirubin:　　　　　　　　0.6 mg%
　　alkaline phosphatase:　　　　　164 IU
　　glucose:　　　　　　　　　　　82 mg%
Chest films:　　　　　　　　　　negative
Plain films - abdomen: dilated
loops of small bowel　　　　　　(Fig. 4.1)

QUESTIONS

1.　Which one of the following studies would be most helpful at this time in management?
　　A.　Complete blood count, sedimentation rate
　　B.　Intravenous pyelogram
　　C.　Upper gastrointestinal series
　　D.　Barium enema
　　E.　Proctoscopy

2.　Based on the previous laboratory and radiological data, which of the following is the probable diagnosis?
　　A.　Pyloric stenosis
　　B.　Intussusception
　　C.　Malrotation with midgut volvulus
　　D.　Annular pancreas
　　E.　Meconium ileus

3.　The usual clinical features, some evident in this patient, include which of the following?
　　A.　Vomiting (formula, bile-stained or not)
　　B.　Abdominal distention
　　C.　Hematemesis
　　D.　Malabsorption
　　E.　Ascites

Questions 4 and 5:　Answer true (T) or false (F).

4.　Malrotation is associated with other anomalies in 25 to 30% of cases.

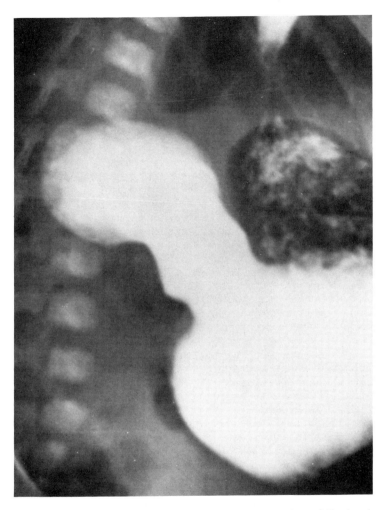

Figure 4.1   Barium swallow. Abrupt termination of the barium outline is evident in the proximal duodenum, first portion.

5.   When the diagnostic evaluation indicates the presence of volvulus in addition to malrotation, surgical intervention is mandatory.

6. More common problems or complications associated with
   this condition's surgical treatment include which of the fol-
   lowing?
   A. Recurrent volvulus
   B. Recurrent abdominal pain/constipation
   C. Duodenal stenosis
   D. Intussusception
   E. Intestinal pseudo-obstruction

ANSWERS AND COMMENTS

1. (C) Plain films of the abdomen may reveal no abnormality
in midgut volvulus in some cases or may reveal gaseous distention of stomach and proximal small intestine. Small amounts of
air may also be present in the lower abdomen. Barium enema
will usually reveal the malposition of the incompletely rotated
colon (failure of descent of cecum), but this does not imply a
symptomatic condition or the presence of other anomalies. (1-3)
The upper gastrointestinal series will demonstrate an obstructive pattern, generally with a compressed or twisted contour and
narrowing in the duodenojejunal region. Little or no barium
flows by this narrowed area. This patient provides an excellent
example of such a situation.

2. (C) Malrotation of the intestine relates to its abnormal
(faulty) movement around the superior mesenteric artery during
embryological development. (3,4) There is an upper duodenojejunal portion and a lower or colic portion (cecum downward)
which rotate sequentially. A rotational arrest can involve one
or both portions. This is a failure to complete the required
270º counterclockwise rotation, occurring between 10 to 12
weeks of gestation. (3-5) If both are affected, volvulus of the
midgut can result. Also involved is faulty fixation of the mesentery. (3,4) In addition, partial or complete obstruction of the
duodenum by peritoneal bands can evolve. Usually these bands
obstruct the second or third portions of the duodenum. (1-5)
Kinking of the duodenum can also result.

3. (A,B) Of symptomatic cases, an intestinal obstructive pattern is found within the first 30 days of life in 70 to 80%. (1-5)
Vomiting may not begin for the first two to three days. Ingested
formula or breast milk and/or bile-stained fluid may be vomited.
The vomiting will usually occur one to two hours after feedings.
(1-6) Abdominal distention will develop in the majority of cases,
but its presence primarily depends on the site of obstruction.

Constipation may ultimately develop. With the presence of volvulus, vascular compromise results, and its manifestations include melena, hematochezia, and, subsequently, signs of perforation and sepsis and/or peritonitis.

If the symptomatic pattern begins later in the first year or thereafter, intermittent obstruction is more characteristic, particularly related to meals. (1-5) In a small percentage of cases, a malabsorption-like picture may even develop, i.e., failure to thrive. (7-11) Lymphatic and vascular (venous) obstruction can be chronic, resulting in chronic diarrhea, steatorrhea, and even chylous ascites, a rare occurrence. (7-11) A recent review of 159 surgically treated cases revealed an incidence of 18% between 1 to 12 months of age and also 18% between 1 to 15 years of age. (11)

4. (T) Intestinal malrotation is associated with other abnormalities in 25 to 30% of cases. (5,9,11) These abnormalities can include annular pancreas, congenital atresia/stenosis (particularly in the duodenum), diaphragmatic hernia, tracheoesophageal fistula, and omphalocele. Moreover, nonrotation also has similar associated abnormalities. In most series, the most common intestinal abnormality is omphalocele or duodenal atresia stenosis. (5,9,11) The most common extraintestinal abnormality is congenital heart disease, e.g., ventricular septal defect. Extraintestinal abnormalities are relatively frequent. (5)

5. (T) When the diagnostic evaluation demonstrates the presence of volvulus of the midgut, surgical intervention is urgent. (3,11,12) Vascular obstruction quickly occurs with possible perforation, secondary sepsis, and peritonitis. (3,11,12) Mortality is high, 18 to 35%, and has been so for many years despite all surgical advances.

Surgical treatment consists of the initial reduction of the volvulus. Any peritoneal bands are divided, and most surgeons also perform prophylactic midgut fixation. (11,12)

6. (A,B) Recurrent volvulus and/or recurrent abdominal pain/constipation may occur, and did so more frequently in previous years because of failure of prophylactic midgut fixation. (5,11, 12) Since vascular obstruction, with resultant gangrene, etc., occurs not infrequently, small intestinal resection of variable length is necessitated, resulting not infrequently in short bowel syndromes. Malrotation has more recently been found to be associated with intussusception and, less so, with Hirschsprung's disease. (4,5,11,12) Treatment may be complicated due to the presence of the two conditions. (5) Intestinal pseudo-obstruction and duodenal stenosis are not encountered with any regularity,

even in a small percentage. Nutritional management may be difficult, possibly requiring enteral or parenteral programs.

REFERENCES

1. Berdon, W.E., Baker, D.H., Bull, S., et al.: Midgut malrotation and volvulus. Radiology 96:375, 1970.

2. Firor, H.V. and Harris, V.J.: Rotational abnormalities of the gut. Am J Roentgenol Radium Ther Nucl Med 120: 315, 1974.

3. Ree, J.R. and Redo, S.F.: Anomalies of intestinal rotation and fixation. Am J Surg 116:834, 1968.

4. Roy, C.C., Silverman, A., Cozzetto, F.J.: Pediatric Clinical Gastroenterology, 2nd Edition. The CV Mosby Co., St. Louis, 1975, p. 62.

5. Filston, H.C., Kirks, D.R.: Malrotation - The ubiquitous anomaly. J Pediatr Surg 16:614, 1981.

6. Pochaczeusky, R., Ratner, H., Leonidas, J.C. et al.: Unusual forms of volvulus after the neonatal period. Am J Roentgenol Radium Ther Nucl Med 114:390, 1972.

7. Verma, T.R. and Bankole, M.A.: Lymphovenous obstruction in anomalous midgut rotation. Arch Dis Child 48:154, 1973.

8. Zachary, R.B.: Intestinal obstruction. Progr Pediatr Surg 2:57, 1971.

9. Young, D.G. and Wilkinson, A.W.: Abnormalities associated with neonatal duodenal obstruction. Surgery 63:832, 1968.

10. Leslie, J.W.M. and Matheson, W.J.: Failure to thrive in early infancy due to abnormalities of rotation of the midgut. Clin Pediatr 4:681, 1965.

11. Stewart, D.R., Colodny, A.L., Daggett, W.C.: Malrotation of the bowel in infants and children. Surgery 79: 716, 1976.

12.   Brennom, W.S. and Bill, A.H.: Prophylactic fixation of
the intestine for midgut nonrotation. Surg Gynecol Obstet
138:181, 1974.

Case 5

ABDOMINAL DISTENTION, VOMITING, AND POOR FEEDING IN A 2-DAY-OLD MALE

HISTORY

A 2-day-old white male presented with abdominal distention, poor feeding, and recurrent vomiting, the vomitus being bile-stained. The patient had passed one meconium stool. There was no associated history of fever, diarrhea, melena, hematochezia, jaundice, lesions, or trauma. The patient was the product of a term pregnancy, normal gestation, and normal delivery, with birth weight 6 lbs 9 oz. The remainder of the past history, developmental history, family history, social history, and review of systems was noncontributory.

EXAMINATION

He was in moderate distress, with abdominal distention, heart rate 180 per minute, respiration 52 per minute, rectal temperature 37.9°C, head circumference 33 cm, length 50 cm, weight 2.85 kg. The remainder of the examination was unremarkable except for prominent abdominal distention, no visible peristalsis, no definite masses, questionably palpable bowel loops, and nonpalpable liver, spleen, and kidneys. Infrequent bowel sounds were present with no bruits.

LABORATORY DATA

Hemoglobin:	15.2 gm%
Hematocrit:	46%
White blood cell count:	10,600/mm^3
PMN's:	51%

lymphocytes:	43%
monocytes:	4%
eosinophiles:	2%
Urinalysis:	negative
Serum:	
sodium:	138 meq/L
potassium:	4.2 meq/L
chloride:	106 meq/L
bicarbonate:	25 meq/L
calcium:	9.4 mg%
glucose:	72 mg%
creatinine:	0.4 mg%
SGOT:	36 KU
alkaline phosphatase:	78 IU
total bilirubin:	0.8 mg%
direct bilirubin:	0.1 mg%
cholesterol:	100 mg%
ECG:	within normal limits for age
Chest films:	negative
Plain films - abdomen:	bubbly appearance in right lower quadrant
Barium enema:	decreased caliber or diameter of the entire colon (Fig. 5.1)

QUESTIONS

1. What probable underlying cause should be looked for in this patient?
   A. Pyloric stenosis
   B. Biliary atresia
   C. Cystic fibrosis
   D. Hirschsprung's disease
   E. Meckel's diverticulum

2. Which are common conditions associated with this disorder?
   A. Volvulus
   B. Intestinal atresia
   C. Hirschsprung's disease
   D. Tracheoesophageal fistula
   E. Pyloric stenosis

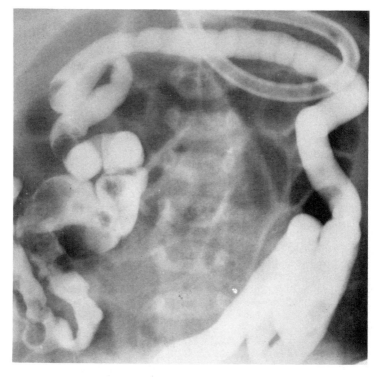

Figure 5.1   Barium enema. A small-diameter colon is evident.

3. Which of the following are the usual clinical features of this disorder?
    A. Abdominal distention
    B. Fever
    C. Bile-stained vomitus
    D. Melena
    E. Minimal or no meconium passage

4. The diagnosis should be established by which of the following studies?
    A. Three-way plain films of the abdomen
    B. Barium enema
    C. Upper gastrointestinal series
    D. CT scan of the abdomen
    E. 99mpertechnetate isotope scan

5. Treatment should usually consist of which of the following?
   A. Gastrografin enemas
   B. Oral acetylcysteine
   C. Pancreatic enzyme supplements
   D. Broad-spectrum antibiotics
   E. Surgery

Question 6: Answer true (T) or false (F).

6. The prognosis of this condition is excellent if early diagnosis and treatment are accomplished.

ANSWERS AND COMMENTS

1. (C) Meconium ileus occurs almost 90% of the time in association with cystic fibrosis. (1-8) Only 8 to 10% of patients with meconium ileus do not have cystic fibrosis. (1-8) The association with cystic fibrosis apparently begins before birth. However, more than one factor may be involved, the end result being abnormal viscosity of the meconium. (1-16) However, only 6 to 20% of newborns with cystic fibrosis have this complication. (1,6) One presumed factor is the markedly decreased to absent pancreatic enzyme production. (1-8) However, other studies indicated an alteration in the small intestinal glands and a more secondary role of the pancreatic status. (1,6) The meconium is thick and viscous, with a high albumin content and decreased water content, resulting in its inspissation. (1-8)

2. (A,B) There is a high incidence of associated anomalies, up to 50%, again suggesting an in utero process. These associations have included volvulus, atresia, secondary peritonitis, pseudocyst formation, and secondary microcolon as a result of proximal obstruction. (1-8,13-16) Local ischemia or kinking due to a twisting of these meconium-filled intestinal loops are thought to be the causes of these associated conditions. (1,6,14)

3. (A,C,E) Usually the infant becomes symptomatic within the first 24 to 72 hours of life. Progressive abdominal distention with associated bile-stained vomiting and decreased appetite develop as a result of the intestinal obstruction. (1-8,13-16) Meconium passage is minimal or absent. A history of hydramnios is found in 10%. (1-8,13-16) Obviously, if there are associated anomalies, such as atresia or volvulus, the clinical picture will develop sooner. (1-8,13-16)
   At birth, if there is ascites, undue distention, tenderness, or fever, antenatal perforation must be suspected. Postnatally,

sudden deterioration is also suggestive of perforation. In older children, similar clinical features may occur. This has been termed "meconium ileus equivalent." (6,7,14)

The usual level of obstruction by meconium is the terminal ileum. (1-8,13-16) Other anatomical abnormalities, such as atresia or stenosis, can be found distal to the involved intestinal segment. (1-8,13-16) In a small percentage, this meconium plug will actually pass spontaneously.

The physical examination usually reveals variable distention, full flanks, and possibly visible peristalsis. A palpable mass (meconium-filled loops) may be present (10 to 30%). (1-8, 13-16) The rectal examination may reveal a small anus and rectum.

4. (A,B) Newborns especially require prompt diagnosis and subsequent therapeutic intervention. Three-way plain films of the abdomen are the essential first step. In meconium ileus, distention of intestinal loops is present, as well as a relative absence of air-fluid levels, and possibly a bubbly granular or "soap bubble" pattern in the lower abdomen, especially the right lower quadrant. (1-8,13-16) Complications, such as perforation and peritonitis or volvulus, may not be evident from these plain films. Recent perforations may be suggested by the presence of free air. Antenatal perforation may be characterized by intra- or extraluminal calcifications, but these are seen in only 10 to 25% of such cases. (1-8,20) Testicular calcifications are an example of such extraluminal location, occurring only in 1-4% of antenatal perforations. (1,6,14) Barium enema examination will usually demonstrate variable microcolon and rule out associated volvulus or other conditions. (1-8,13-16) The meconium plug will be delineated.

5. (E) For almost all newborn infants, surgical exploration must be performed. It is particularly indicated in all complicated cases. The affected segment or segments are resected, and an end-to-side anastomosis is the usual procedure performed. This "Roux-en-Y" anastomosis allows evacuation of the intestine and distal segment. (1-8,13-21) Irrigation with pancreatic enzymes and mucolytic agents, such as acetylcysteine 5 to 10%, has been used, too. (17-19) More recently, Tween 80 administered through the enterostomy orally or rectally has been recommended. (17)

Meconium passed before surgery or obtained at surgery should be saved for subsequent analysis, including albumin content and fecal pancreatic enzyme levels. A number of simple rapid techniques are available, principally colorimetric in type. (11,12)

In some uncomplicated cases, medical treatment may be contemplated. Unfortunately, there are no definite criteria for uncomplicated meconium ileus. For such cases, successful management usually consisted of rectal administration of enemas, gastrografin (diatrizoatemethylglucamine) in particular. (17-19) Care must be used because of the markedly hyperosmolar nature of these enemas, approximately 1,900 mOsm/L. (17-19) Fluid and electrolyte balance must be closely watched, including serum electrolytes, intake and output. More than one enema may be needed. If the obstruction disappears, oral feedings can be reinitiated after a period of 36 to 48 hours. In addition, pancreatic enzyme supplements and usually oral preparations, such as acetylcysteine, are begun, together with oral feedings. (1-8, 13-18) However, for newborns with intestinal obstruction (uncomplicated meconium ileus) unrelieved by medical means per se, Harverg, et al. (4) utilized a T-tube ileostomy with postoperative irrigation of the intestine with pancreatic enzyme, and reported excellent results in a limited series of infants. (10, 11)

6. (F) The immediate mortality (the first 30 days) after operation is essentially the same for the uncomplicated and complicated group. (1-8, 13-16, 20, 21) This mortality rate has ranged between 30 to 80%. (1-8, 13-16, 20, 21) Ultimately, the long-term prognosis is poor, considering the high percentage of cases occurring secondary to cystic fibrosis. Thus, the prognosis will depend more on the pulmonary status than anything else. In those cases without cystic fibrosis, the outlook is good. (1-8, 13-16)

REFERENCES

1. Donnison, A.B., Shwachman, H., Gross, R.E.: Review of 164 children with meconium ileus seen at Children's Hospital Medical Center, Boston. Pediatrics 37:833, 1966.

2. Holsclaw, D.S., Eckstein, H.B., Nixon, H.: Meconium ileus: 20-year review of 109 cases. Am J Dis Child 109: 101, 1965.

3. Jaffe, B.E., Graham, W.P., Goldman, L.: Post-infancy intestinal obstruction in children with cystic fibrosis. Arch Surg 92:337, 1966.

4. Harberg, F.J., Senekjian, E.K., Pokorny, W.J.: Treatment of uncomplicated meconium ileus via T-tube Ileostomy. J Pediatr Surg 16:61, 1981.

5. Hill, J.T., Snyder, W.H., Pollock, W.F.: Uncomplicated meconium ileus. Arch Surg 88:522, 1964.

6. Grand, R.J.: Changing patterns of gastrointestinal manifestations of cystic fibrosis. Survey of recent progress in diagnosis and treatment. Clin Pediatr 9:588, 1970.

7. Cordonnier, J.K. and Izant, R.J., Jr.: Meconium ileus equivalent. Surgery 50:667, 1963.

8. Beck, A.R. and Alterman, K.: Intestinal obstruction and mucoviscidosis. Gastroenterologica 106:84, 1966.

9. Strober, W., Peter, G., Schwartz, R.H.: Albumin metabolism in cystic fibrosis. Pediatrics 43:416, 1969.

10. Shapira, E., Ben-Yoseph, Y., Nadler, H.L.: Decreased formation of alpha-2-macroglobulin-protease complexes in plasma of patients with cystic fibrosis. Biochem Biophys Commun 71:64, 1976.

11. Young, D.M., Schwent, G.W., Harris, J.S.: Viscosity and origin of meconium in meconium ileus. Proc Soc Exp Biol Med 99:673, 1958.

12. Green, M.N., and Schwachman, H.: Presumptive tests for cystic fibrosis based on serum protein in meconium. Pediatrics 41:989, 1968.

13. Leonidas, J.C., Berdon, W.E., Baker, D.H., et al.: Meconium ileus and its complications: A reappraisal of plain film roentgen diagnostic criteria. Am J Roentgenol Radium Ther Nucl Med 108:598, 1970.

14. Berk, R.N. and Lee, F.A.: The late gastrointestinal manifestations of cystic fibrosis of the pancreas. Radiology 106:377, 1973.

15. White, H. and Rowley, W.F.: Cystic fibrosis of the pancreas: The clinical and roentgenographic manifestations. Radiol Clin N Am 1:539, 1963.

16. Grossman, H., Berdon, W.E., Baker, D.H.: Gastrointestinal findings in cystic fibrosis. Am J Roentgenol 97: 227, 1966.

17. Bowring, A.C., Jones, R.F.C., Kern, I.B.: The use of solvents in the intestinal manifestations of mucoviscidosis. J Pediatr Surg 5:338, 1970.

18. Noblen, H.R.: Treatment of uncomplicated meconium ileus by gastrografin enema: A preliminary report. J Pediatr Surg 4:190, 1969.

19. Rowe, M.J., Furst, A.J., Altman, D.H., et al.: The neonatal response to gastrografin enema. Pediatrics 48: 29, 1971.

20. Dey, D.L.: Surgical treatment of meconium ileus. Med J Aus 50:179, 1963.

21. Komi, N., Miyanga, T., Murakami, K.: Meconium ileus and fibrocystic disease of pancreas in Japan. Bull Tokyo M/Dent Univ 13:1, 1966.

Case 6

ABDOMINAL PAIN, IRRITABILITY, AND
VOMITING IN A 10-MONTH-OLD BOY

HISTORY

A 10-month-old white male presented with an 8-day history of
recurrent, severe abdominal pain, associated crying, and frequent vomiting. He had 4 episodes of such abdominal pain during this period of time. Bowel movements were passed after the
attack of severe abdominal pain on three of the four occasions.
The pain lasted 30 seconds to a maximum of two minutes. Between these episodes of abdominal pain, the patient was described as being active and alert with a good appetite and no
symptomatology. Bowel movements were described as dark
brown with no blood and/or melena. The abdomen was described
as somewhat distended and apparently tender to touch. There
was no associated history of diarrhea, fever, hematemesis, melena, hematochezia, jaundice, skin lesions, or trauma. Urine
was described as clear to yellow in color with no bile or blood.
There was no apparent weight loss during this period of eight
days. The remainder of the past history, developmental history,
family history, social history, and review of systems was unremarkable.

EXAMINATION

He was alert, active, and in no apparent distress, with normal
vital signs, head circumference 36.5 cm, weight 8.8 kg, and
length 71 cm. The remainder of the examination was unremarkable, including the abdomen and anorectal area. However, at
the end of this examination the patient had another episode of severe abdominal pain, associated crying and ending with vomiting. Examination during this episode revealed moderate

abdominal distention, marked tenderness of the patient, generalized in nature and no definite mass, although a fullness was
present in the lower aspect of the right upper quadrant and right
midquadrant, and questionable emptiness of the right lower quadrant was noted. This episode of pain subsided with associated
vomiting occurring at the end; no bowel movement was passed
at this time.

LABORATORY DATA

Hemoglobin:	11.7 gm%
Hematocrit:	34%
White blood cell count:	11,900/mm^3
PMN's:	68%
lymphocytes:	26%
monocytes:	5%
eosinophiles:	1%
Urinalysis:	negative
Serum:	
sodium:	136 meq/L
potassium:	4.1 meq/L
chloride:	100 meq/L
bicarbonate:	20 meq/L
creatinine:	0.5 mg%
Plain film - abdomen:	(Fig. 6.1)
Barium enema:	(Fig. 6.2)

QUESTIONS

1. The most likely diagnosis in this infant is
   A. pyloric stenosis
   B. biliary atresia
   C. annular pancreas
   D. intussusception
   E. polyp (colon)

2. Which of the following statements about this disorder are
   correct?
   A. It is more common after 5 years of age
   B. The pain is of gradual onset
   C. Abdominal pain, nausea, vomiting, and bloody stools
      are common complaints
   D. A palpable mass is frequently found
   E. Radiological examination is not helpful

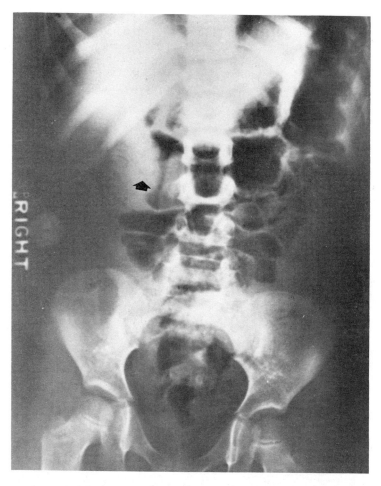

Figure 6.1   Plain film of abdomen. Abrupt termination of air
in colon proximal to hepatic flexure-right colon (arrow).

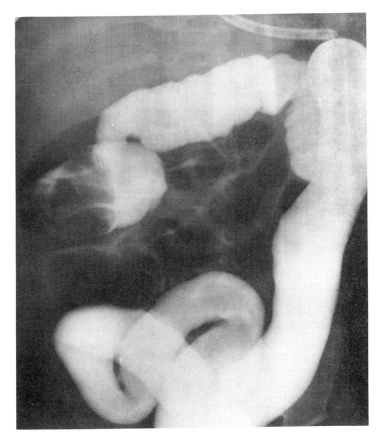

Figure 6.2   Barium enema. Absence of filling of the ascending colon and a coiled spring-like outline are shown.

3. Which of the following statements about treatment for this
    patient are correct?
    A. Hydrostatic pressure (barium enema) may be attempted
        initially
    B. Surgical reduction may be necessary
    C. Corticosteroids may be effective before surgery is con-
        templated
    D. Total parenteral alimentation (TPN) has recently been
        demonstrated to be effective therapy
    E. None of the above are correct

ANSWERS AND COMMENTS

1. (D) This patient has intussusception, with invagination of a
segment of the bowel (ileum) into an adjacent segment (cecum).
Refer to answer 2.

2. (C,D) Intussusception occurs from 3 weeks to 14 years of
age, mainly 2 months to 3 years of age. (1-11) Moreover, 55
to 60% of cases occur from 3 to 11 months of age. (3,7,11) It
is two to three times more frequent in males than in females.
(3,7,11,12) However, intussusception in older children has
been increasingly recognized and reported during recent years.
Turner, et al. (13) confirmed 37 children over the age of 2
years as compared with a composite group of 1,386 cases of intussusception, 77% under the age of 2 years. Only 3 of 37 patients had abdominal pain, lower gastrointestinal bleeding, vomiting, and a palpable abdominal mass. The delay in diagnosis
was longer, at least 48 hours. Thirty of 37 patients were surgically treated, the intussusception in 18 at the ileocecal valve,
and in 12 more proximal. (13)

The cause or causes of intussusception are not completely
settled. Five to fifteen percent of cases are due to anatomic
conditions, such as polyps, tumor, or Meckel's diverticulum.
(1-11) Other proposed etiologies include lymphoid hyperplasia,
especially in the ileocecal region, gastrointestinal allergy, hy-
perperistalsis, autonomic nerve imbalance, and viral agents,
such as adenovirus infection. (1-11) One main observation in
this age group has been the ileocecal valve projection into the
cecum, the small intestinal lumen, and a long mesocolon allowing mobility of the colon. (7,11) In general, the older the patient
the more likely there will be a definable anatomic cause. (1-3,
7,11)

The types of intussusception include ileocolic, the most common (70 to 91%), ileoileal, enteroenteral (jejunal especially),
and colocolic (sigmoid especially). (1-11) The average annual
incidence rate of all types has been 1 to 5 per 1,000 live births.
(3,7,11)

Most patients have abdominal pain, abrupt in onset, colicky
in nature, variable in location (80-95%), plus nausea and vomiting (80-95%). Bloody stools, generally without tenesmus, are
also frequent (40-60%). These stools have frequently been described as currant-jelly in type. Diarrhea, more so than constipation, may be present in some cases. A mass, sausage-
shaped in nature, on the right lower side of the abdomen is
found in 60 to 85% of cases. (1-11) Variable tenderness on abdominal examination is present. There may be a feeling of emptiness in the right lower quadrant (Dance's sign). Rectal

examination may reveal blood and mucus on the finger cot or occasionally a mass.

Laboratory studies, such as the white blood cell count and differential, are usually of little diagnostic merit except that a white cell count of more than 20,000 per cu mm^3 with a shift to the left is associated with a high incidence of vascularly compromised bowel in intussusception. (11) Additionally, barium enema probably should not be performed in these circumstances, and prompt surgical treatment should be considered. (7,11)

The diagnostic approach should also consist of a flat plate of the abdomen, which may reveal a staircase pattern or the obliteration of the usual gas shadows of the cecum and ascending colon with the head of the intussusception visible in the contiguous lumen of the colon. (1-11) Retrograde administration of barium may reveal the following findings: (1) colonic obstruction, usually in the proximal half, although it can be at any level from the anus to the ileocecal valve; (2) a filling defect in the head of the barium column (coiled-spring appearance); and (3) failure of barium to reflux into the ileum (at least 1 to 2 feet). (1-11)

3. (A,B) The duration of the symptomatic pattern and the type of and efficacy of the individual modes of therapy are intimately related. The longer the symptomatic pattern, the greater the need for surgical treatment and the higher the bowel resection rate. (1-11)

The principal forms of treatment are twofold, hydrostatic pressure (barium enema, colonic air or fluid inflation) and surgery (reduction/fixation with or without resection). Infrequently, spontaneous relief of the invagination occurs. Hydrostatic pressure reduction has long been the method of choice in the Scandinavian countries. (5-7,11) The aim of this treatment is slow but gentle reduction under low pressure. This type of treatment is contraindicated in the presence of peritonitis, gangrene, and tumors at the head of the intussusception. (5-7,11) The success rate of hydrostatic reduction has varied widely in series, 18-94%. (5-7,11) Surgical treatment consists of a milking out of the invaginated portion of bowel before strangulation and gangrene occur. If the bowel is in jeopardy or there is definite strangulation and/or gangrene, resection must be performed. As previously mentioned, the duration of symptomatology before treatment is instituted seems to dictate the type of and extent of surgery. If less than 12 hours, hydrostatic reduction can usually be attempted. Surgical treatment, if necessary, will usually consist of reduction and fixation only. (5-7,11) If less than 24 hours, the above is once again applicable. Occasionally, surgery will also consist of a localized resection. (1-11) If over 24 hours, many authors would advise against hydrostatic reduction at all, although this is not a settled issue. Surgical treatment will frequently consist of bowel-resection, usually 25 to 50% of cases. (1-11) The overall mortality in most series has varied from 0 to 10%, while the postsurgery recurrence rate has been 0 to 8%. (1-11)

REFERENCES

1. Peck, D.A., Lynn, H.B., Dushane, J.W.: Intussusception in children. Surg Gynecol Obstet 116:398, 1963.

2. Schoo, B.J.: The story of intussusception in an area of 750,000 people. J Ky Med Ass 68:145, 1970.

3. Cooke, D.C. and Lewis, E.C.: A 30-year survey of acute intussusception in childhood. Lancet 2:1359, 1960.

4. Benson, C.D., Lloyd, J.R., Fischer, H.: Intussusception in infants and children. Arch Surg 86:745, 1963.

5. Ravitch, M.M.: Intussusception in infancy and childhood: An analysis of 77 cases treated by barium enema. N Engl J Med 259:1658, 1958.

6. Santulli, T.V. and Ferrer, J.M., Jr.: Intussusception: An appraisal of present treatment. Ann Surg 143:8, 1956.

7. Ravitch, M.M.: Intussusception. In: Pediatric Surgery, 2nd Edition, Mustard, W.T., et al. (Eds.). Year Book Medical Publishers, Inc., Chicago, 1969, p. 914.

8. Dennison, W.M. and Shaker, M.: Intussusception in infancy and childhood. Br J Surg 57:679, 1970.

9. Farpour, A. and Nourmend, A.: Childhood intussusception. Clin Pediatr 9:210, 1970.

10. Ching, E., Ching, L.T., Lynn, H.B., O'Connell, E.J.: Intussusception in children. Mayo Clin Proc 45:724, 1970.

11. Roy, C.C., Silverman, A., Cozzetto, F.J.: Pediatric Clinical Gastroenterology, 2nd Edition. The CV Mosby Co., St. Louis, 1975, p. 105.

12. Hutchinson, I. F. , Olayiwola, B. , Young, D. G. : Intussusception in infancy and childhood. Br J Surg 67:209, 1980.

13. Turner, D. , Rickwood, A. M. K. , Brereton, R. J. : Intussusception in older children. Arch Dis Child 55:544, 1980.

Case 7

DIARRHEA IN A 4-WEEK-OLD FEMALE

HISTORY

A 4-week-old white female presented with a history of diarrhea since 2 to 3 days of life. The gestational history had been unremarkable except for an ultrasound examination at 34 weeks' gestation which revealed dilated bowel loops; delivery occurred within 3 days of the ultrasound examination, birth weight 2.3 kg. Within the first day of life, surgery was performed, including a small jejunal resection and jejunostomy as well as excision of a duplication of the proximal jejunum. Attempts at feeding, e.g., breast milk, elemental formulas, e.g., Vivonex, were characterized by diarrhea, loose to watery bowel movements, 6 to 13 daily, and inadequate weight gain. There was no history of fever, vomiting, melena, hematochezia, abdominal distention. The remainder of the past, family, and social history, and review of systems was unremarkable.

EXAMINATION

She was alert, in no apparent distress, with normal vital signs, weight 2.36 kg, length 42 cm, and head circumference 31 cm. The remainder of the examination was unremarkable, except for (1) gastrostomy, medial left upper quadrant; (2) minimal abdominal protuberance, no apparent tenderness and/or masses, but active bowel sounds present.

LABORATORY DATA

Hemoglobin: 11.7 gm%
Hematocrit: 34%

White blood cell count:	$12,300/mm^3$
PMN's:	65%
lymphocytes:	24%
monocytes:	10%
eosinophiles:	1%
Urinalysis:	negative
Serum:	
sodium:	136 meq/L
potassium:	3.7 meq/L
chloride:	100 meq/L
bicarbonate:	20 meq/L
creatinine:	0.7 mg%
total protein:	5.1 gm%
albumin:	3.0 gm%
total bilirubin:	3.8 mg%
direct bilirubin:	2.8 mg%
SGPT:	42 units
alkaline phosphatase:	136 IU
amylase:	72 units
Stool:	
smear:	1 to 3 WBC per HPF
hemoccult:	negative
reducing substances:	trace
culture:	negative
ova and parasites:	negative

QUESTIONS

Question 1: Answer true (T) or false (F).

1. The probable diagnosis of this patient is celiac disease.

2. Common conditions associated with short bowel syndrome
    include
    A. intestinal malrotation and volvulus
    B. pyloric stenosis
    C. duodenal ulcer
    D. Meckel's diverticulum
    E. Crohn's disease

3. Clinical features include
    A. diarrhea
    B. constipation
    C. gastric hypersecretion
    D. intestinal hypomotility
    E. malabsorption (carbohydrate, fat, protein)

4. The treatment of this condition may include which of the following?
   A. Diet for age
   B. Elemental diet, formula
   C. Parenteral alimentation
   D. Antibiotics
   E. Steroids

5. Which of the following are important factors influencing the ultimate prognosis?
   A. Age of diagnosis
   B. Birth weight
   C. Extent of resection
   D. Area of small intestinal resection
   E. Preservation or not of ileocecal valve

ANSWERS AND COMMENTS

1. (F) Factors, such as the age of the patient and, most importantly, the lack of exposure to gluten products (gliadin) would eliminate celiac disease (gluten enteropathy) as the diagnosis. Refer to answers 2 through 5.

2. (A, E) The short bowel syndrome comprises alterations of gastrointestinal motility, digestion, absorption, and secretion. These abnormalities occur due to a loss of significant lengths of the small intestine. With extensive loss of the small intestine, there results less time of exposure for digestion (motility) and less area for absorption. With significant loss of small intestinal surface area, loss of enzymes, such as hydrolytic of the brush border, e.g., disaccharidases (particularly, lactase), and loss of bile acids, with loss of the ileum, can occur. (1-5,7)
   In the neonate, conditions leading to extensive loss of the small intestine include intestinal malrotation with volvulus or with bands, atresia of the jejunum and ileum, omphalocele and gastroschisis, duplications, congenital short bowel, and neoplasms. In older infants and children, associated conditions include inflammatory bowel disease, specifically, Crohn's disease, intussusception, intestinal by-pass procedures, e.g., obesity. (1-6) Many of these conditions are caused by vascular accidents, antenatal (gastroschisis, atresias) or postnatal (hypercoagulation), and inflammation (necrotizing enterocolitis, Crohn's disease). (1-7)

3. (A,C,E) The clinical findings of extensive loss of small intestinal surface area are principally failure to thrive (starvation) and diarrhea. (1-7) Generally, there is little or no abdominal discomfort, and the patient's appetite is normal or excessive, unless abdominal distention with or without nausea and vomiting are present. The latter usually signify obstruction, e.g., stricture, stagnant loop. (1-7) As previously mentioned, the diarrhea tends to be quite impressive initially but then will resolve to variable degree as adaptation occurs. The latter would involve an increase in the absorptive area of the remaining small intestine, i.e., diameter, length, and thickness of the wall, as well as an increase in villus size (widening) and length. (1-9) Additionally, the shortened transit time, as measured by a nonabsorbable marker, e.g., carmine red, becomes less marked, as does gastric hypersecretion, present in 30 to 50% of patients. Interestingly, serum gastrin levels have been, and continue to be, normal. (1,2,5) The net result of the decrease in the early negative changes of the short bowel syndrome is a corresponding increase in the absorptive ability for fat, protein, and carbohydrate. This improvement is more evident and more consistently present in the ileum with proximal resections than in the jejunum with distal resections. (1-7) Moreover, with reference to distal resections, the ileum and its microvilli possess specific receptor sites for their role in the absorption of vitamin B_{12} - intrinsic factor complex, calcium, conjugated bile acids, and iron. Therefore, in ileal resections, fecal losses of bile acids may actually exceed the capacity of the liver to maintain critical micellar concentration for micellar solubilization and, thus, affect fat digestion and absorption, resulting in steatorrhea. (1,2,7)

Laboratory features include anemia, hypoproteinemia, low serum carotene and cholesterol levels, as well as low calcium and magnesium levels (tetany). With the resultant steatorrhea, vitamin D and other fat-soluble vitamin values will be low and result in impaired functional capability, e.g., coagulation (vitamin K). Electrolytes, as well as water, may also be lost in excessive amounts, too, e.g., potassium (muscle cramps). (Refer to Table 7.1.)

Lastly, the ileocecal valve acts as a physiological barrier to colonic microflora. Its resection could result in bacterial colonization of the remaining small intestine. Deconjugation of bile acids with increased steatorrhea and diarrhea could then occur. Additionally, vitamin B_{12} could be metabolized, and its deficiency would be increased. The general adaptive response could be compromised, too. (1-7)

TABLE 7.1   Nutrient Absorption in Small Intestine

Area	Nutrients
Duodenum	iron calcium carbohydrate vitamins (water-soluble)
Jejunum	carbohydrate fat proteins folic acid vitamins (water-soluble, fat- soluble) bicarbonate water, electrolytes
Ileum	vitamin B_{12} bile acids water electrolytes

Note: absorption of water and electrolytes in colon

4. (B,C,D) The patient with extensive loss of small intestine
is a long-term challenge. Information regarding the area and
extent of intestinal resection, the fate of the ileocecal valve,
the anastomosis, presence of infection or not, and condition of
the remaining small intestine should be available to the medical
personnel so as to formulate the most appropriate management
plan.

The overall goal of treatment is to allow the patient to survive until adaptation of the remaining small intestine can occur.
Therefore, selection of a diet is paramount. The diet must be
tolerated and yet supply nutrients in required amounts for
growth and development and adaptation to result. With reference
to carbohydrate, extensive loss of small intestine usually leads
to lactose intolerance (lactase insufficiency) and frequently to
sucrose intolerance, too (sucrase insufficiency). Therefore,
glucose is the most reasonable choice, since it is efficiently absorbed without enzyme hydrolysis. Glucose is an osmotically
active substance, and patients are sensitive to hypertonic feedings. Therefore, isotonic or hypotonic feedings must be used

initially. Glucose polymers, such as Polycose®, seem to minimize even this effect. (1-7,10-12) With regard to fat, intolerance is the usual rule because of bile acid malabsorption and reduced bile acid pool, decreased pancreatic stimulation and resultant secretion, and reduced coefficient of absorption (motility). (1,2,6,7) Therefore, medium chain triglycerides are better tolerated since they essentially do not require bile acids for
digestion and also are partially water-soluble. (1-7,10-12) With
regard to protein, whole protein is not as well absorbed as some
predigested protein or amino acids due to the decreased absorptive surface area. (1-7) Low molecular weight peptides or amino acids are efficiently absorbed, the former by initial hydrolysis at the brush border before transport into the intestinal cells.
(1-7) With regard to other nutrients, such as fat-soluble vitamins, calcium, and magnesium, supplementation is frequently
necessary. If the ileum has been resected, vitamin B_{12} treatment will be necessary, a minimum of 4 to 5 years. (1-7,10-12)

Practically, the combination of protein hydrolysates or amino acids, medium-chain triglycerides with lesser or small
amounts of long-chain triglycerides (essential fatty acid fraction), and monosaccharide with polysaccharides, rather than
disaccharides, can be found in the elemental formula/liquid
e.g., Vivonex, Pregestimil, Vital, Portagen, Modular formula.
One-fourth to one-half strength formula/liquid is used initially,
at a volume of 10 to 50 ml/kg/24 hr, dependent upon the extent
of resection and similar factors, as previously discussed. Usually volume is increased initially, 5 to 15% every 1 to 3 days,
before strength (caloric density) is increased gradually to full
strength, e.g., Pregestimil, 0.67 cal/ml, 350 mosmoles. (Refer to Table 7.2.)

Frequent small feedings are used, as possible, and if not
tolerated, tube or ostomy, e.g., gastrostomy, feedings are attempted, generally continuous drip in type, rather than bolus.
Infusion drip time can be progressively decreased to 12 to 14
hours, e.g., night, for psychosocial purpose, and on an outpatient as well as inpatient basis. Monitoring of stool output (vol-
ume/weight) and reducing substances, intake volume and calories, and patient weight is indicated for evaluation of tolerance
or not. Respiratory hydrogen secretion can be used to further
assess the adaptive response. (13)

Parenteral alimentation is usually necessary when there is
severe malabsorption and inadequate oral caloric intake. For
a time period greater than 2 weeks, central catheter use is usually necessary rather than peripheral vein alimentation, e.g.,
conditions resulting in less than 60 to 80 cm of small intestine
remaining. (1,2,5,10-12) Oral intake is usually maintained even

TABLE 7.2   Selected Special Chemically Defined Diets

Product	Carbohydrate	Fat	Protein
Ensure (Ross)	sucrose corn syrup	corn oil	casein soy
IsoCal (Mead Johnson)	sucrose corn syrup	soy oil medium-chain triglycerides	casein
Nutramigen (Mead Johnson)	sucrose tapioca	corn oil	hydro-lyzed casein
Osmolite (Ross)	corn starch	corn oil medium-chain triglycerides soy oil	casein soy
Pregestimil (Mead Johnson)	corn syrup glucose tapioca	corn oil medium-chain triglycerides	hydro-lyzed casein
ProSobee (Mead Johnson)	corn syrup	soy oil coconut oil	soy
RCF (Ross)	none	soy oil coconut oil	soy
Travasorb (Travenol)	oligosaccharides	medium-chain triglycerides sunflower oil	soy
Vital (Ross)	sucrose glucose oligosaccharides polysaccharides	sunflower oil medium-chain triglycerides	peptides amino acids
Vivonex (Norwich Eaton)	glucose oligosaccharides	safflower oil	amino acids

at low amounts, since luminal nutrition has a definite positive
effect (hastening) on small intestinal mucosal adaptation.

Medication may be necessary in selected patients. Antidiarrheal agents, e.g., anticholinergics, opiates, should not be
used. Antacids and H_2 receptor antagonists, e.g., cimetidine
(Tagamet®), have been tried in infants and children with mar-
ginal results in regard to gastric hypersecretion. Cholestyramine (Questran®), generally 4 to 12 grams daily (divided doses,
with meals), can be useful in treating the diarrhea caused by
bile acid losses and their action on colonic mucosa (cholerrheic).
Aluminum hydroxide salts should be an alternative to cholestyramine for bile acid binding. (1,2,5,6) Antibiotics, broad-spectrum (aerobic, anaerobic), may be helpful if the contaminated
small bowel is suggested or confirmed. Bacteria overgrowth is
present, and appropriate antibiotic choices will ensure a positive
response, i.e., control of bacterial colonization. However,
the underlying cause, e.g., stagnant loop, must be identified.
Steroids have essentially no clinically proven role in the adaptive response per se. (1,2,5,6)

5. (C,D,E) The outcome after extensive loss of small intestine is dependent predominantly on the following factors: (1) extent of resection; (2) area of the small intestine removed, e.g.,
jejunum, ileum; (3) functional capability of remaining small intestine; (4) preservation of the ileocecal valve; and (5) adaptive
response of remaining small intestine (degree of). (1,2,5,14,
15) The presence of associated anomalies, significant prematurity, post resection symptomatology, e.g., abdominal distention, vomiting, adds to the risk of survival.

Rickham, et al. (14) reported on a 10- to 18-year follow-up
of 9 patients, 8 of 9 being normal. Most patients become
"asymptomatic" by 20 to 24 months of age, and can consume a
relatively normal diet, except for fat. (1,2,5,6,9) Developmental delay is common, but its relationship to the short bowel syndrome is tenuous. (1,2,5) Therefore, the overall consensus is
early, aggressive treatment in patients with significant small intestinal resection, since survival is likely. (1,2,5,14,15)

For additional dietary information, refer to Tables 7.3 and
7.4.

TABLE 7.3 Recommended Daily Dietary Allowances[a]

Age (years)	Energy (cal/kg)	Protein (grams)	Fluid (ml/kg)
0-1	100-115	1.7-2.2	80-150
1-3	90-110	1.5-2.0	80-125
4-6	80-100	1.2-1.8	75-100
7-12	75-90	1.0-1.5	60-90
over 12-13	60-75	0.75-1.2	25-60

[a]Adapted from the recommendations of the National Academy of Sciences and American Dietetic Association

TABLE 7.4 Nutritional Assessment of Pediatric Patients

History
    Previous growth record
    Illness(es)
    Social/Family history
    Medication

Diet
    Feeding history
    Socioenvironmental factors
    Content
    Food intolerances

Anthropometrics
    Recumbent length/height, weight, head
        circumference (less than 3 years)
    Triceps skinfold thickness (fat)
    Midarm circumference
    Midarm muscle circumference (muscle mass)

TABLE 7.4   Nutritional Assessment of Pediatric Patients (Cont'd)

Laboratory
　　Hemoglobin, hematocrit
　　Total lymphocyte count (visceral protein)
　　　creatinine (urine)/height index
　　　serum albumin, prealbumin, and transferrin levels

Physical Examination
　　Skin
　　Mucous membranes
　　Dentition
　　Muscle
　　Nervous system

REFERENCES

1.   Daum, F., Silverberg, M.: Effect of congenital anomalies of the gastrointestinal tract on infant nutrition. In: Textbook of Gastroenterology and Nutrition in Infancy. E. Lebenthal (ed). Raven Press, New York, 1981, p. 921.

2.   Klish, W.J., Putnam, T.C.: The short gut. Am J Dis Child 135:1056, 1981.

3.   Williamson, R.C.N.: Intestinal adaptation. N Engl J Med 298:1393, 1443, 1978.

4.   Greenberger, N.J.: The management of the patient with short bowel syndrome. Am J Gastroenterol 70:527, 1978.

5.   Silverman, A., Roy, C.C.: Pediatric Clinical Gastroenterology, 3rd Edition. The CV Mosby Company, St. Louis, 1983, p. 287.

6.   Compston, J.E., Creamer, B.: The consequences of small intestinal resection. Q J Med 46:485, 1977.

7.   Krejs, G.J.: The small bowel. I. Intestinal resection. Clin Gastroenterol 8:373, 1979.

8.   Rickham, P.P.: Subtotal intestinal resection in the newborn. Ann Chir Infant 18:173, 1977.

9. Weser, E.: Intestinal adaptation after small bowel resection. Viewpt Dig Dis 10:1, 1978.

10. Bohane, T.D., Haka-Ikse, K., Biggar, W.D., et al.: A clinical study of young infants after small intestinal resection. J Pediatr 94:552, 1979.

11. Buts, J.P., Morin, C.L., Ling, V.: Influence of dietary components on intestinal adaptation after small bowel resection in rats. Clin Invest Med 2:59, 1979.

12. Tefas, J.J., MacLean, W.C., Kolbach, S., et al.: Total management of short gut secondary to midgut volvulus without prolonged total parenteral alimentation. J Pediatr Surg 13:622, 1979.

13. Shermeta, D.W., Ruaz, E., Fink, B.B., et al.: Respiratory hydrogen secretion: A simple test of bowel adaptation in infants with short gut syndrome. J Pediatr Surg 16:271, 1981.

14. Rickham, P.P., Irving, I., Shmerling, D.H.: Long-term results following extensive small intestinal resection in the neonatal period. Prog Pediatr Surg 10:65, 1977.

15. Wilmore, D.W.: Factors correlating with a successful outcome following extensive intestinal resection in newborn infants. J Pediatr 80:88, 1972.

Case 8

RECURRENT RECTAL BLEEDING IN A 2-YEAR-OLD GIRL

HISTORY

A 2-year-old white female presented with a recurrent history of hematochezia for a duration of 12 months, increasingly severe and recurrent during the last 2 to 3 weeks. Bowel habit pattern consisted of one bowel movement daily, firm to soft in nature, and there was no associated history of melena, abdominal pain, fever, diarrhea, anorexia, dysuria, skin lesions, vomiting, jaundice, or trauma. Her private physician's evaluation included a barium enema which was negative, upper GI-small bowel series which was also negative, and anoscopy which was negative. Her treatment included Colace for stool softening and Anusol-Hydrocortisone suppositories without apparent improvement. Her activity had been unchanged. Two prior stool studies for culture only had been performed, which were negative. The remainder of the past history, developmental history, family social history, and review of systems was unremarkable.

EXAMINATION

She was alert, active, and in no distress, with normal vital signs, weight 14 kg, height 88 cm, and head circumference 48.5 cm. The remainder of the examination was unremarkable, including the abdomen and anorectal area.

LABORATORY DATA

Hemoglobin:	11.6 gm%
Hematocrit:	34%

White blood cell count:	$10,500/mm^3$
PMN's:	48%
lymphocytes:	50%
monocytes:	1%
eosinophiles:	1%
Reticulocyte count:	1.3%
Sedimentation rate:	10 mm/hr
Urinalysis:	negative
Serum:	
carotene:	150 μg%
folate:	14 ng/ml
total protein:	6.0 gm%
albumin:	4.2 gm%
total bilirubin:	0.7 mg%
direct bilirubin:	0.4 mg%
alkaline phosphatase:	140 IU
SGPT:	18 units
IgG:	720 mg%
IgA:	48 mg%
IgM:	98 mg%
creatinine:	0.6 mg%
Stool:	
reducing substances:	negative
culture:	negative
ova and parasites:	negative
Proctosigmoidoscopy:	negative
Rectal biopsy:	negative
$99m$Pertechnetate isotope scan:	(Fig. 8.1)
Barium enema:	negative
Upper GI - small bowel series:	negative

QUESTIONS

Questions 1-9: Answer true (T) or false (F).

From the history and physical examination you may assume that
1. the probable diagnosis is not Meckel's diverticulum.
2. this anatomical entity is present in 1 to 2% of the population, the majority being asymptomatic.
3. there is equal sex incidence of this condition.
4. the presence of heterotopic tissue is unusual.
5. the chief complaint is abdominal pain.
6. rectal hemorrhage is frequent and can be bright red, dark red, or tarry in nature.
7. complications include intestinal obstruction, diverticulitis, perforation, or severe rectal hemorrhage.

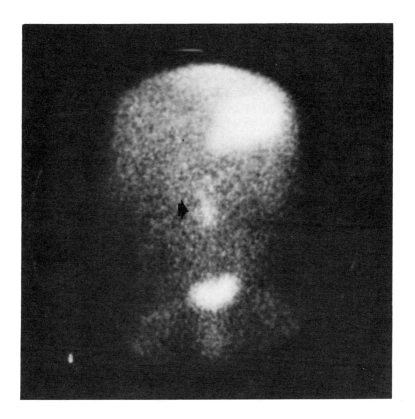

Figure 8.1 99m Tc-Pettechnetate scan. Accumulation of
dye (arrow) is present in the midabdomen at the same time as
the gastric outline is seen.

8. the main diagnostic study is upper gastrointestinal series.
9. surgery is the treatment of choice.

ANSWERS AND COMMENTS

1. (F) The probable diagnosis is Meckel's diverticulum. Refer to answers 2 to 9.

2. (T) Meckel's diverticulum is the vestigial remnant of the
omphalomesenteric duct and is present in 1 to 3% of the population. (1-3) The vast majority are asymptomatic. Meckel's

diverticulum is located in the distal ileum, usually within 3 to 4 feet of the ileocecal valve. (1-3) It is antimesenteric in course, has its own blood supply, and has a narrower lumen than base. (1-4)

3. (F) In toto, Meckel's diverticulum is two to three times more frequent in males than females. (1-3) Complications of this disease entity are three to five times more frequent in males than females. (1, 2)

4. (F) Heterotopic tissue is present in 50 to 70% of cases, and this likelihood is increased eight to tenfold in symptomatic cases. (1-3) The majority of cases with heterotopic tissue have gastric mucosa (50 to 80%), the rest being in order of frequency, pancreatic, jejunal, and colonic. (1-6) Meckel's diverticulum has also been noted to have an increased incidence in association with other malformations, e.g., esophageal atresia, anorectal agenesis, neurological and cardiovascular abnormalities. (3) The vast majority of such cases present in the first two years of life. (1-6)

5. (F) Rectal bleeding is the chief complaint, occurring in 40 to 70% of symptomatic cases. (1-6) Refer to answer 6.

6. (T) Rectal bleeding is the chief complaint in Meckel's diverticulum. As previously mentioned, the vast majority present in the first two years of life either as profuse asymptomatic (painless) rectal bleeding or as recurrent bleeding. The predominant form of bleeding is bright red only, 5 to 10%; dark red only, 25 to 50%; both bright and dark, 15 to 25%; tarry only, 5 to 10%; or in combination with the other types, 5 to 10%. (1-5) Severe anemia and/or shock is not infrequent. In those patients with recurrent bleeding, the majority have had their episode or episodes within a year, the amounts being smaller than the one being investigated. (1-5) In the overwhelming majority of those with hemorrhage, gastric mucosa with erosive or ulcerating change(s) is found. (1-5)

7. (T) Intestinal obstruction occurs in 10 to 20% of symptomatic cases of Meckel's diverticulum. (1-3) One of two main forms of obstruction is volvulus, the twisting of bowel around a fibrous remnant of the omphalomesenteric duct, connecting the diverticulum to the abdominal wall. (1, 2) Infarction of such is usually present. (1, 2) The predominant form is intussusception, the diverticulum acting as the leadpoint, and presenting the symptomatic pattern of ileocolic intussusception. (1, 2) Once again, infarction rapidly and frequently ensues. (1, 2) On physical

examination a mass can frequently be palpated in the right lower quadrant, in addition to frequent signs of tenderness, localized and/or generalized. Other forms of obstruction have included strangulation in an inguinal hernia, adhesions secondary to prior diverticulitis, and involvement of a mesodiverticular band, vascular in nature, to the tip of the diverticulum from the base of the mesentery. (1,2)

Diverticulitis occurs in 1 to 10% of cases and can be indistinguishable from acute appendicitis. (1-5) In addition, the nature of pain and the physical findings, including the Rovsing's psoas and obturator signs, may precisely mimic acute appendicitis. Perforation with peritonitis may also occur. (1-5)

8. (F) The differential diagnosis, dependent upon age, may include anal fissure, volvulus, intussusception, colonic polyp, ulcerative colitis, intestinal parasitosis, and blood dyscrasia. Thus, a rectosigmoidoscopy, coagulation profile, and stool examination (gram stain, culture, ova and parasites) should be considered and performed as the situation dictates. In many cases the child's clinical status must first be stabilized, including transfusion(s), before further diagnostic and/or therapeutic measures can be enacted.

Radiological examination, small bowel series, or barium enema in particular, is seldom helpful (diagnostic). (1-6) However, radiological demonstration by enteroclysis, selective antegrade small intestinal enema, has been quite reliable in diagnosis in 13 of 15 patients. (7) As previously mentioned, hemorrhage from Meckel's diverticulum almost invariably occurs as a result of ulceration or erosion of small bowel mucosa adjacent to heterotopic gastric mucosa in the diverticulum. This gastric mucosa contains chief and parietal cells and has the capacity to secrete hydrochloric acid and, therefore, has the capacity to concentrate the isotope ^{99m}Tc sodium pertechnetate. (4,8) Furthermore, an abdominal scan after administration of this isotope will show activity over the stomach as well as uptake over the diverticulum. (8-11) Rectolinear scanning is performed at 30 minutes, 4 hours, and 24 hours. This timing does place a limitation on its diagnostic value in the acutely bleeding child. Thus, gamma camera scanning is more useful in the acutely ill child. (6-8) The isotope begins to concentrate within 5 minutes after injection; the optimum time for gastric tissue visualization is 30 to 45 minutes after isotope injection. (5-8) To minimize confusion by gastric secretion or bladder accumulation, nasogastric suction or fasting and bladder emptying can be accomplished. Since barium absorbs pertechnetate, prior barium contrast studies may negate the value of the scan. (6-8) False negative results have been reported in 10 to 30% of proven cases,

while false positive results occur in few cases, usually 1 to 8%.
(8-10) The latter have occurred in intussusception, small intestinal obstruction, abdominal abscess with ileal perforation, and
telangiectasia of the jejunum. (8-10)

To improve (decrease) the incidence of false negative results, several authors have recommended the use of cimetidine
(Tagamet), 20 mg/kg/24 hr, for 24 to 72 hours before the scan.
This H_2-receptor antagonist would block acid (secretion) by parietal cells and aid in isotope accumulation. (11,14) Ranitidine
(Zantac), another H_2 receptor antagonist, has not been evaluated
adequately. Despite such limitations, this represents a major
advance in diagnosis and is the most useful diagnostic modality
in this disorder.

Visceral angiography can occasionally be of significant aid
and should be considered in selective cases when other studies
are negative or equivocal. An area of persistent density (staining) may be demonstrated, presumably due to the increased vas-
cularity of gastric mucosa. (12,13)

9. (T) The preoperative management is directed toward correction of the hypovolemic state with blood or other colloid
agents, dependent upon the magnitude of such deficit. In addition, control of injection is important if obstruction or imflam-
mation is present, and broad-spectrum antibiotic administration
(ampicillin/gentamycin or similar combination) should be initiated.

Exploratory laparotomy is then performed, and the diverticulum is restricted. In addition, inspection of the ileum proximal to and distal to the diverticulum is performed in order to
identify further heterotopic tissue and/or ulcerations. (1-5,14)

REFERENCES

1. Seagram, C.G.E., Louch, R.E., Stephens, C.A., et al.:
    Meckel's diverticulum: A ten-year review of 218 cases.
    Can J Surg 11:369, 1968.

2. Rutherford, R.B. and Akers, D.R.: Meckel's diverticu-
    lum: A review of 148 pediatric patients, with special ref-
    erence to the pattern of bleeding and to mesodiverticular
    vascular bands. Surgery 59:618, 1966.

3. Simms, M.H., Corkery, J.J.: Meckel's diverticulum: Its
    association with congenital malformation and the signifi-
    cance of atypical morphology. Br J Surg 67:216, 1980.

4. Liebman, W.M., Bujanover, Y.: Group I, II pepsinogens in Meckel's diverticulum. J Histochem Cytochem 26:867, 1978.

5. Dalinka, M.K. and Wunder, J.E.: Meckel's diverticulum and its complications, with emphasis on roentgenologic demonstration. Radiology 106:295, 1972.

6. Meguid, M.M., Wilkinson, R.H., Canty, T., et al.: Futility of barium sulfate in diagnosis of bleeding Meckel's diverticulum. Arch Surg 108:361, 1974.

7. Maglinte, D.D.T., Elmore, M.F., Isenberg, M., et al.: Meckel's diverticulum: Radiologic demonstration by enteroclysis. Am J Roentgenol 134:925, 1980.

8. Harden, R.M., Alexander, W.D., Kennedy, I.: Isotope uptake and scanning of stomach in man with 99m Tc-pertechnetate. Lancet 1:1305, 1967.

9. Jewett, T.C., Jr., Duszynski, D.O., Allen, J.F.: The visualization of Meckel's diverticulum with 99m Tc-pertechnetate. Surgery 68:567, 1970.

10. Kilpatrick, Z.M., Aseron, C.A., Jr.: Radioisotope detection of Meckel's diverticulum causing acute rectal hemorrhage. N Engl J Med 287:653, 1972.

11. Chaudhuri, T.K., Chaudhuri, T.K., Christie, J.H.: False positive Meckel's diverticulum scan. Surgery 71:313, 1972.

12. Bree, R.J. and Reuter, S.R.: Angiographic demonstration of a bleeding Meckel's diverticulum. Radiology 108:287, 1973.

13. Muroff, L.R., Casarella, W.J., Johnson, P.M.: Preoperative diagnosis of Meckel's diverticulum: Angiographic and radionuclide studies in an adult. J Am Med Ass 229:1900, 1974.

14. Pellerin, D., Harouchi, T., Delmas, P.: Meckel's diverticulum: Review of 250 cases in children. Ann Chir Infant 17:157, 1976.

Case 9

LACK OF BOWEL MOVEMENTS IN A 3-DAY-OLD BABY

HISTORY

A 3-day-old white male presented with a history of no bowel movements since birth. There was no history of fever, vomiting, diarrhea, skin lesions, or birth trauma. Urination was normal. Gestational and delivery history was unremarkable. Birth weight was 3.4 kg. The remainder of the past, family, and social history, and review of systems was unremarkable.

EXAMINATION

He was alert and in no apparent distress, with normal vital signs, weight 3.4 kg, length 47 cm, and head circumference 33 cm. The remainder of the examination was unremarkable, except for an apparent shortened rectal vault, terminating in a blind ending.

LABORATORY DATA

Hemoglobin:	14.8 gm%
Hematocrit:	45%
White blood cell count:	11,400/mm^3
PMN's:	58%
lymphocytes:	37%
monocytes:	3%
eosinophiles:	2%
Urinalysis:	negative
Serum:	
sodium:	139 meq/L
potassium:	4.2 meq/L

chloride:	103 meq/L
bicarbonate:	23 meq/L
creatinine:	0.5 mg%
total protein:	6.3 gm%
albumin:	4.7 gm%
total bilirubin:	7 mg%
direct bilirubin:	0.8 mg%
SGPT:	20 units
alkaline phosphatase:	160 IU
Colon follow through (barium):	(Fig. 9.1)
IVP:	negative

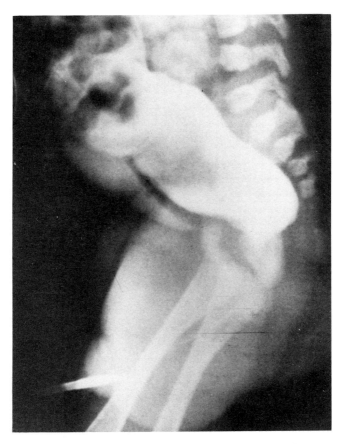

Figure 9.1   Barium enema.   Abrupt termination of rectum is present with barium seen below the pubococcygeal line.

QUESTIONS

1. The probable diagnosis of this patient is
   A. imperforate anus (anorectal anomaly)
   B. Hirschsprung's disease
   C. intussusception
   D. fistula-in-ano
   E. amebiasis (dysentery)

Question 2: Answer true (T) or false (F).

2. At least one-third of patients with this disorder have associated congenital malformations.

3. Which of the following is the most common type of imperforate anus (anorectal anomaly)?
   A. Rectal atresia
   B. Anal membrane
   C. Anorectal agenesis
   D. Fistula-in-ano
   E. Anal stenosis

4. The usual clinical presentation includes
   A. failure of passage of meconium
   B. vomiting
   C. abdominal pain
   D. straining with defecation
   E. hematochezia

5. Which of the following are important factors influencing the ultimate prognosis?
   A. Type of anomaly
   B. Associated congenital malformations
   C. Birth weight
   D. Age of diagnosis
   E. Weight at time of treatment

Questions 6 and 7: Answer true (T) or false (F).

6. All types of anorectal anomalies (imperforate anus) are treated surgically.

7. Fecal incontinence is a significant problem in this disorder, particularly in those with "high" defects.

ANSWERS AND COMMENTS

1.   (A) The most probable diagnosis is an anorectal anomaly
(imperforate anus). Refer to answers 2 to 7.

2.   (T) At least one-third of patients have associated congenital
malformations. (1-4) Genitourinary malformations are most
common, including exstrophy of the bladder and hypospadias.
(1-4) Equally common are anomalies of the sacrum, but the majority of these patients do not have normal innervation of the levator ani muscles, resulting in possible urinary and fecal incontinence, depending upon the extent of the neurological deficit.
(1-3) Gastrointestinal anomalies are next in frequency, particularly esophageal atresia with or without accompanying tracheo-
esophageal fistula. (1-3) Other gastrointestinal anomalies include small and large intestinal atresia, annular pancreas, and
intestinal malrotation. (1-5) Anomalies of other organs include
cardiac, such as a ventriculoseptal defect (VSD).

3.   (C) Anorectal agenesis accounts for at least 75% of anorectal anomalies. (1-3) The embryonic development of the anus,
lower rectum, and urogenital tract occurs between the end of
the first month and the sixth month. (6) The cloaca is separated
by the urorectal septum into the anterior urogenital sinus (ure-
thra, bladder) and the posterior hindgut (rectum). (6) The hindgut moves posteriorly and superiorly and eventually joins with
the lower anal canal. The cloacal membrane (anal urogenital
membrane) disappears, allowing separate openings of the urogenital sinus and hindgut and tubercles but then encircles the
hindgut's terminal end, producing a central depression, the
proctodeum. The inferior part of the proctodeum becomes the
lower anal canal.
    Anorectal agenesis results from the defective embryonic de-
velopment of the anorectal region. In anal agenesis, the anal
dimple is present, the bowel extends below the pubococcygeal
line, and fistulous tracts are frequent. These fistulas are perineal or vulvar in females, while being perineal or urethral in
males. (1-7) In rectal agenesis, the rectal segment can be at
or above the pubococcygeal line, and fistulas are particularly
frequent. (1-7) These fistulas may not be visualized easily and
consist of vestibular, vaginal (high/low), or cloacal types in females, while being rectourethral or rectovesical in males. (1-7)

4.   (A,D) In anal stenosis, there is a small opening, filled with
meconium. Defecation is quite difficult, and stools, if passed,
are thin or ribbon-like. Abdominal distention is not uncommon,

nor is fecal impaction. Secondary megacolon can eventually develop. In the anal membrane type, there is a failure of passage of meconium, and a fistulous connection with the perineum is possible. (1-7) In anorectal agenesis, failure of meconium passage, intestinal obstruction (no fistula) or passage of meconium and stool in the urine or to the skin surface comprise the usual presenting picutre. In rectal atresia, there is no fistula, but the presenting symptomatology depends upon the degree of completeness of this anorectal anomaly. Thus, intestinal obstruction or difficult defecation are the usual presenting patterns. (1-7)

Radiological evaluation of this group of disorders is an important facet in management. A lateral X-ray with the patient in the upside-down position for 5 minutes, lower extremities at right angle to the trunk, and radiopaque marker fixed to anal location, will reveal the terminal end of the bowel. Air in the bladder, vertebral anomalies, and meconium accumulation may be shown too. (1-7) The location of air or gastrografin in relation to the imaginary pubococcygeal line may also aid in determining the extent of the defect, as well as the type. Intravenous pyelography and/or cystourethrography should be considered too, for demonstrating associated anomalies. (1-7)

5. (A,B,C) Birth weight and the absence or presence of associated malformations are more important determinants of the ultimate prognosis than the type of anomaly or the presence or absence of a fistula. (1-10) In prematures and small-for-gestational-age infants, the mortality will be higher, as much as 50 to 60%. (1-10) With associated malformations, the mortality is higher too. (1-10) The actual functional result of treatment is proportionally more dependent on the type of anorectal anomaly, being better in low as opposed to high anomalies. This is related to control of defecation, urination, and flatus passage. One apparent reason is the association of neurological defects and fistulas with the high anomalies. (1-10)

6. (F) Anal stenosis accounts for 7 to 10% of cases of anorectal anomalies and usually is successfully managed by digital dilatations at varying time intervals. (1-10) Usually, several months of dilatations are required. In a small percentage of cases, extensive anal stenosis is present, and surgical excision of tissue, as well as rectal mobilization and attachment to the lower anal canal or perineum, are necessary. (1-10) This anomaly has the best prognosis of all because the remainder of the anorectal area is normal. (1-10)

Treatment of imperforate anal membrane consists of excision. This leads to normal anorectal and sphincter function, unless an extensive fistulous tract is present. (1-10)

Treatment of anal agenesis involves either anoproctoplasty (no fistula) or colostomy if, as occurs in males especially, there is a fistula or significant interruption of bowel function. Definitive anoplasty can be performed at 9 to 12 months of age. (1-10)

Treatment of rectal agenesis depends to some extent upon the presence or absence of a fistula. In these high anomalies (at or above the pubococcygeal line), a colostomy should be performed in the neonatal period, and the definitive procedure, abdominoperineal repair, performed at 9 to 12 months of age. (1-10) Recently, Ito, et al. (11) suggested that the colon could be safely pulled through within the puborectalis sling by the Rehbein procedure without sacral dissection (endorectal pull-through), i.e., actually better clinical scores with the endorectal pull-through procedure than the abdominoperineal pull-through procedure.

Treatment of rectal atresia is the same as for a high anomaly, and in particular, that described for rectal agenesis. Fortunately, this type does not have associated fistulas.

7. (T) The functional results, in general, are significantly better in those patients with low anomalies. Associated neurological defects, as well as fistulous communications in high anomalies, necessitate more complex procedures, and the functional results are not as good. (1-12) Thus, fecal incontinence continues to be a significant problem. Continence is achieved in 75 to 90% of those patients with the low types, but in only 30 to 70% of those with high types. (11-14) Sensory awareness of rectal fullness is decreased, although frequently improves with age, even over several years. (11,12) Important factors are the functional presence or not of the puborectalis sling and of the internal sphincter. (1-3,8-10) Postoperative incontinence can be aided to a variable extent by medical measures, such as bulk production, daily evacuation by suppository or enema, and more recently, by training programs involving biofeedback techniques. Lastly, the puborectalis sling may be surgically reconstructed. (8,10,12)

REFERENCES

1. Kiesewetter, W.B., Turner, C.R., Sieber, W.K.: Imperforate anus: Review of a 16-year experience with 146 patients. Am J Surg 107:412, 1964.

2. Santulli, T.V., Kiesewetter, W.B., Bill, A.H., Jr.: Anorectal anomalies: A suggested international classification. J Pediatr Surg 5:281, 1970.

3. Wilkinson, A.W.: Congenital anomalies of the anus and rectum. Arch Dis Child 47:960, 1972.

4. Kiesewetter, W.B., Sukarochana, K., Sieber, W.K.: The frequency of aganglionosis associated with imperforate anus. Surgery 58:877, 1965.

5. Cremin, B.J., Cywes, S., Louw, J.H.: A rational radiological approach to the surgical correction of anorectal anomalies. Surgery 71:806, 1972.

6. Stephens, F.D.: Embryologic and functional aspects of "imperforate anus." Surg Clin North Am 50:191, 1970.

7. Manny, J., Schiller, M., Horner, R., et al.: Congenital familial anorectal anomaly. Am J Surg 125:639, 1973.

8. Eisner, M.: Functional examination of rectum and anus in normals, in disturbances of continence and defecation and in congenital malformation. Scand J Gastroenterol 7: 305, 1972.

9. Kiesewetter, W.B.: Imperforate anus: The rationale and technic of the sacro-abdominal perineal operation. J Pediatr Surg 2:106, 1967.

10. Taylor, I., Duthie, H.L., Zachary, R.B.: Anal continence following surgery for imperforate anus. J Pediatr Surg 8:497, 1973.

11. Ito, Y., Yokoyama, J., Hayashi, A., et al.: Reappraisal of endorectal pull-through procedure I. Anorectal malformations. J Pediatr Surg 16:476, 1981.

12. Haberkorn, H., Chrispin, A., Nixon, H.H.: Assessment of fecal incontinence by manometric and radiological techniques. J Pediatr Surg 9:43, 1974.

13. Engel, B.T., Nikoomanesh, P., Schuster, M.M.: Operant conditioning of recto-sphincteric responses in the treatment of fecal incontinence. N Engl J Med 290:646, 1974.

14. Symposium on ano-rectal congenital malformations - Bologna 21-22 October 1977. Rass Ital Chir Pediatr 20:3, 1978.

Case 10

JAUNDICE FOR 3 WEEKS IN A 6-WEEK-OLD MALE

HISTORY

A 6-week-old white male presented with jaundice of 3 to 4 weeks' duration. The pregnancy was full-term, birth weight 6 lb 5 oz, with no apparent history of difficulty during gestation. The patient apparently had no problems in the immediate postnatal period. His diet consisted of breast milk, with no difficulties being noted. The mother noticed jaundice of the patient at 2-1/2 weeks of age. However, a well-baby examination was performed, and no jaundice was noted at that time. At 5 weeks of age, apparent jaundice was noted by the patient's physician. Laboratory studies at this time revealed total bilirubin level of 7.4 mg/100 ml (no direct or indirect fraction determined). At 6 weeks of age, the repeat total bilirubin value was 8.6 mg/100 ml, direct 6.6 mg/100 ml. Other laboratory studies revealed SGPT 49 units, SGOT 133 units, alkaline phosphatase 881 IU, total protein 5.6 gm/ml, albumin 3.6 gm/100 ml, and triglycerides 535 mg/100 mg/100 ml. The stools supposedly were yellow-white in color. The baby's appetite and activity had been good. The previously mentioned breast feedings had been supplemented with apple sauce and cereals. There was no history of associated fever, vomiting, diarrhea, constipation, melena, hematochezia, lethargy, or other difficulties.

EXAMINATION

He was relatively alert, well-nourished, and in no apparent distress, with normal vital signs, weight 3.7 kg, height 54 cm, head circumference 38 cm. The remainder of the examination was unremarkable except for (1) scleral and conjunctival icterus, (2) grade II systolic, ejection murmur present over the lower

left precordium only, and (3) liver, palpable 3.0 cm below the
right costal margin in the midclavicular line, not tender or nodular, and firm in consistency, total span being 6.0 cm by percussion. No abdominal bruits were noted.

LABORATORY DATA

Hemoglobin:	10.8 gm%
Hematocrit:	31%
White blood cell count:	8,800/mm^3
PMN's:	44%
lymphocytes:	54%
monocytes:	1%
eosinophiles:	1%
Platelet count:	250,000/mm^3
Sedimentation rate:	10 mm/hr
Serum:	
SGOT:	99 KU
SGPT:	34 KU
total protein:	5.9 gm%
albumin:	3.9 gm%
total bilirubin:	9.8 mg%
direct bilirubin:	7.5 mg%
alkaline phosphatase:	800 IU
alpha-fetoprotein:	negative
alpha-1-antitrypsin:	450 mg%
cholesterol:	375 mg%
Prothrombin time:	15.0 seconds (11.0 seconds)
Partial thromboplastin time:	37 seconds (less than 36 seconds)
VDRL:	negative
Torch titers:	negative
HbsAg:	negative
AntiHbs:	negative
HbcAg:	negative
AntiHbc:	negative
Sweat test:	
Cl:	10 meq/L
Na:	10 meq/L
Urinalysis:	negative
Urine amino acid screen:	negative
Echocardiogram:	negative
^{131}I Rose Bengal isotope study:	3.5% (72-hr stool excretion)
Percutaneous liver biopsy:	(Fig. 10.1)

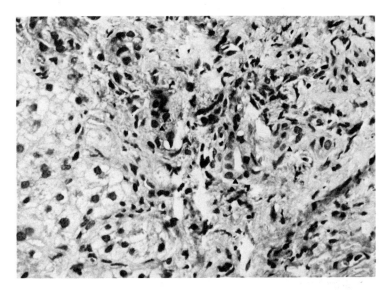

Figure 10.1   Liver. Numerous bile duct-like structures (arrows) are present amidst few chronic inflammatory cells and connective tissue elements (H&E, X 250).

QUESTIONS

1. The clinical course, laboratory studies, and the liver biopsy (see Fig. 10.1) are most compatible with which of the following conditions?
    A. Neonatal hepatitis
    B. Alpha-1-antitrypsin deficiency
    C. Hereditary fructose intolerance
    D. Intrahepatic biliary hypoplasia
    E. Extrahepatic biliary atresia

2. Which of the following would be most appropriate in the treatment of this patient?
    A. Phenobarbital
    B. Cholestyramine
    C. Idoxuridine (IDU)
    D. Steroids
    E. Surgery

Question 3: Answer true (T) or false (F).

3. Despite newer methodology in treatment of this condition, the prognosis remains poor.

ANSWERS AND COMMENTS

1. (E) Extrahepatic biliary atresia continues to account for 30 to 60% of all cases of prolonged "obstructive" jaundice in neonates, although the estimated incidence is only 1:8,000 to 1:15,000 live births. (1-5) Four to 5 times greater incidence has been reported in Orientals. (1-5) The specific etiology of this abnormality remains unknown, although certain hypotheses have been proposed. These include (1) congenital malformation of the bile duct system (abnormal development), (2) progressive obliterative cholangiopathy, ascending in type, (3) progressive obliterative cholangiopathy, descending in type, and (4) recanalization defect (failure). (1-5)

As illustrated by this patient's history, the jaundice usually appears at 2 to 3 weeks of age, the urine is dark, and the stools light or without color. (1-8) The infant does not appear to be particularly ill, and the onset of failure to thrive is gradual. Later in the course of this disease, digital clubbing, cyanosis, xanthomas, firm, significant hepatomegaly and splenomegaly occur. The latter heralds the presence of portal hypertension. Pruritus may become noticeable. Signs of vitamin D deficiency may become noticeable, too, such as rachitic rosary.

The laboratory studies performed in the evaluation of prolonged obstructive jaundice have been discussed to some extent in the prior case study. In extrahepatic biliary atresia, the serum transaminases (SGOT, SGPT) are variably elevated, usually below 400 to 500 units; the alkaline phosphatase markedly elevated, frequently over 450 international units; the serum 5' nucleotidase greater than 25 international units; and the presence of a direct (conjugated) hyperbilirubinemia. (1-8) Isoenzyme analysis of alkaline phosphatase is not particularly helpful, hepatic versus bone, for example. Serum bile acids are elevated in patients with cholestasis of whatever etiology. Therefore, their pattern must be scrutinized carefully, i.e., cholate/chenodeoxycholate ratio, less than 2 with nonpatent bile ducts. Additionally, administration of phenobarbital, lowering serum bile acid concentration with patency of bile ducts, or cholestyramine, preferentially binding chenodeoxycholate in the small intestine, can be accomplished. The red blood cell peroxide hemolysis test, dependent on vitamin E integrity, does not offer increased sensitivity of disease discrimination. (1-8) Serum vitamin E can be measured before and after oral α-tocopherol administration, increasing in neonatal hepatitis but not in biliary atresia. (3,8) Lipoprotein-X measurement has been discussed previously, i.e., more elevated in biliary atresia. (3,8) The [131]I Rose Bengal isotope excretion test, if less than 5% excretion in 72 hours, is diagnostic of biliary atresia. (3,7,8) More recently, ^{131}I-RB scanning has been replaced by the use of newer isotopes, e.g., Technetium-99M-N, or 12,6 diethylacetanilide iminodiacetic acid (99M-Tc-PIPIDA). The advantages of the newer agents include rapid hepatic uptake and excretion, reduced hepatic radiation dose, improved imaging and diagnostic accuracy. (9,10) Regardless, the level of direct bilirubin is a major factor in interpreting radionuclide biliary imaging examinations with all of the tracers. (9,10)

Finally, the percutaneous liver biopsy in combination with the other studies will provide the correct diagnosis in 90 to 95% of patients with extrahepatic biliary atresia. (2,3,8) The histologic features strongly suggestive of the diagnosis include bile duct proliferation, portal fibrosis, perilobular fibrosis, bile lakes, and intralobular and canalicular cholestasis. (2,3,8) This pattern, however, develops at a variable rate, although usually developing by 3 to 4 months of age. (2,3,8) A potential alternative to open (general anesthesia) versus percutaneous liver biopsy is the mini-lap procedure, an integrated procedure consisting of transhepatic cholangiography, liver biopsy, and omentoportography, performed under local anesthesia through a subxiphoid incision. (3,6,8) However, this technique has seldom been used in children.

The laboratory studies and the liver biopsy in this patient are most compatible with extrahepatic biliary atresia. The liver biopsy findings are not compatible with hepatitis and cholestasis only. The alpha-1-antitrypsin level was normal, virtually eliminating a deficiency of such with associated liver disease. The patient had never consumed sucrose- (glucose, fructose) or fructose-containing liquids and foods, and the biopsy findings are also not compatible with fructose intolerance. The biopsy findings demonstrate bile duct proliferation, not a paucity of bile ducts, as in intrahepatic hypoplasia.

2. (E) Once the diagnosis is strongly suggested, as in the present case, surgery is required. If significant malnutrition has occurred, a period of nutritional replenishment is preferable, including vitamins, such as fat-soluble D and K. (9-19) If the gallbladder is identified, aspiration is performed (normal bile or not). Operative cholangiography is then done in order to observe the distal biliary system. If the gallbladder is atretic or absent, most surgeons would dissect the porta hepatis to the

hilus of the liver in order to identify a possible bile duct for
anastomosis to bowel. This possibility is only realized in 10
to 25% if the gallbladder is absent or atretic. (9-19) Fibrous
remnants of the bile ducts are also dissected for the purpose of
finding a possible channel. A dissecting microscope is frequently used during this procedure. If a patent portion of the extrahepatic biliary system is found, an anastomosis is attempted,
in particular, a choledochoduodenostomy, choledochojejunostomy,
cholecystoduodenostomy, or cholecystojejunostomy. (9-19) As
previously mentioned, this primary anastomosis is only possible
in 10 to 25%. Otherwise, a "noncorrectable" situation exists,
and the current approach is the so-called Kasai procedure, or
hepatoportoenterostomy. (9-19) The distal common duct remnant is ligated, the remaining extrahepatic ductal system is dissected and resected, including a wedge of tissue at the porta
hepatis. (9-19) Bile drainage is established via a hepatic porto-
jejunostomy in a Roux-en-Y arrangement. (9-21) Alternative
techniques of biliary drainage (prevention of ascending cholangitis) have included an ostomy (Sawaguchi technique), cutaneous
enterostomy (Suruga technique). (22-25) Some type of choleretic, such as phenobarbital, is usually used thereafter, as well
as broad spectrum antibiotics for a minimum of 1 to 2 weeks.
(26) Prophylactic antibiotics, e.g., Septra (trimethoprim-sul-
famethoxazole) have been attempted to reduce the incidence of
cholangitis, too, but the results have not been encouraging. (20)
    The final alternative is orthotopic liver transplantation. Al-
though the results are disappointing, the biliary atresia group
has had the best results so far. (20) Complications include rejection and necrosis of the transplanted liver and liver abscesses, as well as superimposed infections (viral, protozoal, and
fungal) due to the routine use of immunosuppressive and anti-
inflammatory agents. (18)

3.   (T) Despite the present surgical methodology, as well as
medical treatment, such as elemental formulas, medium-chain
triglyceride oil, phenobarbital and/or cholestyramine, the prognosis remains poor, in particular only 5 to 10% long-term survival, although Kasai and others are beginning to report higher
survival rates, e.g., 30 to 50%. (20-28) Ascending cholangitis
occurs in at least 50% of successfully operated patients, apparently unrelated to the establishment of good bile flow. The management of ascending cholangitis is a major factor in the survival rate. (20-28) In addition, continued fibrosis and obliteration
of the intrahepatic ductal system occurs, apparently due to the
basic underlying disease process and not to the quality of established bile flow. (11-27) The reversibility of biliary cirrhosis
is obviously dependent on more than the establishment of bile

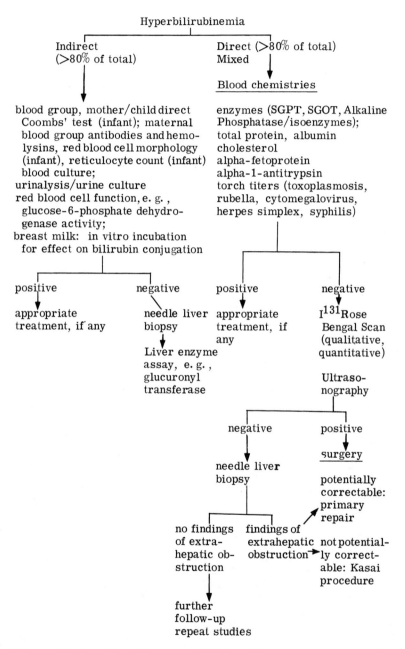

Figure 10.2   Algorithm, neonatal jaundice.

flow. (11-27) However, the degree of fibrosis does correlate to some extent with the age of the patient at operation. Conversely, the stage (timing of operation) at which biliary cirrhosis is stopped, or even reversed, is not known, although Kasai continues to state that the majority of patients with noncorrectable biliary atresia may be cured if the modified hepatoportoenterostomy is accomplished by 10 weeks of age. (25)

For additional information, see Figure 10.2.

REFERENCES

1. Stowens, D.: Congenital biliary atresia. Am J Gastroenterol 32:577, 1959.

2. Brough, A.J. and Bernstein, J.: Liver biopsy in the diagnosis of infantile obstructive jaundice. Pediatrics 43: 519, 1969.

3. Thaler, M.M.: Neonatal hyperbilirubinemia. Semin Hematol 9:107, 1972.

4. Thaler, M.M. and Gellis, S.S.: Studies in neonatal hepatitis and biliary atresia. III. Progression and regression of cirrhosis in biliary atresia. IV. Diagnosis. Am J Dis Child 116:257, 1968.

5. Landing, B.H.: Considerations of the pathogenesis of neonatal hepatitis, biliary atresia, and choledochal cyst: The concept of infantile obstructive cholangiopathy. Prog Pediatr Surg 6:113, 1974.

6. Sass-Kortsak, A.: Management of young infants presenting with direct-reacting hyperbilirubinemia. Pediatr Clin North Am 21:777, 1974.

7. Strack, P.R., Newman, H.K., Lerner, A.G., et al.: An integrated procedure for the rapid diagnosis of biliary obstruction, portal hypertension and liver disease of uncertain etiology. N Engl J Med 285:1225, 1971.

8. Thaler, M.M.: Jaundice in the newborn: Algorithmic diagnosis of conjugated and unconjugated hyperbilirubinemia. J Am Med Assoc 237:58, 1977.

9. Sty, J.R., Glicklich, M., Babbitt, D.P., et al.: Technetium-99m biliary imaging in pediatric surgical patients. J Pediatr Surg 16:686, 1981.

10. Miller, J.H., Sinatra, F.R., Thomas, D.W.: Biliary excretion disorders in infants: evaluation using 99M-Tc-PIPIDA. Am J Roentgenol 135:47, 1980.

11. Kasai, M., Kimura, S., Asakura, Y., et al.: Surgical treatment of biliary atresia. J Pediatr Surg 3:665, 1968.

12. Kasai, M.: Treatment of biliary atresia with special reference to hepatic portoenterostomy and its modifications. Prog Pediatr Surg 6:5, 1974.

13. Krovetz, L.J.: Congenital biliary atresia. I. Analysis of 30 cases with particular reference to diagnosis. II. Analysis of the therapeutic problem. Surgery 47:453, 1960.

14. Danks, D.M., Clarke, A.M., Jones, P.G., et al.: Extrahepatic biliary atresia: Further comments on potentially operable cases. J Pediatr Surg 3:584, 1968.

15. Campbell, D.P., Poley, J.R., Bhatia, M., et al.: Hepatic portoenterostomy: Is it indicated in the treatment of biliary atresia? J Pediatr Surg 9:329, 1974.

16. Howard, E.R., Psacharopoulos, H., Mowat, A.P.: Extrahepatic biliary atresia: Results of surgical treatment. Gut 8:A956, 1977.

17. Berenson, M.M., Garde, A.R., Moody, F.G.: Twenty-five-year survival after surgery for complete extrahepatic biliary atresia. Gastroenterology 66:260, 1974.

18. Kobayashi, A., Utsunomiya, T., Ohbe, Y., et al.: Ascending cholangitis after successful surgical repair of biliary atresia. Arch Dis Child 48:697, 1973.

19. Draz, S., Barajas, L., Fonkalsrud, E.W.: Reversibility of biliary cirrhosis due to bile duct obstruction. J Pediatr Surg 6:256, 1971.

20. Silverman, A., Roy, C.C.: Pediatric Clinical Gastroenterology, 3rd Edition. The CV Mosby Co., St. Louis, 1983, p. 438.

21. Silverberg, M. and Davidson, M.: Nutritional requirements of infants and children with liver disease. Am J Clin Nutr 23:604, 1970.

22. Weber, T.R. and Grosfeld, J.L.: Contemporary management of biliary atresia. Surg Clin North Am 61:1079, 1981.

23. Kitamura, T., Sawaguchi, S., Akiyama, H., et al.: Long-term results after operation for congenital biliary atresia in 144 personal cases. Z Kinderchir 31:239, 1980.

24. Weber, T.R., Grosfeld, J.L., Fitzgerald, J.F.: Prognostic determinants after hepatoportoenterostomy for biliary atresia. Am J Surg 141:57, 1981.

25. deVries, P.A. and Cox, K.L.: Surgical treatment of congenital and neonatal biliary obstruction. Surg Clin North Am 61:987, 1981.

26. Stiehl, A., Thaler, M.M., Admirand, W.H.: The effect of phenobarbital on bile salts and bilirubin in patients with intrahepatic and extrahepatic cholestasis. N Engl J Med 286:858, 1972.

27. Hays, D.M. and Snyder, W., Jr.: Untreated biliary atresia. Surgery 54:373, 1963.

28. DeLorimier, A.A.: Jaundiced infants: Problems of surgical management. N Engl J Med 288:1284, 1973.

Case 11

DIARRHEA IN AN 11-WEEK-OLD MALE

HISTORY

An 11-week-old white male presented with a history of diarrhea
since 10 to 11 days of life. The gestational history had been unremarkable, birth weight 1.9 kg. Within the first day of life,
surgery was performed, including a jejunal and ileal resection,
jejunostomy, as well as excision of the ileocecal valve. Attempts
at feeding, e.g., breast milk, elemental formulas, such as
Pregestimil, were characterized by diarrhea, loose to watery
bowel movements, 5 to 12 daily, inadequate weight gain, increased flatus, and variance colic. There was no history of fever, vomiting, melena, hematochezia, abdominal distention.
The remainder of the past, family, and social history, and review of systems was unremarkable.

EXAMINATION

He was alert, in no apparent distress, with normal vital signs,
weight 2.06 kg, length 40 cm, and head circumference 30 cm.
The remainder of the examination was unremarkable, except
for (1) gastrostomy, medial left upper quadrant, (2) minimal abdominal protuberance, no apparent tenderness and/or masses,
but active bowel sounds present.

LABORATORY DATA

Hemoglobin:	11.4 gm%
Hematocrit:	33%
White blood cell count:	10,800/mm^3
PMN's:	55%

lymphocytes:	34%
monocytes:	8%
eosinophiles:	3%
Urinalysis:	negative
Serum:	
sodium:	139 meq/L
potassium:	4.3 meq/L
chloride:	102 meq/L
bicarbonate:	21 meq/L
creatinine:	0.7 mg%
total protein:	5.6 gm%
albumin:	3.2 gm%
total bilirubin:	1.2 mg%
direct bilirubin:	1.0 mg%
SGPT:	53 units
alkaline phosphatase:	173 IU
amylase:	42 units
Stool:	
smear:	1 to 3 WBC per HPF
hemoccult:	negative
reducing substances:	trace
culture:	negative
ova and parasites:	negative

QUESTIONS

Question 1: Answer true (T) or false (F).

1. The probable diagnosis of this patient is cystic fibrosis.

2. Conditions associated with the contaminated small bowel
    syndrome include
    A. gastroesophageal reflux
    B. pyloric stenosis
    C. duodenal ulcer
    D. intestinal stenosis or stricture
    E. Crohn's disease

3. Clinical features of this syndrome include
    A. diarrhea
    B. constipation
    C. abdominal pain
    D. heartburn (pyrosis)
    E. malabsorption (carbohydrate, fat, protein)

4. Diagnosis of this condition can be suggested or confirmed by which of the following?
   A. Small intestinal fluid culture (aerobic, anaerobic)
   B. Small intestinal biopsy
   C. Upper endoscopy
   D. Gastric acid analysis
   E. Breath hydrogen or CO_2 analysis

5. The treatment of this condition may include which of the following?
   A. Elemental diet, formula
   B. Antispasmodic
   C. Anticholinergic
   D. Antibiotics
   E. Steroids

ANSWERS AND COMMENTS

1. (F) Factors, such as the presentation and age relationship, as well as the immediate neonatal course, would make the diagnosis of cystic fibrosis much less likely.

2. (D, E) "Contaminated small bowel syndrome" is a clinical condition characterized by malabsorption associated with the proliferation of excessive numbers of bacteria, chiefly anaerobics, in the small intestine. (1-8) Contaminated small bowel syndrome is a heterogeneous condition with numerous causes. The diseases associated with contamination of the small bowel (bacterial overgrowth) include postoperative phase of intestinal surgery in young infants, chronic diarrhea, persistent or intractable, blind loop due to an end-to-side anastomosis, strictures, stenotic areas, fistulas, Crohn's disease, and chronic idiopathic intestinal pseudo-obstruction. (1-9)

Intestinal microflora of the proximal and mid-small intestine of normals is sparsely populated with bacteria, consisting predominantly of aerobic bacteria (less than 10^4/ml), together with small numbers of Enterobacteriaceae and Bacteroides. (1-9) The upper intestinal flora of people living in tropical countries is more abundant. The distal ileum represents a transition zone between the upper small intestine and colon. Bacterial counts are still modest in the ileum (10^5 to 10^8) in comparison with the colon and feces (10^{11}/ml). In the right colon, the flora is predominantly nonsporeforming anaerobic organisms, such as Bacteroides fragilis (40-50%), and other Bacteroides species along with Bifidobacterium, Eubacterium, and Propionobacterium. These outnumber facultative anaerobic bacteria such as Streptococcus faecalis, Escherichia coli, and lactobacilli. (1-9)

The primary bile acids (cholic and chenodeoxy) are in the lower small intestine and colon and are largely deconjugated and dehydroxylated (to deoxycholic and lithocholic acid, respectively). In the contaminated small bowel syndrome, bacterial transformation of bile acids takes place in the upper intestine. This leads to impairment of fat absorption because free and dehydroxylated bile acids cannot form micelles. (1-10) They now can be passively transported in the upper intestine. As a result, bile acid concentrations may be too low to ensure micellar solubilization. Fat malabsorption also relates to the inhibition of uptake and reesterification of fatty acids by free and secondary bile acids. Unabsorbed fatty acids can be metabolized by intestinal bacteria to produce long-chain hydroxy acids. Hydroxy fatty acids impair water and sodium transport and induce water secretion.

Enteric microorganisms metabolize carbohydrates and transform them into organic acids and hydrogen. Monosaccharide transport can be inhibited by deconjugated bile acids. Hyproteinemia is commonly found in the "blind loop" syndrome. Bacteria can use amino acids. The end products can be absorbed and excreted in urine. This is the basis for indicanuria as a marker of excess bacterial tryptophan metabolism. In addition, dipeptide and amino acid uptake may be inhibited by deconjugated bile acids. (1-9)

Other defects include vitamin B_{12} deficiency, since certain bacteria can bind vitamin B_{12} and compete with intrinsic factor and hyproxaturia. Morphologically, bacterial contamination is not accompanied by villous or epithelial cell structural changes, but infiltration of the lamina propria by inflammatory cells is usual. Ultrastructural changes are more prominent and include damage to microvilli mitochondria, and the Golgi apparatus. (1-7)

3. (A,C,E) Clinically, the patient with contaminated small bowel syndrome usually has symptoms of malabsorption and demonstrates the associated nutritional consequences. Significant growth retardation may be seen if symptoms are longstanding. The history can be that of a primary intestinal disease. It is not unusual for the contaminated small bowel syndrome to start years after such a surgical procedure. (1-10) Clinical findings pointing toward a malabsorption syndrome include recurrent abdominal pain, colicky in nature and associated with abdominal distention. Anorexia, nausea, vomiting, the passage of pale, odorous stools (float in water), are frequent. Megaloblastic anemia is also seen. Children with the contaminated small bowel syndrome often have severe, watery

diarrhea with water, electrolyte, and acid-base imbalance. Hypoproteinemia, hypocalcemia, and hypomagnesemia are common abnormalities. The watery diarrhea is particularly impressive in newborns during the first month or two postsurgery. However, the typical picture is not consistent. Consequently, the diagnosis of contaminated small bowel syndrome should be considered in all patients with malabsorption. (1-10)

4.   (A,E) The diagnosis rests on proving that there is malabsorption. Second, certain criteria must be met before attributing malabsorption to intraluminal bacteria. Available methods for investigation of intestinal bacterial populations fall short of the ideal. Intubations of the small bowel must be carried out, the specimens being obtained under anaerobic conditions. They are serially diluted and cultured on selective media (1-11). One of the most striking consequences of significant proliferation of bacteria in the small intestine is malabsorption of vitamin B_{12}, characterized by an abnormal Schilling test. The absorption of carbohydrate may be abnormal. Evidence of intraluminal bacterial catabolism of carbohydrate can be documented by measurement of breath hydrogen, CO_2, or CO after doses of the carbohydrate. Bile acid deconjugation results from the overgrowth of bacteria. One can demonstrate that a major portion of the bile acids in intestinal contents are not in the aqueous phase. The presence of a significant percentage of free bile acids not normally present in the jejunum can be established by thin-layer chromatography. Large fecal losses of bile acids can be documented similarly. Bacterial overgrowth can be established indirectly by the demonstration of bile acid deconjugation, e.g., breath test (cholyl-^{14}C-glycine). Stable isotopes (13 CO_2) will become increasingly available and used in pediatrics. (12,13) Radiological demonstration of any abnormal anatomy is particularly important. A stenotic area with proximal dilatation or poor propulsive action in a suspected intestinal segment may provide additional evidence.

Small intestinal biopsy provides small intestinal mucosa which is commonly normal. Electron microscopy usually is not helpful. (1-8) Response to antibiotic therapy could be an additional diagnostic feature, but treatment failure does not rule out the diagnosis. As intimated in the previous discussion, procedures for obtaining small intestinal fluid are uncomfortable, invasive, expensive, and frequently require use of sedation and exposure to radiation (fluoroscopy). More recently, the Enterotest-Pediatric or string test has been utilized to obtain a small aliquot of duodenal fluid and has been demonstrated to have

TABLE 11.1   Normal Flora

ORGANISMS CONSISTENT WITH NORMAL GASTROINTESTINAL
   AND RECTAL FLORA
A. Various Enterobacteriaceae except Salmonella sp., Shigella
    sp., Arizona, Yersinia, Vibrio sp., and Campylobacter sp.
B. Non-dextrose-fermenting Gram-negative rods
C. Enterococci
D. Staphylococcus epidermidis
E. Alpha hemolytic and nonhemolytic streptococci
F. Diphtheroids
G. Staphylococcus aureus in small numbers
H. Yeast in small numbers
 I. Anaerobes in large numbers

ORGANISMS CONSISTENT WITH NORMAL GENITAL FLORA
A. Any amount of the following:
    Hemophilus vaginalis
    Corynebacterium sp.
    Lactobacillus sp.
    Alpha hemolytic and nonhemolytic streptococci
    Nonpathogenic Neisseria sp.
B. The following when mixed and not predominant:
    Enterococci
    Enterobacteriaceae and other Gram-negative rods
    Staphylococcus aureus
    Staphylococcus epidermidis
    Candida albicans and other yeasts
    Group B Streptococci
C. Anaerobes (too many species to list); the following are
      reported when in full growth or clearly predominant:
    Bacteroides fragilis group
    Clostridium sp.
    Peptostreptococcus sp.
    Peptococcus sp.

ORGANISMS CONSISTENT WITH ORONASAL FLORA
A. Any amount of the following:
    Diphtheroids
    Nonpathogenic Neisseria sp.
    Alpha hemolytic streptococci
    Staphylococcus epidermidis
    Nonhemolytic streptococci
    Anaerobes (too many species to list: varying amounts of
      Bacteroides sp., anaerobic cocci, diphtheroids, Fuso-
      bacterium sp., etc.

TABLE 11.1   Normal Flora (Cont'd)

B.   Lesser amounts of the following when accompanied by or-
     ganisms listed above:
     Yeasts
     Hemophilus sp.
     Pneumococci
     Staphylococcus aureus
     Gram-negative rods
     Neisseria meninaitidis

ORGANISMS CONSISTENT WITH NORMAL SKIN FLORA

A.   Staphylococcus epidermidis
B.   Staphylococcus aurea (in small numbers)
C.   Micrococcus sp.
D.   Non-pathogenic Neisseria
E.   Alpha hemolytic and nonhemolytic streptococci
F.   Propionibacterium sp.
G.   Peptococcus sp.
H.   Small numbers of other organisms (Candida sp. , Acineto-
     bacter sp. , etc.)

---

comparable accuracy with intestinal intubation and aspiration
(tube). (14-16)

5.   (A,D) The goals of treatment are correction of the nutritional deficits, elimination of the bacterial overgrowth, and, as
feasible, restoration of the small intestinal anatomic and functional integrity. (4-8)
     Correction of acute and chronic nutritional deficiencies is
directed at appropriate administration of nutrients and vitamins.
Steatorrhea and diarrhea can both be helped by a low-fat diet
(10 to 20 gm of long-chain triglycerides) supplemented with medium-chain triglycerides, e.g., medium-chain trigylceride oil.
Parenteral alimentation may have to be used for short time periods, occasionally longer periods (over 1-2 weeks). The carbohydrate content of the formula must be carefully monitored in
young infants recovering from intestinal surgery. Cholestyramine has been helpful on occasions in control of the watery diarrhea secondary to the presence of free bile acids. (4-8) The
author has not found loperamide helpful, however.
     Reduction or elimination of the bacterial overgrowth can be
accomplished by the administration of tetracycline, lincomycin,

TABLE 11.2 Small Intestinal Microflora in Chronic Diarrhea[a,b]

Group	Gram-positive bacteria	Candida	Entero-bacteria	Fecal bacteria	Anaerobes	Total organisms
Aspirate	6	3	5	7	9	27
String	6	3	5	7	9	27
Range of isolates in all patients Aspirate	$0-2.3 \times 10^5$	$0-3 \times 10^4$	$0-5 \times 10^5$	$0-2 \times 10^5$	$0-5 \times 10^5$	$0-7.5 \times 10^6$
String	$0-2 \times 10^4$	$0-4 \times 10^3$	$0-2 \times 10^5$	$0-5.4 \times 10^4$	$0-1.6 \times 10^5$	$0-2.1 \times 10^6$

[a] 18 children and infants 8 months to 16 years with chronic diarrhea.
[b] Duodenal aspirate and string test in all subjects (anaerobic, aerobic).

clindamycin, or metronidazole. These antibiotics are particularly effective against anaerobes that are largely responsible for the spectrum of associated absorptive defects. There are minimal data with respect to what is appropriate for long-term antibiotic therapy. Intermittent therapy, 1 week out of every 2, 2 or 3 weeks out of every 4 weeks, and a change of antibiotic from time to time are recommended. (4-8) Surgical correction of the abnormality causing small bowel stasis is clearly an important goal. Appropriate surgical selection and timing are obviously important.

For additional information on flora, see Tables 11.1 and 11.2.

REFERENCES

1. Borriello, P., Hudson, M., and Hill, M.: Investigation of the gastrointestinal bacterial flora. Clin Gastroenterol 7: 329-349, 1978.

2. Mallory, A., Kern, F., Smith, J., Savage, D.: Patterns of bile acids and microflora in the human small intestine. Gastroenterology 64:26-33, 34-42, 1973.

3. Donaldson, R.M., Jr.: Normal bacterial population of the intestine and their relation to intestinal function. N Engl J Med 170:938, 1964.

4. Donaldson, R.M., Jr.: Small bowel bacterial overgrowth. Adv Intern Med 16:191, 1970.

5. Drude, R.B., and Hines, C.: The pathophysiology of intestinal bacterial overgrowth syndromes. Arch Intern Med 140:1349-1352, 1980.

6. Isaacs, P.T. and Kim, Y.S.: The contaminated small bowel syndrome. Am J Med 67:1049-1057, 1979.

7. Kern, L.: Bacterial contamination syndrome of the small bowel. Clin Gastroenterol 8:397-401, 1979.

8. King, C.E. and Toskes, P.P.: Small intestine bacterial overgrowth. Gastroenterology 76:1035-1055, 1979.

9. Challacombe, D.N., Richardson, J.M., Rowe, B., Anderson, C.M.: Bacterial microflora of the upper gastrointestinal tract in infants with protracted diarrhea. Arch Dis Child 49:270-277, 1974.

10. Ament, M.E., Shimoda, S., Saunders, D.R., Rubin, C.E.: The pathogenesis of steatorrhea in three cases of small intestinal stasis syndrome. Gastroenterology 63: 728-747, 1972.

11. Northfield, T.C., Drasar, B.S., Wright, J.T.: Value of small intestinal bile acid analysis in the diagnosis of the stagnant loop syndrome. Gut 14:341-347, 1971.

12. Caspary, W.F.: Breath tests. Clin Gastroenterol 7:362-364, 1978.

13. Schoeller, D.A., Schneider, J.F., Solomons, N.W., et al., Clinical diagnosis with the stable isotope ^{13}C in CO_2 breath tests. J Lab Clin Med 90:412-421, 1977.

14. Tracey, M., Sunarjono, Sunotui: Use of a simple duodenal capsule to study upper intestinal microflora. Arch Dis Child 52:74, 1977.

15. Rosenthal, P. and Liebman, W.M.: Comparative study of stool examinations, duodenal aspiration, and pediatric Entero-Test for giardiasis in children. J Pediatr 96:278, 1980.

16. Liebman, W.M. and Rosenthal, P.: Comparative study of duodenal aspiration and pediatric entero-test for small intestinal bacterial overgrowth in infants and children. Am J Dis Child 137:1177, 1983.

Case 12

MIDCHEST DISCOMFORT IN A 13-MONTH-OLD MALE

HISTORY

A 13-month-old white male presented with a 1-week history of
apparent midsternal discomfort and refusal to consume fluids
and solids. There was associated excessive salivation but no
history of emesis, hematemesis, fever, diarrhea, constipation,
abdominal pain, fever, melena, or trauma. The mother mentioned the possibility of ingestion of a cleaning liquid, type unknown, at the onset, since there was almost one ounce of her
cleaning liquid missing. The remainder of the past, developmental, family, and social history, as well as review of systems, was unremarkable.

EXAMINATION

He was alert, with normal vital signs, height 77.5 cm, weight
11 kg, and head circumference 46 cm. The remainder of the
examination was unremarkable.

LABORATORY DATA

Hemoglobin:	11.9 gm%
Hematocrit:	35%
White blood cell count:	9,600/mm^3
PMN's:	52%
lymphocytes:	42%
monocytes:	4%
eosinophiles:	2%
Urinalysis:	negative
Serum:	
creatinine:	0.5 mg%

SGOT: 22 KU
  total protein: 6.4 gm%
  albumin: 3.9 gm%
Chest X-ray: negative
ECG: within normal limits for age
Upper GI series: (Fig. 12.1)
Fiberoptic upper endoscopy: mild erythema without ul-
                                      ceration, friability or mem-
                                      brane in the distal 5 cm of
                                      the esophagus

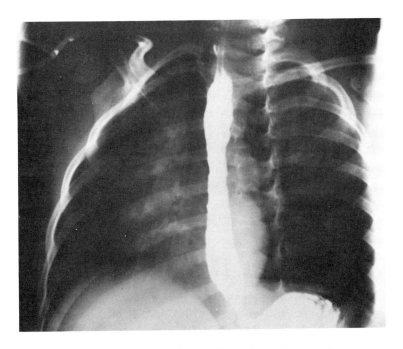

Figure 12.1   Barium swallow. Fine ulcerations and irregularity of the mucosal pattern of the esophageal outline are demonstrated.

QUESTIONS

1. The most likely diagnosis is
    A. peptic esophagitis
    B. achalasia
    C. caustic esophagitis
    D. diffuse spasm

2. The most important cause is
    A. acids
    B. alkalis
    C. solids
    D. liquids
    E. spicy foods

3. Treatment includes
    A. induced vomiting by syrup of ipecac or substitute
    B. antibiotics
    C. steroids
    D. dilatation
    E. surgery

ANSWERS AND COMMENTS

1. (C) The most likely diagnosis is caustic esophagitis, considering the clinical picture, the acute onset and age of presentation.

2. (B) The commonest cause of esophageal stricture in children is the ingestion of corrosive agents. These chemical burns (corrosive esophagitis) are mainly due to alkali caustic agents, such as sodium and potassium hydroxide. Their form can be granular, liquid, or paste. The liquid form requires the smallest amount to cause severe injury. Acids are more likely to cause injury of the stomach and proximal small intestine. (5) Over 80% of such burns occur in children less than 3 years of age, and boys predominate over girls (3:2). (1-8) Associated gastric injury occurs in 10 to 20%. (1-3,5-9)

The contact of these agents with the esophageal mucosa causes varying degrees of inflammation, necrosis, and vascular thrombosis. The resultant injury is graded according to the extent of involvement, in particular, mucosal (first degree), transmucosal (second degree), transmural (third degree), and transmural plus perforation (fourth degree). The esophageal reaction is extensive during the first 4 to 5 days, including possible necrosis, small vessel thrombosis, and later, ulceration and granuloma formation. After about 2 weeks, intensive connective tissue formation occurs, and after 4 to 6 weeks, there is subsequent stricture formation. (5,6)

In a significant number of cases, actual documentation of ingestion cannot be made. Fiberoptic endoscopy must be enacted in all cases in order to determine the presence and/or extent of injury. Oral lesions are frequently present. Substernal or abdominal distress may be present, as well as dyspnea and dysphagia. Radiological examination usually deomonstrates the stricture or strictures. Later, narrowing and shortening of the esophagus will be apparent. Associated gastric injury occurs in 10 to 20%. (1-3,5-9)

3. (B,C,D) The immediate treatment should consist of dilution and neutralization of the caustic ingestion and no induction of vomiting. Parenteral antibiotics are recommended, such as ampicillin, 100 mg/kg/day. Additionally, use of prednisone, 1 to 2 mg/kg/day or its equivalent, should be considered except in fourth degree injuries. Their use in first degree injuries is questionable. Their administration is for 4 weeks. However, good, controlled studies in children are lacking. (5)

If oral intake is not possible, then intravenous fluid administration should be initiated. Within the first 24 hours, fiberoptic endoscopy should be performed in order to assess the presence and extent of injury. If injury is confirmed, the previously mentioned treatment is instituted. By the 7th to 10th day, dilatation (bougienage) can be initiated with extreme caution. If the stricture is particularly tight, then retrograde dilatation through a gastrostomy must be accomplished. Continued dilatation is the rule. Although medical management is usually satisfactory for this condition, occasional patients will require surgical treatment because of severe caustic injury, even mediastinal involvement, and/or stricture formation. Surgical treatment has included substernal colon interposition and gastric tubes. Transthoracic esophagectomy, blunt transmediastinal total esophagectomy with substernal colon interposition have been used infrequently in pediatric patients with caustic injury. (1-13) Intraluminal splints have been used with success in experimental models, e.g., cats, but human studies are lacking. (5)

Long-term consequences, whether medical or surgical treatment has been used, include persistent acid peptic reflux and esophagitis (pain, dysphagia, bleeding/anemia) and possible carcinomatous transformation after 25 to 40 years. The epithelium overlying the cicatrix is most frequently the origin of the neoplastic change. (13)

REFERENCES

1. Giffin, C.A.: Management of children with suspected esophageal burns. Postgrad Med 35:611, 1964.

2. Haller, J.A., Andrews, H.G., White, J.J., et al.: Pathology and management of acute corrosive burns of the esophagus: Results of treatment in 285 children. J Pediatr Surg 6:578, 1971.

3. Holinger, P.H.: Management of esophageal lesions caused by chemical burns. Ann Otol 77:819, 1968.

4. Leape, L.L., Ashcraft, K.W., Scarpelli, D.G., et al.: Hazard to health: Liquid lye. N Engl J Med 284:578, 1971.

5. Toccalino, H., Licastro, R., Guastavino, E., et al.: Caustic oesophagitis. Clin Gastroenterol 6(2):273, 1977.

6. Yarington, C.T., Jr.: Ingestion of caustic: Pediatric problem. J Pediatr 67:674, 1965.

7. Kinman, J.E.: Management of severe lye corrosions of the esophagus. J Laryngol 83:899, 1969.

8. Aschcraft, K.N. and Simon, J.L.: Accidental caustic ingestion in childhood: A review. Pathogenesis and current concepts of treatment. Texas Med 68:86, 1972.

9. Temple, A.R., Lovejoy, F.H., Jr. (Eds), Cleaning Products and their Accidental Ingestion. The Soap and Detergent Association, New York, 1980, p. 11.

10. Boyce, H.W., Jr. and Palmer, E.D.: Techniques of Clinical Gastroenterology. Charles C. Thomas, Springfield, 1975, p. 261.

11. Silverman, A., Roy, C.C.: Pediatric Clinical Gastroenterology, 3rd Edition. The CV Mosby Co., St. Louis, 1983, p. 145.

12. Thomas, A.N. and Dedo, H.H.: Pharyngogastrostomy for treatment of severe caustic stricture of the pharynx and esophagus. J Thorac Cardiovasc Surg 73:817, 1977.

13. Rodgers, B.M., Ryckman, F.C., Talbert, J.L.: Blunt transmediastinal total esophagectomy with simultaneous substernal colon, interposition for esophageal caustic strictures in children. J Pediatr Surg 16:184, 1981.

Case 13

GAGGING, UPPER ABDOMINAL DISCOMFORT
IN A 6-YEAR-OLD BOY

HISTORY

A 6-year-old white male presented with a history of recurrent
gagging of 5 months duration with associated upper abdominal
discomfort. There was variable frequency of this gagging,
which occurred with the ingestion of solids or liquids, generally within seconds to 2 minutes after actual swallowing, but without associated nausea or actual vomiting. Regurgitated material
was similar to the ingested foods. Activity and appetite remained unchanged. He had no excessive salivation, eructation,
pyrosis, hematemesis, diarrhea, constipation, melena, hematochezia, fever, lethargy, or trauma. Recent medication included Donnatal Elixir without significant improvement. Bowel
habit pattern was once daily to once every 2 days, with stools
firm to soft in nature. Birth weight was 6 lbs 2 oz, delivery
being at 35 weeks gestation. There was neonatal Rh incompati-
bility with subsequent exchange transfusions (two). The subsequent developmental and neonatal history was unremarkable.
The family history revealed a maternal grandmother with peptic
ulcer disease and maternal uncle with diabetes mellitus. The
past history, developmental history, family history, social history, and review of systems were unremarkable.

EXAMINATION

He was alert, cooperative, active, and in no apparent distress,
with normal vital signs. Height was 107 cm and weight 22.5 kg.
The remainder of the examination was unremarkable, including
the abdomen and chest. Stool hemoccult examination was negative.

98

LABORATORY DATA

Hemoglobin:	13.0 gm%
Hematocrit:	40%
White blood cell count:	6,400/mm^3
PMN's:	46%
lymphocytes:	59%
monocytes:	1%
eosinophiles:	3%
Urinalysis:	negative
Serum:	
SGPT:	21 units
alkaline phosphatase:	140 IU
total protein:	6.2 gm%
albumin:	4.6%
creatinine:	0.6 mg%
carotene:	160 μg%
Upper GI series:	(Fig. 13.1)
Esophageal manometry:	
mean LES (lower esophageal sphincter) pressure:	30 mmHg
minimal relaxation of LES lack of peristalsis in body of esophagus	
Fiberoptic upper endoscopy:	nonperistaltic contractions slight erythema at the gastroesophageal junction tight gastroesophageal junction

QUESTIONS

Questions 1-7: Answer true (T) or false (F).

From the historical and radiological details you may assume that
1. the probable diagnosis is achalasia.
2. this disease entity frequently occurs in the first decade of life.
3. difficulty in swallowing solids occurs for months to years before difficulty in liquids.
4. radiological examination is not helpful in achalasia.
5. esophageal motility and manometry are specific for aschalasia.
6. the initial treatment consists of hydrostatic dilatation.
7. if intractable, surgery is the treatment of choice, including Nissen fundoplication.

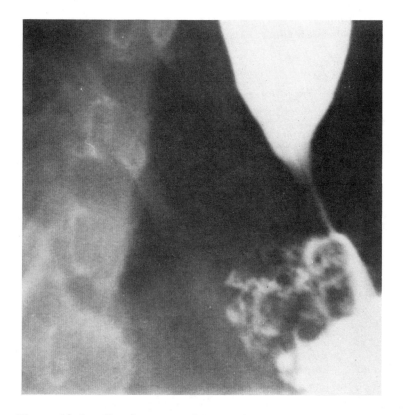

Figure 13.1 Esophagram. A tapered narrowing of the distal esophagus with proximal dilation is shown.

ANSWERS AND COMMENTS

1. (T) Achalasia of the esophagus is a disease of unknown cause, characterized by a decrease or degeneration of ganglion cells in Auerbach's (myenteric) plexus. The result is a failure of relaxation of the lower esophageal sphincter and a lack of peristalsis in the body of the stomach. The site of alteration of the postganglionic parasympathetic innervation has been postulated to be primarily in Auerbach's plexus (esophagus), the vagus, or even in the central nervous system (dorsal motor nucleus of the vagus). (1-3) Thus, the primary site remains

controversial. Secondary forms of achalasia can occur, including trypanosomiasis (Chagas' disease) and vitamin B_1 deficiency. Additionally, achalasia has been associated with volvulus and malrotation. (7)

2. (F) Achalasia is uncommon in children less than 5 years of age and is only occasionally seen in teenagers. However, the clinical history will frequently go back for many years before the diagnosis is made. (3,6,7)

3. (T) Swallowing difficulty is the major manifestation of achalasia. Intermittent difficulty in swallowing of solids may be present for years. This dysphagia can be accompanied by sternal or retrosternal pain. The food seems to stick in the upper chest and is relieved by repeated swallowing, bending forward, or vomiting. Regurgitation occurs early in the clinical course but only gradually becomes persistent. Failure to thrive, anemia, and pulmonary complications secondary to aspiration may occur, although in the minority. (3,6,7)

4. (F) The esophagram will demonstrate varying dilatation of the esophagus, a tapered narrowing of the distal esophagus, and little or no peristaltic activity. The cine-esophagram will show the above, too, as well as the failure of relaxation of the lower esophageal sphincter area. However, in infants and young children and during the early phases of the disease, the esophagram may be normal. (3,6,7)

5. (T) Esophageal manometry records the lower esophageal sphincter (LES) pressure at rest and with swallowing. In achalasia, LES pressure is usually significantly higher than in normals (15-30 mmHg), and there is failure or diminished relaxation of the LES during swallowing. The esophageal motility pattern will confirm the absence of primary peristaltic contraction in the body of the esophagus. The upper esophageal sphincter (UES) is normal, i.e., pressure, relaxation. (1-8)

Subcutaneous injection of a small dose of a parasympathomimetic drug, methacholine (Mecholyl) in particular, induces an exaggerated response of the entire esophagus (spastic response). This response is specific. (2-8)

Upper endoscopy (esophagoscopy) does allow a direct inspection of the esophagus with regard to the size of the distal esophagus (narrowing) and failure of the gastroesophageal junction to be open or degree of retention of food, size of the proximal esophagus, and the presence or not, as well as degree, of esophagitis. Specificity is not usually attainable, however. (8,9)

6. (T) The initial treatment should be hydrostatic (pneumatic) dilatation. This brusque rupture of the LES is performed under local anesthesia and with fluoroscopic control. The pressure in the inflatable balloon, positioned fluoroscopically in the LES area, is adapted for each patient according to the operator's assessment of resistance and patient response. Esophageal perforation occurs in approximately 1% of the cases. (1, 6, 10, 11)

7. (T) For intractable lesions, surgery is the treatment of choice. The surgical procedure most commonly used is the Heller procedure. The muscle coats are split longitudinally down to the mucosa; this incision extends from above the LES into the cardiac region of the stomach. The rate of success is 90 to 95%. A complication of this procedure is LES incompetence with gastroesophageal reflux and peptic esophagitis. (3, 4, 7, 11, 12) Assessment of treatment outcome has, however, been based mainly on symptomatology. More objective criteria have been suggested but not implemented to any extent, e.g., lower esophageal sphincter pressure measurements, postsurgical endoscopy. (9) Correlation with symptoms will be necessary. In an initial correlative study, Holloway, et al. (13) utilized radionuclide esophageal emptying of a solid meal (egg salad sandwich labeled with 99m-Tc-sulfur colloid and compared such with lower esophageal sphincter (LES) pressure measurements and a graded symptom scoring in assessing treatment outcome. They concluded that this method could be a practical alternative to more cumbersome methodology, e.g., LES manometry. Unfortunately, the youngest patient was 12 years of age. Future pediatric study is awaited.

REFERENCES

1. Asch, M.J., Liebman, W.M., Lachman, R.S.: Esophageal achalasia: Diagnosis and cardiomyotomy in a newborn infant. J Pediatr Surg 9:911, 1974.

2. Cohen, S. and Lipshutz, W.: Lower esophageal sphincter dysfunction in achalasia. Gastroenterology 61:814, 1971.

3. Elder, J.B.: Achalasia of the cardia in childhood. Digestion 3:90, 1970.

4. Tachovsky, T.J., Lynn, H.B., Ellis, F.H.: The surgical approach to esophageal achalasia in children. J Pediatr Surg 3:226, 1968.

5. Vaughan, W.H. and Williams, J.L.: Familial achalasia with pulmonary complications in children. Radiology 107: 407, 1973.

6. Willich, E.: The function of the cardia in childhood. Progr Surg 3:141, 1972.

7. Silverman, A. and Roy, C.C.: Pediatric Clinical Gastroenterology, 3rd Edition. The CV Mosby Co., St. Louis, 1983, p. 158.

8. Arvanitakes, C.: Achalasia of the cardia. Am J Dig Dis 20:841, 1975.

9. Toccalino, H., Licastro, R., Guastavino, E., et al.: Vomiting and regurgitation. Clin Gastroenterol 6:274, 1977.

10. Liebman, W.M., Applebaum, M., Thaler, M.M.: Achalasia of the esophagus: Pneumatic dilatation in a four-year-old boy. Am J Gastroenterol 70:73, 1978.

11. Yon, J. and Christensen, J.: An uncontrolled comparison of treatments for achalasia. Ann Surg 187:672, 1975.

12. Effler, O., Loop F., Grooes, L., et al.: Primary surgical treatment for esophageal achalasia. Surg Gynec Obstet 132:1057, 1971.

13. Holloway, R.H., Krosin, G., Lange, R.C., et al.: Radionuclide esophageal emptying of a solid meal to quantitate results of therapy in achalasia. Gastroenterology 84: 771, 1983.

Case 14

ABDOMINAL PAIN AND CRYING IN A 2-MONTH-OLD GIRL

HISTORY

A 2-month-old girl presented with a 6-week history of recurrent abdominal pain, associated crying, and variable fussiness. She had these episodes almost daily, and they could recur during the same day, lasting minutes to hours. Bowel movements were described as yellow to yellow-brown, soft to firm in consistency, and without blood and/or melena. There was no associated fever, diarrhea, constipation, vomiting, skin lesions, anorexia, or weight loss. She was described as alert, active, with a good appetite. The remainder of the past history, developmental history, family history, social history, and review of systems was unremarkable.

EXAMINATION

She was alert, active, and in no apparent distress, with normal vital signs, head circumference 36 cm, weight 4.5 kg, and length 56 cm. The remainder of the examination was unremarkable, including the abdomen and anorectal area.

LABORATORY DATA

Hemoglobin:	12.2 gm%
Hematocrit:	37%
White blood cell count:	$9,700/mm^3$
Urinalysis:	negative
Stool:	negative for occult blood
Plain film-abdomen:	negative

QUESTIONS

1. The most likely diagnosis in this infant is
   A. pyloric stenosis
   B. biliary atresia
   C. polyp (colon)
   D. duodenal ulcer
   E. infantile colic

2. Presenting symptomatology usually includes
   A. fever
   B. vomiting
   C. diarrhea
   D. abdominal pain
   E. crying

3. Which of the following are reported causes of this disorder?
   A. Food allergy
   B. Carbohydrate intolerance
   C. Anatomic malformation/obstruction
   D. Collagen-vascular disease
   E. Bacterial overgrowth

4. Treatment should consist of which of the following?
   A. Parental support and counseling
   B. Antacids
   C. Metoclopramide
   D. Broad-spectrum antibiotics
   E. Surgery

ANSWERS AND COMMENTS

1. (E) The most likely diagnosis is infantile colic, since the patient's age and the symptomatic pattern (apparent abdominal pain, crying, irritability) are quite compatible. The age of onset, stool pattern, and lack of diarrhea, fever, vomiting, jaundice, and hematochezia would tend to eliminate the other choices.

2. (D, E) The term "infantile colic" is somewhat imprecise and frequently abused. The usual age of onset is the first 8 to 12 weeks of life, particularly greater than 2 weeks and less than 8 weeks. (1-3) The infant cries continuously for 3 or more hours per day and is quite irritable. (1-5) The upper and/or lower extremities will be flailing. He/she will be described as "gassy, fussy," not sleeping easily, and not being able to be

comforted by rocking or holding. At times, however, walking
or some type of motion, e.g., auto ride, can produce temporary relief. (1-6) Otherwise, this infant is healthy, gaining
height and weight at a normal rate, and is active and alert. (1-6)

3. (A,B) Colic is a self-limiting disorder, with a normal pattern of growth and development, and with no apparent long-term
effects. (1-6) Implicated factors (mechanisms) have included
socioenvironmental variables, such as tension in the home environment, maternal anxiety, and improper feeding techniques.
(1,6,7) Immaturity of the gastrointestinal tract, including neuromuscular dysfunction, e.g., motility, has been a frequent
theme. There obviously have been no substantive objective data
regarding such. Colic also has been regarded as a neonatal-
early-infantile variant of the irritable bowel syndrome, suggesting spasm of the bowel, particularly the colon, as the final pathway. (1,6,7) The role of allergy has been difficult to define objectively and fully, but recent studies on breast-fed infants with
colic have suggested that cow's milk protein sensitivity may be
an important factor. (8,9) Carbohydrate intolerance, particularly lactose, has been frequently implicated as a factor by the
mechanism of fermentation of unhydrolyzed carbohydrate and
hydrogen gas production. (8,10) There has been no affinity for
any one social class, sex, or ethnic group. (1,5) Additionally,
the incidence has varied from 10 to 15% in both premature and
full-term newborns. (1,11)

4. (A) Just as there is no single explanation for colic, there
is no particular medicinal cure. Antispasmodics, anticholinergics, and sedatives have been frequently used, but there is no
objective evidence of their effectiveness. (1,2) Organic disease
must be ruled out. Then feeding techniques must be reviewed
and corrected as necessary. Feedings should be performed in
a calm and comfortable setting, with frequent burping. Breast-
feeding mothers should reduce or eliminate milk and milk products from their diets; a reasonable time period for evaluation of
this dietary elimination should be 2 weeks. A soy formula can
be used in formula-fed babies. Parent education regarding crying, e.g., tension relief, not parental rejection, is very important. Parents can work with the infant, trying to calm for 15 to
30 minutes, then allowing the infant a similar time (15 to 30 minutes) alone without stimulation. Parents should also plan 1 to 2
hours a day away from the "colicky" infant. Lastly, there is no
objective evidence for late sequelae developmentally or otherwise. (1,12)

REFERENCES

1. Paradise, J.L.: Maternal and other factors in the etiology of infantile colic: Report of a prospective study of 106 infants. J Am Med Assoc 197:123, 1966.

2. Brazelton, T.B.: Crying in infancy. Pediatrics 30:579, 1962.

3. Roy, C.C., Silverman, A., Cozzetto, F.J.: Pediatric Clinical Gastroenterology, 2nd Edition. The CV Mosby Company, St. Louis, 1975, p. 32.

4. Oberklaid, F.: Why colic? Med J Aust 2:486, 1979.

5. Waldman, W.H., Sarsgard, D.: Helping parents to cope with colic. Pediatr Basics 33:12, 1982.

6. O'Donnovan, J.D.: Infantile colic, or What to do until the fourth month comes. Compr Ther 6:9, 1980.

7. Davidson, M., Wasserman, R.: The irritable colon of childhood. J Pediatr 69:1027, 1966.

8. Liebman, W.M.: Infantile colic. Association with lactose and milk intolerance. J Am Med Assoc 245:732, 1981.

9. Jakobsson, I., Lindberg, T.: Cow's milk as a cause of infantile colic in breast-fed infants. Lancet 1:437, 1978.

10. Liebman, W.M.: Recurrent abdominal pain in children: Lactose and sucrose intolerance, a prospective study. Pediatrics 64:43, 1979.

11. Meyer, J.E., Thaler, M.M.: Colic in low birth weight infants. Am J Dis Child, 122:25, 1971.

12. White, P.J.: Management of infantile colic. Am J Dis Child 133:995, 1976.

Case 15

ACUTE ONSET OF EPIGASTRIC PAIN
IN AN 11-YEAR-OLD GIRL

HISTORY

An 11-year-old white female presented with a 4-week history of
recurrent abdominal pain, epigastric in location, gnawing in
type, with radiation around to both sides and the adjacent back
area, occurring almost daily for the past 1 to 2 weeks. There
had been associated nausea and vomiting for almost 1 week.
There was no history of fever, hematemesis, diarrhea, melena, hematochezia, skin lesions, anorexia, or trauma. The activity had remained essentially unchanged, although she did
seem to tire more easily. Her bowel habit pattern had generally been once daily, soft and brown in nature. Medication had included Rolaids, without effect. The family history included a
sister and maternal grandmother with diabetes mellitus and an
older brother with possible peptic ulcer disease. The remainder of the past history, family history, social history, developmental history, and review of systems was unremarkable.

EXAMINATION

She was alert, active, and in no apparent distress, with normal
vital signs, height 131 cm and weight 36.2 kg. The remainder
of the examination was unremarkable except for mild tenderness
in the epigastric area of the abdomen.

LABORATORY DATA:

Hemoglobin:	12.4 gm%
Hematocrit:	38%
White blood cell count:	7,700/mm^3
PMN's	61%
lymphocytes:	36%
monocytes:	1%
eosinophiles:	2%
Serum:	
total protein:	6.8 gm%
albumin:	4.8 gm%
SGPT:	20 units
alkaline phosphatase:	195 IU
creatinine:	0.5 mg%
amylase:	106 units
carotene:	170 mg%
Urinalysis:	negative
Urine amylase (diastase)	2,500 units/24 hr

QUESTIONS

1. Which studies would be in order at this point?
   A. Electrocardiogram
   B. Chest X-ray
   C. Barium swallow
   D. Lumbar puncture
   E. Direct laryngoscopy

2. After the studies in question 1, which of the following tests would be indicated?
   A. Echocardiography
   B. CT scan-abdomen
   C. Esophageal manometry
   D. Gastric analysis
   E. Serum gastrin measurement

3. After the studies in question 2, which of the following tests would be indicated?
   A. Cine-esophagram
   B. Intravenous pyelogram
   C. Acid reflux test with pH probe
   D. Esophagoscopy/biopsy
   E. Serum amylase measurement

ANSWERS AND COMMENTS

1. (B,C) Vomiting/spitting-up is one of the most common complaints in pediatric practice; estimated significant organic etiology for this problem has generally been about 5%. (1-3) These causes have included disaccharidase deficiency, cow's milk protein intolerance, and urinary tract infection. The incidence of associated hiatus hernia has been quite variable, usually 5-45%. (1-3)

In infants and children with gastroesophageal reflux, vomiting/spitting-up is the most common manifestation. (1-3) The vomitus usually consists of undigested food or formula. This vomiting can be projectile, although usually is effortless, can occur minutes to hours after meals, and is more likely when the patient is lying down. Older children may experience substernal burning, acidic or bitter taste due to gastric contents in the mouth, nocturnal cough or wheezing (1-4%), pneumonitis (4-10%), hematemesis (10-25%), occult blood in stools (10-50%), or anemia (1-4%). Failure to grow may occur due to the reduced caloric intake (30-50%). (1-3)

The diagnostic evaluation should include (1) complete history and physical examination, as well as longitudinal height/weight profile; (2) complete blood count; (3) urinalysis; (4) occult blood testing of stools; (5) chest X-ray; and (6) barium swallow or cineradiography of the esophagus. The latter is more sensitive for detecting gastroesophageal reflux than the barium swallow; the positive results have varied from 59 to 80%. (1-5) Further tests are in order and will be discussed in answers 2,3.

2. (C) The main tests for evaluation of gastroesophageal reflux can be broadly classified into two groups on the basis of the abnormality being assessed (Table 15.1). The first group is concerned with an assessment of the function, i.e., dysfunction of the lower esophageal sphincter (LES) and esophageal motility. These tests include the barium swallow and cineradiography of the esophagus, previously discussed in answer 1, and esophageal manometry and motility. Manometry of the esophagus involves three of four perfusion tubes with distal openings, a perfusion pump for water perfusion, and a recorder. The perfusion tubes are connected to pressure transducers, which convert mechanical energy to electrical energy; the latter is then recorded. The tubes (openings) are placed into the stomach, and then are slowly pulled from the stomach into the esophagus over 15- to 30-second intervals. Constant recording is performed. The intragastric pressure is used as the zero point (reference), and the positive deflection height is the pressure of the lower esophageal sphincter. At least three determinations are made with

TABLE 15.1 Diagnosis of Gastroesophageal Reflux
(positive, negative)

Reflux (positive, negative)
  Barium swallow
  Scintigraphic reflux study
  pH probe test (standard or Tuttle)
  pH probe test (24 hour intraesophageal monitoring)
  String test (Enterotest-Pediatric)

Reflux (degree of)
  Ph probe test (24 hour intraesophageal monitoring)
  Endoscopy

Reflux (sequelae)
  Chest X-ray
  Scintigraphic reflux study
  Barium swallow
  Endoscopy/esophageal biopsy
  Apnea monitor

each of the distal three openings. One of the distal openings is
anchored in the lower esophageal sphincter, and relaxation of
the sphincter is assessed by asking the patient to swallow spontaneously or with water. Motility of the body of the esophagus
is assessed (contraction waves) by recording from distal openings located in the esophagus while swallowing. (1-5) In infants
and children, the normal LES pressure is 15 to 30 mmHg, while
in those with gastroesophageal reflux, the pressure is frequently, but not always, below normal. (1-5) There is a good correlation with an incompetent LES when the LES pressure is less
than 10 mmHg. (6) The other choices do not apply to GER.

3. (C,D) The second group is concerned with the detection of
reflux of acid into the esophagus (Table 15.1). These tests include the gastroesophageal scintiscan, acid reflux test (modified
Tuttle test), string test, 24-hour pH monitoring, and esophagoscopy with biopsy. (1-15) Gastroesophageal scintiscan measures the reflux of technetium 99m-sulfur colloid after its instillation into the stomach. This radioisotope is nonadsorbable and
nonabsorbable with minimal radiation exposure. The scintiscan
seems to be very sensitive, with 90+% correlation with the pH-
probe results (positivity). (8) The acid reflux test (modified

Tuttle test) measures the acid reflux from the stomach by placement of a pH probe above the lower esophageal sphincter and instillation of 0.1 N HCl into the stomach. (3,5-7) The lower
esophageal sphincter must be determined manometrically before
this test. The pH electrode is passed into the esophagus and
placed at a position above the LES, 13% of the length of the body
of the esophagus. (3,5-7) After the HCl instillation into the
stomach, constant determination of intraluminal pH is performed for 10 minutes, then for 5 minutes along with measures
to increase the intragastric pressure, such as manual abdominal compression. If necessary, these procedures are performed in the right lateral, left lateral, and prone positions.
A positive test consists of finding a pH less than 3.0 on two occasions. Euler and Ament (6) more recently reported on 65 Tuttle tests in children with symptoms of gastroesophageal reflux,
28 being positive (26 required surgery), and 37 being negative
(2 required surgery). Due to a need for improved correlation
between symptoms and GER, 24-hour esophageal pH monitoring
was developed and applied in children. In a manner similar to
pH probe test, the probe was accurately placed intraesophageal-
ly and taped to the nares for the duration of the study, 24 hours.
(7,8) The pH is continuously recorded throughout the 24 hours
(rest, feedings, sleep). Normals usually have 0 to 1 reflux episodes per hour, and 0 to 1 during sleep (5-8%, time). (7,8)
Symptoms and/or sequelae, e.g., cyanosis, apnea, are correlated with the pH pattern (quantitative plus qualitative).

The more recent availability of smaller fiberoptic endoscopic instruments has permitted direct visualization of the esophageal mucosa, i.e., presence of esophagitis. (2,4,11,12) Grasp
or suction biopsies (blindly performed) should be carried out to
confirm the presence of esophagitis. The suggestive findings
on biopsy include basal-cell hyperplasia, basal-zone thickness
greater than 15% of the epithelial height, papillae height greater
than 2/3 of the epithelial height, and the presence of an inflammatory reaction, including the presence of eosinophiles.
(2,11-14)

Cine-esophagram would not add to the information from the
barium swallow examination, while the other choices do not apply to GER.

REFERENCES

1. Pope, C.E.: Pathophysiology and diagnosis of reflux esoph-
    agitis. Gastroenterology 70:445, 1976.

2. Euler, A.R. and Ament, M.E.: Gastroesophageal reflux in children: Clinical manifestations, diagnosis, pathophysiology, and therapy. Pediatr Ann 5:678, 1976.

3. Behar, L.J., Sheehan, D.G., Biancani, P., et al.: Medical and surgical management of reflux esophagitis. N Engl J Med 293:263, 1975.

4. Benz, L.J., Hootkin, L.A., Margalies, S., et al.: A comparison of clinical measurements of gastroesophageal reflux. Gastroenterology 62:1, 1972.

5. Tuttle, S.G., Bettarello, A., Grossman, M.J.: Esophageal acid perfusion test and a gastroesophageal reflux test in patients with esophagitis. Gastroenterology 38:861, 1960.

6. Euler, A.R. and Ament, M.E.: Detection of gastroesophageal reflux by Tuttle test. Pediatrics 60:65, 1977.

7. Berquist, W.E.: Gastroesophageal reflux in children: Clinical review. Pediatr Ann 11:135, 1982.

8. Sondheimer, J.M.: Continuous monitoring of distal esophageal pH: A diagnostic test for gastroesophageal reflux in infants. J Pediatr 96:804, 1980.

9. Fisher, R.S., Malmud, L.S., Roberts, G.S., et al.: Gastroensophageal (GE) scintiscanning to detect and quantitate GE reflux. Gastroenterology 70:301, 1976.

10. Liebman, W.M., Rosenthal, P.: The string test for gastroesophageal reflux. Am J Dis Child 134:775, 1980.

11. Liebman, W.M.: Fiberoptic endoscopy of the gastrointestinal tract in infants and children. I. Upper endoscopy in 53 children. Am J Gastroenterol 68:362, 1977.

12. Ismail-Beizi, F., Horton, P.F., Pope, C.E.: Histological consequences of gastroesophageal reflux in man. Gastroenterology 58:163, 1970.

13. Winter, H.S., Madara, J.L., Stafford, R.J., et al.: Intraepithelial eosinophils: A new diagnostic criterion for reflux esophagitis. Gastroenterology, 83:818, 1982.

14. Leape, L.L., Bhar, I., Ramenofsky, M.: Esophageal biopsy in the diagnosis of reflux esophagitis. J Pediatr Surg 16:379, 1981.

15. Arasu, T.S., Wyllie, R., Fitzgerald, J.F., et al.: Gastroesophageal reflux in infants and children: Comparison of diagnostic methods. J Pediatr 96:798, 1980.

Case 16

RECURRENT WHEEZING IN AN 11-MONTH-OLD GIRL

HISTORY

An 11-month-old white female presented with a 5-month history
of recurrent wheezing, associated crying, and vomiting. There
was no history of fever, hematemesis, diarrhea, constipation,
melena, hematochezia, anorexia. The activity had been variable between no change and decreased with irritability. Her
bowel habit pattern had generally been once daily, soft and
brown in nature. Medication had included Marax and Alupent
without significant effect. The family history included a maternal aunt with bronchial asthma. The remainder of the past history, family history, social history, developmental history, and
review of systems was unremarkable.

EXAMINATION

She was alert, active, and in mild respiratory distress, height
71 cm and weight 8.4 kg. The remainder of the examination
was unremarkable, except for mild substernal retractions and
coarse breath sounds in the anterior and posterior lung fields.

LABORATORY DATA

Hemoglobin:	11.0 gm%
Hematocrit:	33%
White blood cell count:	10,300/mm^3
PMN's:	48%
lymphocytes:	38%
monocytes:	8%
eosinophiles:	6%

Serum:
   total protein: 6.0 gm%
   albumin: 3.6 gm%
   creatinine: 0.6 mg%
   amylase: 68 units
   gastrin: 71 pg/ml
Urinalysis: negative
Chest X-ray: slight hyperinflation
Barium swallow: moderate reflux
Esophageal manometry (LES
 pressure):   12 mmHg
Tuttle (acid probe test):   positive (spontaneous)
Intraesophageal pH monitoring
 (24 hr):   abnormal % (12)
Fiberoptic upper endoscopy: moderate erythema with increased friability of distal esophagus
Distal esophageal biopsy: (Fig. 16.1)

QUESTIONS

Question 1: Answer true (T) or false (F).

1. From the historical, radiological and laboratory details, you may assume that the probable diagnosis is gastroesophageal reflux (GER).

2. Medical management of this condition includes which of the following?
   A. Upright position (over 60°) for 24 hours a day
   B. Antacids if esophagitis is present
   C. Anticholinergics
   D. Antibiotics
   E. Metoclopramide

3. Surgical treatment would be indicated under which of the following circumstances?
   A. Apnea
   B. Failure of response to medical management after 3 weeks
   C. Failure of response to medical management after 6 weeks
   D. Associated upper gastrointestinal hemorrhage
   E. Nocturnal asthma

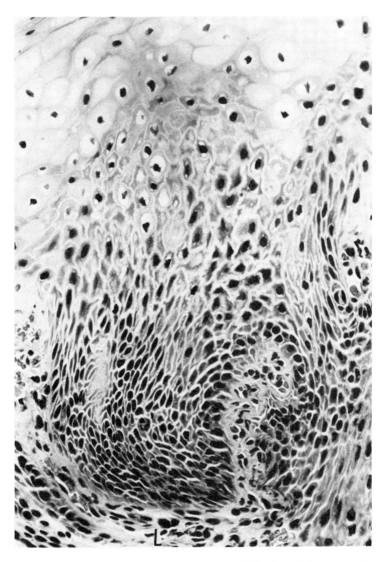

Figure 16.1 Esophagus. Thickening of the basal layer, extension of the dermal pegs, and inflammatory reaction (round cells) in the lamina propria (L) are shown (H&E, X250).

118 / Case 16

ANSWERS AND COMMENTS

1. (T) The probable diagnosis is gastroesophageal reflux
(GER). The barium swallow demonstrated GER, while the pH
probe test (Tuttle) also confirmed acid reflux. The 24-hr intraesophageal pH monitoring also demonstrated acid reflux, abnormal in amount (%), and the upper endoscopy/biopsy demonstrated
the presence of esophagitis, presumably secondary to GER (peptic). (1-3)

2. (A,B,E) (Table 16.1) In infants, the medical regimen consists of an increased number of feedings, specifically, every 2
to 3 hours, limited volume per feeding, and maintaining an upright position, at least 45^0 to 60^0, 24 hours a day, for a minimum of 4 to 6 weeks. Most infants will respond favorably to
such a regimen. However, the results have not been as favorable in older infants and children. An increase in LES pressure
and a decrease in reflux cannot be anticipated, however. (1,2)
Variable success with reference to growth and general well-
being has been documented; moreover, a variable rate of stricture formation, usually 3 to 6%, but as high as 33% (3,4) has
been reported. Other indicated measures include avoidance of
food or liquids after supper, tight clothing, bending at the waist,
and lifting. Antacids, 15 to 30 ml every hour, should be administered during waking hours if esophagitis is present, and the
head of the bed should be elevated 4 to 6 inches with wooden
blocks or bricks. The combination of alginate and antacid (Gavi-
scon®) has also been utilized in order to provide a coating or
mechanical barrier in the esophagus, as well as the antacid action. The role of antacids, as well as acid suppressants, e.g.,
H^2-receptor antgonists (cimetidine, ranitidine) is pain relief but
may not prevent continued esophageal injury. (1-4)
  Pharmacologic treatment has not been extensively investigated in children. In adults, cholinergic agents, such as Bethanechol and Metoclopramide, have been demonstrated orally to
increase lower esophageal sphincter pressure and, thereby, to
decrease gastroesophageal reflux. (4-7) Bethanechol, 8.7 mg/
m^2/d (divided doses; a.c.), has been useful in the majority of
infants and children and may allow an adequate interval of time
for maturity. Only one controlled series in children, however,
has been performed. (6) In infants and children, metoclopramide has been used in a dose of 0.5-0.6 mg/kg/d (divided doses;
a.c.), particularly in those with respiratory symptoms, e.g.,
wheezing, since Bethanechol is a cholinergic agent (author's
note). This treatment, even if successful, reflects a control,
not a cure.

TABLE 16.1   Treatment of Gastroesophageal Reflux

Step I (4-6 weeks)
   Feedings - increased frequency and decreased amounts per
      feeding

   Thickening, cereal/fruits

   Positioning, upright (after meals, night vs. 24 hours a day)
   30 degree angle
   Prone board

Step II (2-4 weeks)
   Medication

      Bethanechol (Urecholine), 8.7 mg/m^2 surface area/24 hr,
      before meals

      Metoclopramide (Reglan), 0.5-0.75 mg/kg bodyweight/24
      hr, before meals

Step III
   Surgery

      Stricture, esophageal

      Respiratory symptoms
         Recurrent pneumonia
         Apnea
         Other, e.g., cough, choking, unresponsive at Step I, II

      Failure to thrive, unresponsive at Step I, II

      GI bleeding, life-threatening or unresponsive at Step I, II

---

3. (A, C) The presence of an associated hiatus hernia, hematemesis, and respiratory complications should not alter the de-
cision for medical management. However, the presence of associated apnea or a stricture should result in a surgical approach.
   Various surgical approaches for gastroesophageal reflux
have been used. These include the Allison procedure, repair of
the phrenoesophageal ligament, the Belsey procedure, anterior
fundoplication, the Hill procedure, posterior gastropexy, and

the Nissen fundoplication (anterior). (2,8,13) A new surgical approach has been the Angelchik procedure, consisting of the insertion of an inert device to provide tightening of the gastro-esophageal junctional zone. (13) This procedure is simple, flexible or adaptive for growth, and consumes less surgical anesthesia time. No comparative studies are available yet in children. The Nissen procedure has been particularly popular and consists of the mobilization of the esophagus and upper stomach; the upper stomach is wrapped about the distal esophagus and sutured anteriorly to the esophagus. (1,2,9) The rate of success in children has varied from 80 to 100%. The mortality rate is very low, and the recurrence rate is also quite low. (1,2,11) Vomiting ceases, growth is evident, and pulmonary complications disappear. Esophagitis heals, as do any ulcerations. (1, 2,11) Postsurgical manometric studies reveal significant elevation of the lower esophageal sphincter pressure, and acid reflux tests become negative. (1,2,11) Esophagrams are normal too. (2,9,11)

As previously mentioned (in 4), the rate of success is high, 80 to 100%, and the recurrence is low, 0 to 20%, usually 6 to 8%. (1,2,11) Pulmonary infections do cease, while growth rapidly ensues, normal weight usually being achieved within 6 months postoperatively. (1,2,11) Healing of esophagitis and esophageal ulcerations occurs. (1,2,11,12)

Pyloric stenosis or obstruction has been found in some series, necessitating a pyloroplasty. (2) In the author's experience, this has been necessary in only one case.

REFERENCES

1. Berquist, W.E.: Gastroesophageal reflux in children: A clinical review. Pediatr Ann 11:135, 1982.

2. Baswell, D.L. and Lebenthal, E.: Gastroesophageal Reflux. In: Textbook of Gastroenterology and Nutrition in Infancy. Lebenthal, E. (Ed). Raven Press, New York, 1981, p. 911.

3. Christie, D.L., O'Grady, L.R., Mack, D.V.: Incompetent lower esophageal sphincter and gastroesophageal reflux in recurrent acute pulmonary disease of infancy and childhood. J Pediatr 93:23, 1978.

4. Behar, J., Biancani, P., Sheahan, D.G., et al.: Cimetidine in the treatment of symptomatic gastroesophageal reflux. A double-blind controlled trial. Gastroenterology 74:441, 1978.

5. Farrell, R.L., Roling, G.T., Castell, D.O.: Cholinergic therapy of chronic heartburn. Ann Intern Med 80:573, 1974.

6. Euler, A.R.: Use of bethanechol for the treatment of gastroesophageal reflux. J Pediatr 96:321, 1980.

7. McCallum, R.W., Kline, M.M., Curry, N., et al.: Comparative effects of metoclopramide and bethanechol on lower esophageal sphincter pressure in reflux patients. Gastroenterology 68:1114, 1975.

8. Lipshutz, W.H., Eckert, R.J., Gaskins, R.D., et al.: Normal lower esophageal sphincter function after surgical treatment of gastroesophageal reflux. N Engl J Med 291: 1107, 1974.

9. Euler, A.R., Fonkalsrad, E.W., Ament, M.E.: Effect of Nissen fundoplication on the lower esophageal sphincter reflux pressure of children with gastroesophageal reflux. Gastroenterology 72:260, 1977.

10. Kaye, M.D. and Showalter, J.P.: Pyloric incompetence in patients with symptomatic gastroesophageal reflux. J Lab Clin Med 83:198, 1974.

11. Fonkalsrad, E.W., Ament, M.E., Byrne, W.J., et al.: Gastroesophageal fundoplication for the management of reflux in infants and children. J Thorac Cardiovasc Surg 76: 655, 1978.

12. Wilkinson, J.D., Dudgeon, D.L., Sondheimer, J.M.: A comparison of medical and surgical treatment of gastroesophageal reflux in severely retarded children. J Pediatr 99:202, 1981.

13. Angelchik, J.P. and Cohan, R.: A new surgical procedure for the treatment of gastroesophageal reflux and hiatal hernia. Surg Gynecol Obstet 148:246, 1979.

Case 17

PALLOR, POOR APPETITE, AND WEAKNESS IN A 29-MONTH-OLD GIRL

HISTORY

A 29-month-old white female presented with a history of recurrent pallor, weakness, and decreased appetite of almost two years' duration. There was no associated history of fever, nausea, vomiting, diarrhea, constipation, melena, hematochezia, jaundice, skin lesions, dysuria, headache, incoordination, or trauma. There was no associated loss of consciousness nor any history of recurrent purulent infection. The family history included a mother with a history of spastic colitis. Past history, developmental history, family history, social history, and review of systems were unremarkable.

EXAMINATION

She was alert and in no apparent distress, with normal vital signs, head circumference 49 cm, weight 12 kg, and height 89 cm. The remainder of the physical examination was unremarkable except for mild pallor of nail beds and of mucous membranes. Abdominal examination was unremarkable with no palpable liver, spleen, and kidneys. Neurological examination was felt to be within normal limits.

LABORATORY DATA

Hemoglobin:	9.2 gm%
Hematocrit:	27%
White blood cell count:	10,000/mm^3
PMN's:	38%
lymphocytes:	50%

122

monocytes:	1%
eosinophiles:	1%
Sedimentation rate:	13 mm/hr
Urinalysis:	negative
Serum:	
sodium:	136 meq/L
potassium:	4.1 meq/L
chloride:	100 meq/L
bicarbonate:	23 meq/L
creatinine:	0.4 mg%
total protein:	6.2 gm%
albumin:	4.2 gm%
SGOT:	18 KU
alkaline phosphatase:	170 IU
total bilirubin:	0.6 mg%
direct bilirubin:	0.4 mg%
amylase:	88 units
carotene:	128 μg%
folate:	11 ng/ml
vitamin B_{12}:	90 mg%
Parietal cell antibodies:	negative
Intrinsic factor (IF) antibodies:	negative
Schilling test:	
without IF:	1.7%
with IF:	12.8%
Gastric analysis:	
basal output:	1.4 meq/hr
stimulated (Histalog) output:	15.3 meq/hr
ECG:	within normal limits for age
Chest films:	negative
Upper gastrointestinal series:	negative

QUESTIONS

1. The most likely diagnosis of this patient is which of the following?
   A. Hiatus hernia
   B. Pernicious anemia (PA)
   C. Celiac disease
   D. Cystic fibrosis
   E. Crohn's disease

2. Which of the following studies would be most helpful in establishing the diagnosis?
   A. Serum vitamin B_{12} level
   B. Vitamin B_{12} absorption (Schilling test)
   C. Esophagram
   D. Gastric analysis
   E. Fiberoptic endoscopy

3. The cause of this condition is which of the following?
   A. Absence of intrinsic factor
   B. Hypergastrinemia
   C. Small intestine mucosal defect
   D. Deficiency of endogenous intestinal binder, e.g., transcobalamin II
   E. Altered intestinal motility

4. Associated conditions include which of the following?
   A. Thyrotoxicosis
   B. Idiopathic hyperparathyroidism
   C. Addison's disease
   D. Chronic active liver disease
   E. None of these

5. Specific treatment includes which of the following?
   A. Antacids
   B. Anticholinergics
   C. Trasylol
   D. Oral elemental diet
   E. Vitamin B_{12}

Question 6: Answer true (T) or false (F).

6. After a period of 6 to 12 months of treatment, a certain percentage of patients no longer require treatment.

ANSWERS AND COMMENTS

1. (B) The most likely diagnosis in this patient is pernicious anemia, juvenile in type. The age of onset, the lack of relationship to food types or new food introduction, and the lack of diarrhea, blood in stools, or abdominal pain, as well as the normal intestinal absorptive studies, would mitigate against the other possibilities, such as celiac disease, cystic fibrosis, and Crohn's disease. The type of anemia, megaloblastic and not hypochromic/microcytic, as well as the lack of regurgitation/vomiting and apparent abdominal/lower chest pain, would mitigate against hiatus hernia (secondary gastroesophageal reflux).

2. (A,B,C) Pernicious anemia is a megaloblastic anemia which is caused by a deficiency of vitamin B_{12}. (1-5) The specific mechanism will be discussed in answer 3. The usual age of onset is between 3 to 36 months of age. (1-5) Symptomatology includes pallor, fatigue, anorexia, failure to thrive, and neurological sequelae, e.g., ataxia, speech defects. (1-5)

Megaloblastic anemia is rare in children and results from a deficiency of folic acid, vitamin B_{12}, or both. (1-5) The assay of serum vitamin B_{12} is now available in most centers, and in PA the value is low or negligible, less than 100 ng/ml, normal being 300-400. (1-5) However, megaloblastic anemia with vitamin B_{12} deficiency can be due to small intestinal bacterial overgrowth, ileal disease, especially distal, exocrine pancreatic insufficiency, D. latum infestations, and absent intrinsic factor production. (6-10) Therefore, the Schilling test, using ^{57}Co-cyanocobalamin orally, nonradioactive vitamin B_{12} intramuscularly, and a 48-hour urine collection may be quite helpful. (1-5) Vitamin B_{12} deficiency is confirmed by low excretion (less than 10% per day); excretion of vitamin B_{12} is normal in folate deficiency. (1-5) In intestinal disorders, the excretion is low, but usually over 3%, while being low and less than 3% in those patients with pernicious anemia. (1-5) In patients with low values, the test can be repeated after the administration of intrinsic factor plus vitamin B_{12}. An increase in urine excretion is highly suggestive of pernicious anemia. (1-5)

Gastric analysis can be helpful in distinguishing between the juvenile (congenital) and adult (acquired) types of pernicious anemia. (1-5) In the latter type, acid and pepsin production, basal (fasting) and poststimulation (histamine, pentagastrin) are low to absent. (1-5) In the juvenile type, the values are normal. (1-5) Histologically, the stomach is normal in the juvenile type, while demonstrating variable atrophy and inflammation (atrophic gastritis) in the adult type. (1-5) In the latter, parietal cell and intrinsic factor antibodies are found. (1-5) (Table 17.1)

Radiology and endoscopy are not particularly helpful, although endoscopy with biopsy through the endoscope would allow obvious histological assessment.

3. (A) As previously mentioned in answer 2, PA is due to a deficiency of vitamin B_{12} as a result of defective vitamin absorption. (1-5) Furthermore, the diminished absorption is caused by low or absent intrinsic factor (IF) secretion by the stomach, the basic underlying defect. (1-5) Intrinsic factor (IF) is a glycoprotein, 45,000 molecular weight, which binds cobalamin (vitamin B_{12}) with high affinity and plays an important role

TABLE 17.1   Pernicious Anemia: Adult and Juvenile Types

Condition	Age (Onset)	Gastric Acid/ Pepsin	Intrinsic Factor	Anti- bodies	Associated Entities
Adult	10-20 years	↓	0	+	+ (Thyroiditis, Addison's disease, hyperthyroidism)
Juvenile	4-28 months	→	0	0	0

Key: 0 = not present (absent)

   ↓ = decreased

   ↑ = increased

   → = unchanged (normal)

   + = present

Modified from Roy, C.C., Silverman, A., Cozzetto, F.J. (16)

in cobalamin absorption.   The site of synthesis of IF is the stomach, the parietal cells.   Its secretion is significantly stimulated by gastrin, histamine, and cholinergic agents. (1-6) It has the property of binding vitamin B_{12}, forming a vitamin B_{12}-IF complex. B_{12} binds to two molecules of IF.   This complex moves into the small intestine, is absorbed onto the microvilli, attaching to receptor sites, and is then released intracellularly.   This takes place principally in the distal ileum.   Additionally, the presence of pancreatic proteolytic enzymes, e.g., trypsin, facilitates ileal uptake. (1-11) Once inside the enterocyte, the vitamin is freed and then taken up by endogenous binders, specifically Transcobalamin I and II. (1-11) These binders are responsible for plasma transport and delivery to tissues. (1-11) However, recent studies have demonstrated that there is another cobalamin-binding protein in gastric juice, R protein, which binds dietary cobalamin entering the jejunum, not bound to IF, until the R protein complex is partially degraded by pancreatic proteases in the small intestine. At this time, the IF-cobalamin complex is formed in the upper jejunum and then remains intact until the distal ileum where it binds to specific receptors and is released intracellularly. The ileal surface must be intact.

4. (E) The juvenile or congenital type has been characterized by no consistently associated conditions, immune, allergic, chromosomal or otherwise. (1-16) Conversely, the adult or acquired type has been found in association with immunodeficiency states, e.g., a-or hypogammaglobulinemia, multiple endocrine disease, such as Addison's disease, idiopathic hyperparathyroidism, and cystic fibrosis. (11-16)

5. (E) When the diagnosis is established, i.e., vitamin B_{12} deficiency, specific treatment with vitamin B_{12} is administered. Vitamin B_{12} must be given in therapeutic doses, specifically up to 1,000 micrograms (μg) each day for 7 to 10 days by the parenteral route. (1-5,16) Thereafter, doses up to 1,000 μg are administered monthly. (1-5,16) Doses will vary according to the necessary amount for maintenance of normal hematological values and neurological status.

6. (F) As previously mentioned, juvenile PA is a rare condition in the pediatric population. Once this diagnosis is established, treatment (vitamin B_{12}) must be instituted. This treatment must be maintained for life for continued normalcy of hematological and neurological status. (1-5,16)

REFERENCES

1. Castle, W.B.: Current concepts of pernicious anemia. Am J Med 48:541, 1970.

2. Lampkin, B.C. and Schubert, W.K.: Pernicious anemia in the second decade of life. J Pediatr 72:387, 1968.

3. Lillibridge, C.B., Brandborg, L.L., Rubin, C.E.: Childhood pernicious anemia. Gastroenterology 52:792, 1967.

4. McIntyre, O.R., Sullivan, L.W., Jeffries, G.H., et al.: Pernicious anemia in childhood. N Engl J Med 272:981, 1965.

5. Miller, D.R., Bloom, G.E., Streigg, R.R., et al.: Juvenile congenital pernicious anemia: Clinical and immunologic studies. N Engl J Med 275:978, 1966.

6. Allen, R.H.: Cobalamin (vitamin B_{12}) absorption and malabsorption. Viewpt Dig Dis 14:17, 1982.

7. Toskes, P.P. and Deren, J.J.: The role of the pancreas in vitamin B_{12} absorption: Studies of vitamin B_{12} absorption in partially pancreatectomized rats. J Clin Invest 51: 216, 1972.

8. Schade, S.G., Feick, P., Muckerheide, M., et al.: Occurrence in gastric juice of antibody to a complex of intrinsic factor and vitamin B_{12}. N Engl J Med 275:528, 1966.

9. Donaldson, R.M., Jr., MacKenzie, I.L., Trier, J.S.: Intrinsic factor-mediated attachment of vitamin B_{12} to brush borders and microvillous membranes of hamster intestine. J Clin Invest 46:1215, 1967.

10. Okuda, K.: Enhanced vitamin B_{12} absorption from rat intestine by proteases in the absence of intrinsic factor. Proc Soc Exp Biol Med 124:79, 1967.

11. Webb, D.I., Chodos, R.B., Mahar, C.O., et al.: Mechanism of vitamin B_{12} absorption in patients receiving colchicine. N Engl J Med 279:845, 1968.

12. Imerslund, O. and Bjornstad, P.: Familial vitamin B_{12} malabsorption. Acta Haematol 30:1, 1963.

13. Twomey, J.J., Jordan, P.H., Jarrold, T., et al.: The syndrome of immunoglobulin deficiency and pernicious anemia. Am J Med 47:340, 1969.

14. Wuepper, K.D. and Fudenberg, H.H.: Moniliasis, "autoimmune" polyendocrinopathy and immunologic family study. Clin Exp Immunol 2:71, 1967.

15. Whittingham, S., MacKay, I.R., Ungar, B., et al.: The genetic factor in pernicious anemia: A family study in patients with gastritis. Lancet 1:951, 1969.

16. Roy, C.C., Silverman, A., Cozzetto, F.J.: Pediatric Clinical Gastroenterology, 2nd Edition. The CV Mosby Co., St. Louis, 1975, pp. 170, 219, 703.

Case 18

CHRONIC ABDOMINAL PAIN IN A 12-YEAR-OLD BOY

HISTORY

A 12-year-old white male presented with a history of abdominal pain of 11 months' duration. The pain was located in the right, left, and midupper abdomen, as well as in the lower quadrants. The pain could occur in one area or in all areas. There was no other radiation of this pain. There was no association of this pain with activity, position, meals or food types, nor any with bowel movements. The pain occurred more commonly in the morning, especially when preparing to leave for school. The pain lasted as long as 4-5 hours. The patient had associated nausea and vomiting occurring once or twice weekly. If the vomiting coincided with the pain, there was some degree of improvement of the pain after the episode of vomiting. The bowel habit pattern was once daily but bore no relationship to the pain. There was no history of associated fever, diarrhea, melena, hematochezia, weight loss, or inactivity. There was no disturbance of the sleep pattern. The family history included a maternal grandfather with history of duodenal ulcer disease. Social history included frequent absence from school, almost 4-5 weeks in toto, due to the previously mentioned pain as well as to actual purposeful missing of classes. The patient supposedly related well to his mother but poorly with his father, especially in obtaining his attention. The father had two jobs and when he had free time, spent it with his older brother. He was described as increasingly aggressive during the last 1-2 years and prior to that time as happy-go-lucky. Undue pressure in attaining grades or performing other educational or social endeavors was frequent.

EXAMINATION

He was alert, active, and cooperative, in no distress, with normal vital signs, height 150 cm and weight 40.3 kg. The remainder of the examination was unremarkable, including the abdomen.

LABORATORY DATA

Hemoglobin:	12.5 gm%
Hematocrit:	38%
White blood cell count:	$8,200/mm^3$
PMN's:	60%
lymphocytes:	36%
monocytes:	3%
eosinophiles:	1%
Sedimentation rate:	8 mm/hr
Serum amylase:	83 units
Urine:	
examination:	negative
amylase (diastase):	1,800 units/24 hr
Upper GI - small bowel series:	(Fig. 18.1)

QUESTIONS

1. The most likely diagnosis in this child is
   A. duodenal diverticulum
   B. duodenal polyp
   C. duodenal ulcer
   D. giardiasis
   E. annular pancreas

2. Which of the following statements about this condition are
   correct?
   A. Pain is worsened by eating
   B. Pain at night or in the early morning hours may be fre-
      quent
   C. Melena and/or hematemesis is uncommon
   D. Vomiting is present in less than 50%
   E. Incidence is equal in males and females

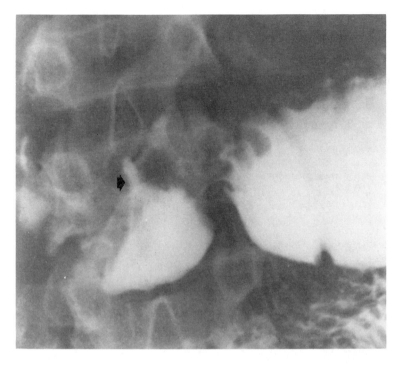

Figure 18.1 Barium swallow. A collection of barium (niche) (arrow) with edema of folds converging toward this area is seen (duodenal bulb).

3. Which of the following laboratory values are frequently present in this disorder?
   A. Basal gastric acid output greater than 10 to 15 meq/hr
   B. Stimulated gastric acid output (Histalog) less than two to three times the basal output
   C. Stimulated gastric acid output (Histalog) greater than normal
   D. Normal basal serum gastrin levels
   E. Elevated basal serum gastrin levels

4. Which of the following radiological findings are character-
   istic of this disorder?
   A. Niche in the duodenal bulb
   B. Delayed gastric emptying
   C. Thickened mucosal folds in the duodenum
   D. Pylorospasm
   E. Segmentation in the duodenum

5. If the barium X-ray examination is negative or equivocal,
   which of the following studies may lead to a diagnosis of an
   ulcer in the duodenum?
   A. Gastric analysis
   B. Basal serum gastrin level
   C. Small intestinal biopsy (peroral)
   D. Sedimentation rate
   E. Fiberoptic panendoscopy

6. Proven effective medical treatment of this disorder includes
   which of the following?
   A. Antacids
   B. Diet (exclusion, such as tea, coffee)
   C. Anticholinergics
   D. H$_2$ receptor antagonists
   E. Radiation (low-dose)

7. Which of the following are indications for surgical treatment
   of this disease?
   A. Obstruction (gastric outlet)
   B. Intractable pain
   C. Major hemorrhage
   D. Perforation
   E. All of these

ANSWERS AND COMMENTS

1. (C) Duodenal ulcer is the most likely diagnosis, considering the clinical history. Refer to answer 2.

2. (B,C) In school-age and adolescent patients, the clinical
findings are more typical of the picture described in adults.
The overall incidence is still low, usually 0.05 to 0.5% of this
age population. (1-12) This disease accounts for only 1.8 to
3.4 per 10,000 patient admissions. Males outnumber females,
2:1 to 4:1. (1-12) The peak age is 12 to 18 years. (1-12) Chronic duodenal ulcers are significantly more frequent than gastric
ulcers, 5:1 to 7:1. (1-12) A family history can be found in 25 to

50% of cases. (1-13) Hyperpepsinogenemia I (group I pepsinogens, precursor zymogens of pepsin) has been reported in one subset of the ulcer population, approximately 25%. (1-13) The most common symptom is pain, usually burning or gnawing in nature, most frequently in the epigastrium. This pain occurs at night or in the early morning hours, in the fasting state, and is frequently relieved by consuming milk or solids. Other symptomatology frequently encountered includes vomiting, 25 to 45%; nausea, 30 to 60%; melena and/or hematemesis, 5 to 25%. Anorexia, with or without significant weight loss, occurs in less than 25 to 30%. (1-12) Occult bleeding or anemia, with or without other typical symptomatology, occurs not infrequently, 10 to 20%. (1-12) Altered bowel habit pattern is infrequent.

So-called secondary ulcers are outnumbered by primary ulcers in a ratio of 1:5 to 1:6. (1-12) The former comprise an almost equal incidence of ulcers in the stomach and duodenum. In addition, certain chronic conditions are associated with duodenal ulcers in children, including rheumatoid arthritis, Crohn's disease, hyperparathyroidism, and, less commonly, cystic fibrosis. (1,11)

3. (C,D) Gastric acidity is determined by collection of gastric contents before stimulation (basal output) and after stimulation with agents, such as Histalog (betazole) or pentagastrin, a synthetic peptide resembling gastrin. The majority of children with a duodenal ulcer will demonstrate high peak acid outputs, but nondiagnostic in nature. In addition, the acid outputs are frequently variable and overlap into the normal range. (1,11,13-15) These augmented gastric analyses are performed with Histalog (betazole, 1.5 mg/kg body weight) or pentagastrin (Peptavlon, 2 to 6 μg/kg body weight. (1,11,13,14)

Gastrin is a gastrointestinal hormone, the c-terminal tetrapeptide being the active part of this agent. It has been localized predominantly in the gastric antrum, but also is found in other areas, such as the proximal duodenum and pancreas. (15,16) It is the most potent factor known in the stimulation of gastric acid secretion and is thought to play a critical role in the regulation of human acid secretion. (15-17) As previously mentioned, increased rates of gastric acid secretion are frequently found in patients with duodenal ulcer. Several studies have demonstrated the interdependency of gastric acid (HCl) and serum gastrin levels. (15,16) The relationship has been an inverse one, low to normal serum gastrin levels associated with elevated rates of basal and augmented (stimulated) gastric acid secretion. (15-17) Furthermore, an interesting, consistent finding has been that there are greater increases in serum gastrin levels of patients with duodenal ulcer than in controls in response to administering pentagastrin, or other similar stimuli. (15-17) Despite the absence of fasting hypergastrinemia, the potential important role of gastrin in the "hypersecretory state," frequently characterizing duodenal ulcer disease, remains.

4. (A) Radiological examination remains the hallmark method of diagnosis of peptic ulcer disease. The purpose continues to be demonstration of the crater. The diagnosis of duodenal ulcer cannot be made unless a persistent crater or niche is demonstrated. (1-12,18)

Duodenal irritability is a frequent radiological finding in asymptomatic children as well as in patients with duodenal ulcer disease. Sometimes, significant irritability may be an indication for closer survey of the bulb area for a possible ulcer niche. Deformity of the duodenal bulb without a crater is usually an indication of a prior ulcer and scar formation. (1-12,18) Thickened mucosal folds in the duodenum may represent an ulcer-equivalent, but this is seen in many asymptomatic children. (1-12) Delayed gastric emptying does not necessarily imply structural or functional pathology in the pyloric or prepyloric area and, thus, is an unreliable sign of peptic ulcer disease or otherwise.

5. (E) Also refer to answer 3. The development of smaller fiberoptic instruments has permitted the direct visualization of the upper gastrointestinal tract in children. These fiberoptic instruments consist of thousands of thin glass fibers, bound in a flexible bundle with identical spatial arrangement at both ends. The length and diameter of each instrument is variable. For children, the instrument's examining-end diameter is 7.2 to 8.4 millimeters. Premedication is usually necessary in order to prevent movement and possible complications. This premedication may include atropine, meperidine, diazepam, chlorpromazine, or promethazine. These are administered 45 to 60 minutes before the procedure. In children less than 10 to 12 years of age, adequate relaxation and cooperation may not be possible by parenteral medication and, therefore, general anesthesia may be necessary. With general or parenteral anesthesia, topical preparations, such as cetacaine spray or viscous xylocaine, frequently may not be necessary. In several studies in patients with recurrent abdominal pain, vomiting, or other symptomatology and prior negative studies, including radiological examination, fiberoptic endoscopy has disclosed a gastric or duodenal ulcer in 11 to 21%. (19) Thus, the value of endoscopic examination has been confirmed.

6. (A,C,D) Peptic ulceration in children has a tendency to spontaneously heal as well as to recur. In adults, bed rest, but only in the hospital, has been shown to hasten the healing rate of ulcers. This has not been studied in children. (11,20) Furthermore, this type of restriction is difficult to accomplish in children and seems to be unnecessary.

With reference to diet, foods that produce pain should be avoided. Usually, the patients are advised to avoid foods that may augment gastric acid secretion, such as tea, spices, and beef broth, but this regimen has not been proven to hasten the healing rate or prevent recurrence in a controlled study. (11, 20)

Antacids, 12 to 30 ml, 1 and 3 hours after meals and at bedtime, remain the cornerstone of treatment. Their efficacy has continued to be contested despite widespread clinical acceptance. However, a recent multicenter study in adults has confirmed improvement in ulcer healing but, at the same time, demonstrated no effect on symptomatology, such as pain (placebo vs. antacids). (21) A second study by the same multicenter group also confirmed the efficacy in healing by the administration of cimetidine. Cimetidine is an H_2-receptor (histamine) antagonist. Histamine stimulates secretion of gastric acid, increases heart rate, and inhibits uterine contractions. (22) These actions have not been antagonized (blocked) by conventional antihistamine drugs (H_1-receptor antagonism), such as diphenhydramine (Benadryl). (22) The pharmacological receptors involved in the previously mentioned actions have been designated as histamine H_2-receptors. However, these actions have been antagonized by another group of drugs, designated H_2-receptor antagonists, including metiamide and now cimetidine. These H_2-receptor antagonists are hydrophilic molecules, with an imidazole ring and an uncharged but polar side chain. A newer agent, ranitidine (Zantac®), also has been demonstrated to be as effective as cimetidine but with fewer side effects at this time. Ranitidine, a a derivative of histamine, was produced by altering the nucleus of a furan ring and possessing a different side chain from that of histamine. (23) Several studies have demonstrated their efficacy in healing of duodenal ulcers (75 to 95%), as well as in preventing recurrences by lower dose, long-term maintenance therapy, e.g., at bedtime for 6 to 12 months. (23-25)

With reference to the usage of anticholinergic medication, such as propantheline bromide (Probanthine, 0.25 to 0.30 mg/kg/dose 4 times daily), widespread controversy continues to exist. A recent American Gastroenterological Association symposium in May 1977, attempted to review this particular matter. K. Ivey reported that anticholinergics demonstrated substantial benefit in treatment in 6 controlled studies, while 10 controlled

studies demonstrated no substantial effect on healing rate, symptomatology, recurrence or complication rate (AGA Symposium,
1977). These drugs, however, must be administered in effective doses, usually causing at least minimal side effects, such
as dryness of mouth and visual blurring. (20) Their current usage seems to be for those patients with continued pain, demonstrated elevated gastric acid secretion, and high recurrence
rate. (20) They are especially prescribed for nocturnal pain
and suppression of nocturnal gastric acid secretion. (20) (See
Table 18.1.)
   Gastric irradiation (low-dose amounts) has not been used in
children and, additionally, would not seem to be warranted.

TABLE 18.1   Control of Gastric Acid Secretion

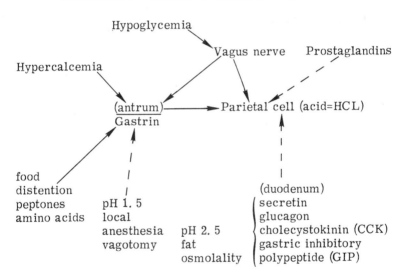

Key: – – – ► = inhibitory effect
       ————————► = stimulatory effect

7.   (E) Surgical treatment of duodenal ulcers in children is reserved for patients with complications; this includes those with
pain resistant to maximized treatment in type and duration and
those with perforation, severe hemorrhage, or obstruction (gastric outlet). (1-12,18,20,25,26) In general, in children, the
need for surgical treatment has varied between 10 and 40%.

(1-12,18,25,26,27) These figures reflect both acute ulcers, including the spontaneous ulcer of the neonate, drug-related ulcers, and chronic ulcers, including the presence of a history of chronic, recurrent abdominal discomfort. The former are generally associated with a higher incidence of surgical intervention. (1-12,25,26)

The incidence of intractability of pain has varied between 5 to 20% in several series. (1-12,18,25,26) This symptomatic indication for surgery has been essentially limited to the chronic ulcer type. As to the duration of medical treatment before labeling as intractable: there is no agreement and widespread variability, i.e., a minimum of 3 to 6 weeks and maximum of 6 to 12 months. (1-12,18,25,26)

The incidence of hemorrhage, melena, or hematemesis varies from 40 to 80% in acute ulcers and from 25 to 50% in chronic ulcers. (1-12) If appropriate monitoring of the vital signs, clinical status, and hematocrit, with or without transfusions, indiciate surgical intervention, then it must be performed promptly, usually involving a suturing of the bleeding point. In acute ulcer cases, surgery is performed in 25 to 75%. (1-12,25,26) Conversely, in chronic ulcers, this indication for surgery results in only 0 to 30% requiring surgical intervention. Utilization of criteria, such as recurrence of bleeding after a 24-hour period of no bleeding or requirement of more than one unit replacement every 8 hours, has not been routinely enacted in children.

Obstruction (gastric outlet), symptomatically, radiologically, or endoscopically confirmed, has been relatively frequent in chronic ulcers, 10 to 30%, while being infrequent in acute ulcers, 1 to 10%. (1-12) Fortunately, medical measures, including gastric suction, intravenous fluid therapy initially, have usually been successful in amelioration of the obstructive pattern, suggesting that edema and spasm were responsible for the problem (1-12,18) However, surgical intervention is occasionally necessary, i.e., in 0 to 5% of acute ulcers and 3 to 10% of chronic ulcers. (1-12,25,26)

Perforation is more frequently encountered in acute than chronic ulcers, 20 to 40% and 5 to 15%, respectively. (1-12,25, 26) Essentially all require surgery. The usual procedures include a drainage procedure and closure (suture) in acute ulcers, while more extensive procedures have been performed in chronic ulcers, such as vagotomy and drainage (pyloroplasty) or definite gastric resection (2/3 to 3/4) with drainage, Billroth I or II. (1,8,11,20,25,26) There continues to be considerable controversy and variable surgical procedural preference, especially in chronic ulcers, in particular drainage (pyloroplasty) with vagotomy versus gastric resection with or without vagotomy. (1,8,11,25,26) A definitive answer in children is wanting. Malignant degeneration is basically not applicable in children.

REFERENCES

1. Tudor, R.B.: Gastric and duodenal ulcers in children. Gastroenterology 62:823, 1972.

2. Robb, J.D.A., Thomas, P.S., Orszulok, J., et al.: Duodenal ulcer in children. Arch Dis Child 47:686, 1972.

3. Karlstrom, F.: Peptic ulcer in children in Sweden during the years 1953-1962. Ann Paediatr 202:218, 1964.

4. Habbick, B.F., Melrose, A.G., Grant, J.C.: Duodenal ulcer in childhood: A study of predisposing factors. Arch Dis Child 43:23, 1968.

5. Sultz, H.A., Schlesinger, E.R., Feldman, J.G., et al.: The epidemiology of peptic ulcer in childhood. Am J Public Health 60:492, 1970.

6. Thomson, N.B., Jewett, T.C., Jr.: Peptic ulcers in infancy and childhood. J Am Med Assoc 189:539, 1964.

7. Baida, M., McIntyre, J.A., Deitel, M.: Peptic ulcer in children and adolescents. Arch Surg (Chicago) 99:15, 1969.

8. Curci, M.R., Little, K., Sieber, W.K., et al.: Peptic ulcer disease in childhood re-examined. J Pediatr Surg 11:329, 1976.

9. Nuss, D. and Lynn, H.B.: Peptic ulceration in childhood. Surg Clin North Am 51:945, 1971.

10. Rosenlund, M.L. and Koop, C.E.: Duodenal ulcer in childhood. Pediatrics 45:283, 1970.

11. Tudor, R.B.: Peptic ulcerations in childhood. Pediatr Clin North Am 14:109, 1967.

12. Schuster, S.R. and Gross, R.E.: Peptic ulcer disease in childhood. Am J Surg 105:324, 1963.

13. Christie, D.L. and Ament, M.E.: Gastric acid hypersecretion in children with duodenal ulcer. Gastroenterology 7:242, 1976.

14. Kopel, F.B. and Barbero, G.: Gastric acid secretion in infancy and childhood. Gastroenterology 52:110, 1967.

15. Liebman, W.M.: Gastric acid secretion and serum gastrin levels in children with gastric and duodenal ulcers. J Clin Gastroenterol 2:243, 1980.

16. Trudeau, W.L. and McGuigan, J.E.: Serum gastrin levels in patients with peptic ulcer disease. Gastroenterology 59:6, 1970.

17. Korman, M.G., Soveny, C., Hansky, J.: Serum gastrin in duodenal ulcer. I. Basal levels and effect of food and atropine. Gut 12:899, 1971.

18. Deckelbaum, R.J., Roy, C.C., Lussier-Lazaroff, J., et al.: Peptic ulcer disease: A clinical study in 73 children. Can Med Assoc J 111:225, 1974.

19. Liebman, W.M.: Fiberoptic endoscopy of the gastrointestinal tract in infants and children. I. Upper endoscopy in 53 children. Am J Gastroenterol 68:362, 1977.

20. Schiff, E.R.: Treatment of uncomplicated peptic ulcer disease. Med Clin North Am 55:305, 1971.

21. Ippoliti, A.F., Sturdevant, R.A.L., Isenberg, J.J., et al.: Cimetidine versus intensive antacid therapy for duodenal ulcer. A multicenter trial. Gastroenterology 74:393, 1978.

22. Ganellin, C.R., Durant, G.J., Emmett, J.C.: Some chemical aspects of histamine H_2-receptor antagonists. Fed Proc 35:1924, 1976.

23. Feely, J. and Wormsley, K.G.: H_2 receptor antagonists-cimetidine and ranitidine. Br Med J 286:695, 1983.

24. Gray, G.R., Smith, I.S., MacKenzie, I., et al.: Long-term cimetidine in the management of severe duodenal ulcer dyspepsia. Gastroenterology 74:397, 1978.

25. Ravitch, M.M. and Duremdes, G.D.: Operative treatment of chronic duodenal ulcer in childhood. Ann Surg 171:641, 1970.

26. Seagram, C.G.F., Stephens, C.A., Cunning, W.A.: Peptic ulceration at the Hospital for Sick Children, Toronto, during the 20-year period, 1949-69. Pediatr Surg 8:407, 1973.

27. Nord, K.S., Rossi, T.M., Lebenthal, E.: Peptic ulcer in children: The predominance of gastric ulcers. Am J Gastroenterol 75:153, 1981.

Case 19

RECURRENT ABDOMINAL PAIN IN A 16-YEAR-OLD BOY

HISTORY

A 16-year-old white male presented with history of recurrent abdominal pain of almost 6 weeks' duration. The pain was located in the epigastric region, without radiation and sometimes related to meals but not related to food type, position, time of day, and/or bowel movements. When related to meals, the pain would start between 20 and 30 minutes after meals. The pain generally would last 1/2 to 2 hours and could recur during the same day. The patient initially had noted the pain every three to four days, but during the last two weeks it had been almost daily in occurrence. It was infrequently associated with nausea, but there was no history of vomiting, diarrhea, constipation, melena, hematochezia, dysuria, jaundice, fever, anorexia, fatigue, and/or trauma. The pertinent family history included maternal grandmother and grandfather with supposed history of peptic ulcer disease. The remainder of the past history, developmental history, family history, social history, and review of systems was unremarkable.

EXAMINATION

He was alert, active, cooperative, and in no apparent distress, with normal vital signs, height 171 cm, weight 63 kg. The remainder of the examination was unremarkable except for mild tenderness in the epigastric region with no rebound tenderness, distention, masses, or palpable liver, spleen, and kidneys. Active bowel sounds were present but no bruits.

142

LABORATORY DATA

Hemoglobin:	12.1 gm%
Hematocrit:	38%
White blood cell count:	7,800/mm^3
PMN's:	64%
lymphocytes:	30%
monocytes:	5%
eosinophiles:	1%
Sedimentation rate:	18 mm/hr
Urinalysis:	negative
Serum:	
sodium:	138 meq/L
potassium:	4.1 meq/L
chloride:	103 meq/L
bicarbonate:	24 meq/L
creatinine:	0.4 mg%
SGOT:	20 KU
alkaline phosphatase:	150 IU
total bilirubin:	0.7 mg%
direct bilirubin:	0.5 mg%
total protein:	6.9 gm%
albumin:	4.8 gm%
serum gastrin:	1,100 pg/ml (basal)
Gastric analysis	
basal:	18 meq
maximal:	24 meq/hr

QUESTIONS

1. Which of the following studies would be most helpful in establishing diagnosis at this point?
   A. Upper gastrointestinal series
   B. Barium enema
   C. Liver-spleen scan
   D. Gastric acid analysis (basal, stimulated)
   E. Basal serum gastrin measurement

2. Based on the new data, which one of the following studies would be most indicated in establishing the diagnosis?
   A. CT scan of abdomen
   B. Abdominal ultrasonography
   C. Selective visceral angiography
   D. Fiberoptic upper endoscopy
   E. Calcium infusion test

3. Current accepted treatment for this condition includes which of the following?
   A. Antacids
   B. Anticholinergics
   C. Steroids
   D. Cimetidine (H_2-receptor antagonist)
   E. Surgery

Question 4: Answer true (T) or false (F).

4. In the vast majority of cases, a tumor in the pancreas is found at surgery.

ANSWERS AND COMMENTS

1. (A,D,E) The presence of abdominal pain as the predominant symptom in this patient, accompanied by vomiting, and additionally, the relief of pain by eating, suggests peptic ulcer disease. However, the recurrent nature of the symptomatic pattern raises the possibility of the Zollinger-Ellison syndrome. In 1955, Zollinger and Ellison (1) described a clinical entity, consisting of peptic ulceration, gastric hypersecretion, and a non-beta islet cell tumor (benign or malignant) of the pancreas. The peptic ulceration has now been recognized to be more often multiple, duodenal and/or jejunal in location rather than gastric, intractable in nature, and possibly fatal. (1-8) More than 25 cases have been reported in children, the youngest being 7 years of age. (7,9,10) There is a male preponderance (3-4:1). (1-10) Associated tumor sites have included pancreas, parathyroid, thyroid, and adrenal glands. (5-7,9) Diagnosis has been confirmed within 1-2 weeks or as long as 5-7 years after the onset of symptoms. (5-7,9)

As in the present case, the predominant symptom is abdominal pain, variable in location, crampy to sharp, usually recurrent, relieved by eating, and frequently accompanied by nausea and vomiting. Other common symptoms are melena and hematemesis and, less frequently, diarrhea and steatorrhea. (1-7, 9,10) Infrequently, massive hematemesis, anemia, and perforation may occur. (1-7,9,10)

Upper gastrointestinal series is usually informative, i.e., determines single or multiple ulcers, duodenal or jejunal, less so, gastric. (1-7,12,13) Rugal hypertrophy and duodenal deformity, i.e., cicatricial changes and dilation, may also be visualized. (1-7,12,13) However, this study is frequently not diagnostic.

Gastric (acid) analysis is usually more reliable than upper gastrointestinal series. (7,11) A 12-hour gastric juice collection will usually reveal increased volume (range, 600 to 2,550 ml), as well as increased acidity (23 to 164 meq/L). (7,9,11) Basal acid output is high, over 15 meq/hr. (7,9-11) Histologic (betazole) stimulation, in contrast to normals, produces little further hydrochloric acid secretion or rate of flow. (7,9-11) Apparently gastrin has already produced maximal stimulation.

Measurement of circulating blood gastrin level may be diagnostic, too. A basal serum gastrin level over 500 picograms (pg)/ml in a patient secreting excessive acid is very, very suggestive of gastrinoma. (14,15) Unfortunately, a significant percentage of such patients have elevated but nondiagnostic gastrin levels, over 200 pg/ml and under 500 pg/ml. (14,15)

Barium enema and liver-spleen scan would not provide diagnostic confirmation.

2. (E) As mentioned in answer 1, a basal acid output/maximal output ratio greater than 0.6 is highly suggestive of gastrinoma, but false positives and negatives do occur. (7,9-11) Additionally, nondiagnostic basal serum gastrin levels, i.e., less than 600 pg/ml, occur not infrequently, too. (14,15)

Thus, another, more reliable test was necessary. Serum gastrin was found to increase in patients with gastrinoma in response to intravenous calcium or secretin infusion. (16-18) The former is continuously administered intravenously as calcium gluconate, 4 mg Ca^{2+}/kg body weight, and blood is drawn at 30-minute intervals for three hours; calcium and gastrin levels are measured. A twofold increase or more over basal levels, an increase of 395 pg/ml or more, or an absolute level over 1,000 pg/ml would be characteristic of gastrinoma. (16-18) The peak response is usually achieved at the end of the infusion. (16-18) Also secretin, 2 μ/kg body weight, can be administered intravenously as a single bolus, rather than calcium. (2,16,17) Blood for gastrin level is drawn at 0, 5, 10, 15, 30, and 60 minutes. (16,17) A similar peak response, as with the calcium infusion test, is achieved, but the peak is within the first 10 to 15 minutes. (16,17) Specifically, a rise of 110 pg/ml or more, with secretin stimulation, would be characteristic. (16,17) Utilizing the previously mentioned criteria for the calcium and secretin stimulation tests, false positive responses are virtually eliminated, although false negative responses are infrequently achieved. (16-18)

The CT scan of the abdomen, abdominal ultrasonography, and selective visceral angiography could disclose the primary lesion, i.e., pancreatic tumor in some cases, or even metastatic foci in others, but the overall yield would be significantly less than with the stimulation tests previously described. Fiberoptic upper endoscopy could disclose single or multiple ulcers in potentially visualized areas, proximal duodenum and stomach, but these findings would certainly be nondiagnostic.

3. (D,E) The most accepted treatment is surgery. Total gastrectomy is performed in those cases with metastatic disease, such as liver or lymph nodes. After total gastrectomy, metastases, as well as the primary tumor, may regress or fail to progress. The keynote seems to be the removal of the target or end organ for gastrin. The use of subtotal gastrectomy is characterized by progression of tumor and death in the vast majority of patients. (7,19,24) At operation, metastatic foci are removed as possible, too. Replacement therapy is necessary postoperatively, in particular, vitamin B_{12} by injection (1,000 μg monthly).

Recently, histamine H_2-receptor blockers (competitive inhibition) have been demonstrated to virtually eliminate gastric acid secretion and to augment healing of duodenal and gastric ulcers. (25,26) These findings led to the use of similar agents, i.e., cimetidine, in the treatment of the Zollinger-Ellison syndrome. (27-29) Several reports have been published, emphasizing encouraging short-term responses. (27) A recent longer-term report has also been published, demonstrating symptomatic relief, ulcer healing in almost all patients, and essentially no adverse effects. McCarthy, et al. (26) further emphasized that Zollinger-Ellison syndrome can be managed medically, and apparently little gain is achieved from the extra risks associated with total gastrectomy (13%) or subtotal gastrectomy (47%). (19-24) However, there are now several cases in which histamine H_2-receptor antagonist therapy has apparently failed. (30-32) With good control (medical treatment), the failure rate should be approximately 15 to 20%, according to McCarthy. (27) The mortality rate for untreated patients is reported to be 78%. (7, 19-24)

4. (F) In the majority of children with Zollinger-Ellison syndrome, the primary (original) pancreatic tumor is not found. (7,19,23) At surgery, metastases to liver or lymph nodes are usually found. (7,19,23) The metastatic foci are removed as possible, and total gastrectomy is performed. As previously mentioned, histamine H_2-receptor antagonist treatment, e.g., cimetidine, ranitidine, may offer an acceptable alternative form of treatment. See answer 3.

For a classification of gastrointestinal and pancreatic endocrine cells, see Table 19.1.

TABLE 19.1   Classification of Gastrointestinal and Pancreatic Endocrine Cells

Cell	Site	Hormone
A	Stomach fundus, pancreas (islets)	Glucagon
B	Pancreas (islets)	Insulin
D	Antrum, upper intestine	Somatostatin
D_1	Stomach, small intestine, pancreas (islet, nonislet)	Vasoactive intestinal polypeptide (VIP)
D_2	Pancreas (predominantly nonislet)	Pancreatic polypeptide (PP)
EC_1 (enterochromaffin)	Gastrointestinal tract	Motilin
EC_2 (enterochromaffin)	Small intestine	Substance P
ECL (enterochromaffin-like)	Stomach fundus	
EG	Small, large intestine	Enteroglucagon
G	Antrum, duodenum	Gastrin
H	Small, large intestine	Vasoactive intestinal polypeptide (VIP)
H	Stomach, duodenum	Bombesin-like
I	Duodenum, jejunum	Cholecystokinin (CCK)

148 / Case 19

TABLE 19.1   Classification of Gastrointestinal and Pancreatic
Endocrine Cells (Cont'd)

Cell	Site	Hormone
K	Small intestine	Gastric inhibitory polypeptide (GIP)
S	Small intestine	Secretin
X	Stomach, duodenum	

Modified from Pearse, A.G.A., et al.: Gastroenterology 72: 746, 1977.

REFERENCES

1. Zollinger, R.M. and Ellison, E.H.: Primary peptic ulcerations of the jejunum associated with islet cell tumors of the pancreas. Ann Surg 142:709, 1955.

2. Cawkwell, W.L.: The Zollinger-Ellison syndrome. N Engl J Med 59:466, 1960.

3. Davis, C.E., Smith, P., Davalos, X.S.: Ulcerogenic tumor of the pancreas. Ann Surg 155:669, 1962.

4. Ellison, E.H. and Wilson, S.D.: The Zollinger-Ellison syndrome and evaluation of 260 registered cases. Ann Surg 160:512, 1964.

5. Hallenbeck, G.A.: The Zollinger-Ellison syndrome. Gastroenterology 54:426, 1968.

6. Ellison, E.H. and Wilson, S.D.: Ulcerogenic tumor of the pancreas. Prog Clin Cancer 3:225, 1967.

7. Rosenlund, M.L.: The Zollinger-Ellison syndrome in children: A review. Am J Med 245:884, 1967.

8. Gregory, R.A., Tracy, H.J., French, J.M., et al.: Extraction of gastrin-like substance from a pancreatic tumor in a case of Zollinger-Ellison syndrome. Lancet 1:1045, 1960.

9.   Judd, D.R., Heimburger, I.L., Vellios, F., et al.: Zol-
     linger-Ellison syndrome in adolescents. Surgery 54:676,
     1963.

10. Cathcart, R.S., III, Webb, C.M., Othersen, H.B.: Zol-
     linger-Ellison syndrome in a seven-year-old boy. Surgery
     66:401, 1969.

11. Kopel, F.B. and Barbero, G.: Gastric acid secretion in
     infancy and childhood. Gastroenterology 52:1101, 1967.

12. Zboralske, F.F. and Amberg, J.R.: Detection of the Zol-
     linger-Ellison syndrome: The radiologist's responsibility.
     Am J Roentgenol 104:529, 1968.

13. Christoforidis, A.J. and Nelson, S.W.: Radiological man-
     ifestation of ulcerogenic tumors of the pancreas. J Am
     Med Assoc 198:97, 1966.

14. Yalow, R.S. and Berson, S.A.: Radioimmunoassay for
     gastrin. Gastroenterology 58:1, 1970.

15. Sanchez, R.E. and Passaro, E. Jr.: Correlation of serum
     gastrin and acid secretory levels in patients with the Zol-
     linger-Ellison syndrome. Surg Forum 20:314, 1969.

16. Iolts, B.E., Herbst, C.A., McGuigan, J.E.: Calcium
     and secretin-stimulated gastrin release in the Zollinger-
     Ellison syndrome. Ann Intern Med 81:758, 1974.

17. Deveney, C.W., Deveney, K.S., Jaffe, B.M., et al.: Use
     of calcium and secretin in the diagnosis of gastrinoma (Zol-
     linger-Ellison syndrome). Ann Intern Med 87:680, 1977.

18. Schwartz, D.L., White, J.J., Saulsbury, F., et al.: Gas-
     trin response to calcium infusion: An aid to the improved
     diagnosis of Zollinger-Ellison syndrome. Surg Gynecol
     Obstet 140:721, 1975.

19. Thompson, J.C., Reeder, D.D., Villar, H.V., et al.:
     Natural history and experience with diagnosis and treat-
     ment of the Zollinger-Ellison syndrome. Surg Gynecol
     Obstet 140:721, 1975.

20. Cameron, A.J. and Hoffman, H.N.: Zollinger-Ellison
     syndrome. Clinical features and long-term follow-up.
     Mayo Clin Proc 49:44, 1974.

21. Isenberg, J.L., Walsh, J.H., Grossman, M.I.: Zollinger-Ellison syndrome. Gastroenterology 65:140, 1973.

22. Way, L., Goldman, L., Dunphy, J.E.: Zollinger-Ellison syndrome. An analysis of 25 cases. Am J Surg 116:293, 1968.

23. Buchta, R.M. and Kaplan, J.M.: Zollinger-Ellison syndrome in a nine-year-old child: A case report and review of this entity in childhood. Pediatrics 47:594, 1971.

24. Wilson, S.D., Schulte, W.J., Meade, R.C.: Longevity studies following total gastrectomy in children with the Zollinger-Ellison syndrome. Arch Surg 103:108, 1971.

25. Blackwood, W.S., Pickard, R.G., Maudgal, D.P., et al.: Cimetidine in duodenal ulcer: Controlled trial. Lancet 2: 174, 1976.

26. McCarthy, D.M., Olinger, E.J., May, R.J., et al.: H_2-histamine receptor blocking agents in the Zollinger-Ellison syndrome. Experience in seven cases and implications for long-term therapy. Ann Intern Med 87:668, 1977.

27. McCarthy, D.M.: Report on the United States' experience with cimetidine in Zollinger-Ellison Syndrome and other hypersecretory states. Gastroenterology 74:453, 1978.

28. Mignon, M., Vallot, T., Mayeur, S., et al.: Ranitidine and cimetidine in Zollinger-Ellison Syndrome. Br J Clin Pharmacol 10:173, 1980.

29. Feely, J., Wormsley, K.G.: H_2 receptor antagonists - cimetidine and ranitidine. Br Med J 286:695, 1983.

30. Stabile, B.E., Ippoliti, A.F., Walsh, J.H., et al.: Failure of histamine H_2 receptor antagonist therapy in Zollinger-Ellison Syndrome. Am J Surg 145:17, 1983.

31. Groarke, J.F., Haggstrom, G.D., Halpern, N.B., et al.: Zollinger-Ellison Syndrome unresponsive to cimetidine. Am J Gastroenterol 72:168, 1979.

32. Danilewitz, M., Tim, L.O., Hirschowitz, B.: Ranitidine suppression of gastric hypersecretion resistant to cimetidine. N Engl J Med 306:20, 1982.

Case 20

ACUTE DIARRHEA IN A 1-YEAR-OLD GIRL

HISTORY

A 1-year-old white female presented with a history of looser, more frequent bowel movements of 2-1/2 weeks' duration. The bowel habit pattern had changed from 1 to 2 bowel movements daily to 4 to 6 bowel movements daily, loose to watery in nature. There was an initial associated increased temperature up to 101°F rectally for 3 to 4 days, then returning to normal. There was no associated vomiting, melena, hematochezia, skin lesions, jaundice, dysuria, or constipation. The appetite was initially decreased and more recently had returned to normal. The activity was initially decreased but had returned to normal. There was no relationship to food types; milk elimination caused no apparent effect. There was no apparent weight loss during this time. The remainder of the past history, developmental history, family history, social history, and review of systems was non-contributory.

EXAMINATION

She was alert, active, and in no apparent distress, with normal vital signs, weight 9.8 kg, height 75 cm, and head circumference 45.5 cm. The remainder of the examination, including the abdomen and anorectal area, was unremarkable, and stool hemoccult testing was negative.

LABORATORY DATA

Hemoglobin:	11.9 gm%
Hematocrit:	35%

White blood cell count:	9,600/mm^3
PMN's:	36%
lymphocytes:	60%
monocytes:	3%
eosinophiles:	1%
Sedimentation rate:	13 mm/hr
Serum:	
sodium:	139 meq/L
potassium:	4.6 meq/L
chloride:	104 meq/L
bicarbonate:	23 meq/L
creatinine:	0.4 mg%
total protein:	6.3 gm%
albumin:	4.1 gm%
SGOT:	20 units
alkaline phosphatase:	140 IU
cholesterol:	132 mg%
glucose:	92 mg%
carotene:	100 μg%
calcium:	9.8 mg%
Urinalysis:	negative
Stool:	
occult blood:	negative
reducing substances:	negative
culture:	negative
ova and parasites:	negative

QUESTIONS

1. This disorder's cause could be determined by which of the
   following studies?
   A. Electron microscopy of stools
   B. Blood culture
   C. Serology (complement-fixing antibody)
   D. Rectal biopsy (histology)
   E. Immunoelectrophoresis

Question 2: Answer true (T) or false (F).

2. Transmission of these agents seems to be from contaminated food or water.

3. Which of the following mechanisms seem to be involved in the resultant clinical disease?
   A. Mucosal invasion
   B. Enterotoxin production
   C. Interruption of enterohepatic circulation
   D. Altered small intestinal transit (faster)
   E. Blood vessel involvement (vasculitis)

4. Treatment of this condition includes which of the following?
   A. Fluid and electrolyte replacement
   B. Anticholinergics
   C. Antibiotics
   D. Cholestyramine
   E. Antacids

ANSWERS AND COMMENTS

1. (A,C) The examination of feces from children with acute gastroenteritis by negative-contrast stain (phosphotungstic acid) electron microscopy has revealed several possible viral agents as culprits. (1-6) These have included orbivirus, duovirus, and "reovirus." Estimates of their responsibility in producing acute gastroenteritis, especially during the winter months, have ranged between 40 and 90%. (1-11) Other studies in adult volunteers have implicated similar agents as well as others, such as Norwalk agent and astrovirus. In both adults and children, enteroviruses, adenovirus, and coronavirus have been implicated, too. (1-11) The former's role has been questioned, particularly since normals have adenovirus in their stools, too. (1-11)

Acute gastroenteritis is particularly prevalent during the winter months and has resulted in the speculation of the proposed predominant causative role of rotavirus-orbivirus-reo-like-virus-duovirus. The rotavirus has been characterized as a spherical 27-30 nm particle in stool isolates. It contains segments of double-stranded RNA. (1-11) Middleton, et al. (6) have further characterized 4 forms of rotavirus: (1) particles with entire edges of greater diameter, (2) particles of lesser diameter with scalloping of edges, (3) stain-penetrated centers with entire edges, and (4) stain-penetrated centers with scalloping of edges. The "true" rotavirus has a diameter of 70 nm, while the mini-reovirus has a diameter of only 30 nm. (6) Characteristics of other proposed viral agents include adenovirus, isohedral in configuration, with a diameter of 75 nm; picornavirus, with a diameter of 22-30 nm, spherical in configuration; and astrovirus, with a diameter of 28 nm, spherical in configuration. The total virus isolate yield during the winter months has ranged between

50 to 90%, but is 30 to 50% during the warmer months. (1-11)
Besides temperature, low humidity seems to favor rotavirus
and similar agents. (1-11) Interestingly, the vast majority of
cases occur in children below 2-3 years of age and over 6
months, with a slight male preponderance 3:2. (1-11) The increased resistance in children over 2 years of age may reflect
functional maturation of intestine and of immunity and/or active
immunity from prior HRVLA exposures.

Further investigation has employed electron microscopy combined with immunological methodology. Antiserum (antibody) to
isolated viral particles in stool has been prepared in animal species, such as guinea pig. (4-6) Serum samples, as well as stool
specimens, have been surveyed, and antigen (virus)-antibody aggregates have been identified. (4-6) Conversely, viral antigen
(particles from stool or other sources) can be incubated with
serum or other involved organ material, and reactions of iden-
tity (aggregates) identified. Additionally, immunofluorescent
techniques can be applied for identification of viral antigens,
too. (4-6)

Serological assessment of acute and convalescent serum
samples has also been used. Complement-fixing antibodies in
serum have been assessed, using stool filtrate or a related virus, such as Nebraska calf diarrhea virus. (4,6,9) A fourfold
or greater rise is highly significant. (4,6,9) The prevalence of
serum complement-fixing antibodies to HRVLA increases from
10 to 30% at 6 months of age to 50 to 90% by 2 years of age. (4,
6,9) More recently, the technique of enzyme immunoassay (EIA)
has been applied successfully for diagnosis, i.e., enzyme-linked
immunosorbent assay (ELISA). (12)

No specific changes are found by histological examination of
involved areas, or by assessment of immunoglobulin patterns.
Obviously, blood cultures are unrevealing.

2. (F) The route of transmission is fecal-oral in nature. (1-
11) Experimental transmission of illness has occurred in man
with certain of these viruses, such as the Norwalk agent, by bac-
teria-free stool filtrates from infected persons. (1-11) These
agents can then replicate within the gastrointestinal tract of man.
(1-11) The incubation period of most of these agents seems to
be short, 6 days or less. (6,9) With reference to rotaviruses,
viral replication is accompanied by watery diarrhea, lasting 3
to 10 days. Occasionally, the diarrhea will become chronic,
even "intractable." (12)

3. (A) Virus particles have been identified within duodenal, jejunal, and, less so, ileal mucosa during the acute infection.
(6,9-14) Mucosal inflammation, varying degrees of villous

shortening, crypt hypertrophy, and increased mitotic activity in intestinal epithelial cells have been identified. (11,14) In addition, disaccharidase activity assays have revealed normal to markedly decreased levels of sucrase, maltase, and lactase. (14) The diminished disaccharidase activity lasts until histological repair occurs. During the period of injury, functional studies, such as d-xylose excretion tolerance (urine, blood) and fat absorption (72-hour stool fat collection) may be abnormal, dependent upon the extent of damage.

In piglets with transmissible gastroenteritis (TGE), Kerzner, et al. (15) have found a defect in glucose-mediated sodium transport in the jejunum. Sodium transport became abnormal within hours of the experimentally induced infection, maximally so after about 40 hours, and then gradually disappeared. Abnormality of villous epithelial cells was felt to be the major cause of this functional abnormality. In a further study, they clarified this abnormality as being at least partly due to the migration of relatively undifferentiated cells from crypt to villus. Thus, functionally immature cells would be present in the villi, resulting in defective sodium transport. (6,15,16) The result is a net intraluminal secretion of water and electrolytes. Intestinal mucosal adenyl cyclase levels have been normal, while sodium-potassium ATPase levels have been decreased in these animal models. (16) In addition, no abnormalities of the mucosa were visualized on light or electron microscopy, making decreased surface area unlikely as a significant factor in the altered sodium transport. (15,16) The resemblance of TGE to human clinical states, such as acute viral gastroenteritis, is striking, and further correlative studies should clarify a possible link.

4. (A) The typical patient becomes suddenly ill with vomiting and, subsequently, fever, diarrhea, and generalized malaise. Lymphocytosis is usual. This illness usually lasts 1-8 days. (6,16,17) Dehydration may be mild to severe. Usually, this disease is self-limited, but the histological and functional changes may persist for 1-2 weeks after clinical symptomatology disappears. (6,16,17) In addition, disaccharide intolerance, especially to lactose, may persist for 4 to 6 weeks. (6,16,17)

Therefore, the cornerstone of treatment is replacement of fluid and electrolyte losses. The World Health Organization has recommended a rehydrating solution with 90 meq sodium, 20 meq potassium, base, and glucose (monosaccharide). (23) Adequate free water must be provided. The carbohydrate concentration should be in the range of 2% to 5% and can be either glucose or sucrose, the latter equally effective to glucose in approximately 90% of patients. (23,24) If vomiting persists, a period of fasting (24-72 hours) is in order. Antiemetics, such

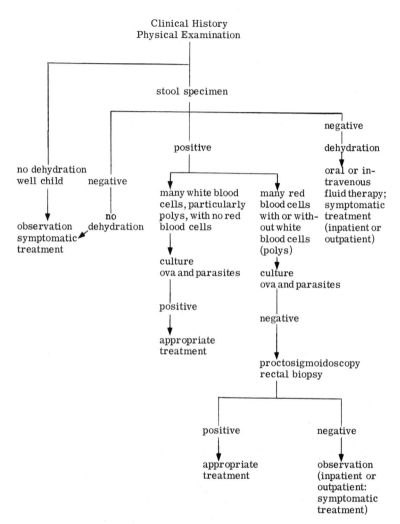

Figure 20.1   Algorithm: Acute diarrhea.

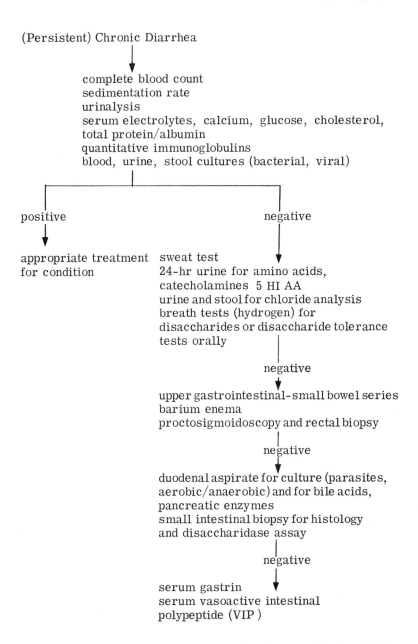

(Persistent) Chronic Diarrhea

complete blood count
sedimentation rate
urinalysis
serum electrolytes, calcium, glucose, cholesterol,
total protein/albumin
quantitative immunoglobulins
blood, urine, stool cultures (bacterial, viral)

positive

negative

appropriate treatment
for condition

sweat test
24-hr urine for amino acids,
catecholamines 5 HI AA
urine and stool for chloride analysis
breath tests (hydrogen) for
disaccharides or disaccharide tolerance
tests orally

negative

upper gastrointestinal-small bowel series
barium enema
proctosigmoidoscopy and rectal biopsy

negative

duodenal aspirate for culture (parasites,
aerobic/anaerobic) and for bile acids,
pancreatic enzymes
small intestinal biopsy for histology
and disaccharidase assay

negative

serum gastrin
serum vasoactive intestinal
polypeptide (VIP)

Figure 20.2   Diagnostic evaluation of patients with intractable
diarrhea.

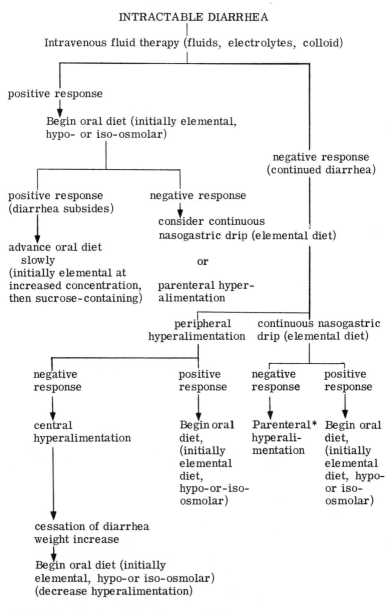

INTRACTABLE DIARRHEA

Intravenous fluid therapy (fluids, electrolytes, colloid)

positive response

Begin oral diet (initially elemental, hypo- or iso-osmolar)

negative response (continued diarrhea)

positive response (diarrhea subsides)

negative response

consider continuous nasogastric drip (elemental diet)

advance oral diet slowly (initially elemental at increased concentration, then sucrose-containing)

or

parenteral hyper-alimentation

peripheral hyperalimentation

continuous nasogastric drip (elemental diet)

negative response

positive response

negative response

positive response

central hyperalimentation

Begin oral diet, (initially elemental diet, hypo-or-iso-osmolar)

Parenteral* hyperali-mentation

Begin oral diet, (initially elemental diet, hypo-or iso-osmolar)

cessation of diarrhea weight increase

Begin oral diet (initially elemental, hypo-or iso-osmolar) (decrease hyperalimentation)

* Parenteral = peripheral or central.

Figure 20.3   Treatment of intractable diarrhea of infancy.

as trimethobenzamide (Tigan), should be used, but with caution, since this type of medication, as well as other types of medication, may mask symptomatology and assessment of clinical severity. Similarly, the use of anticholinergics and antidiarrheal agents does not shorten the illness or diminish the fluid and electrolyte losses and may also mask the clinical severity. (20)

Cholestyramine, a basic anion-exchange resin, has not been demonstrated to have a place in the management of the acute illness. However, excessive bile acid loss of consequence has been confirmed in the acute phase, as has cholestyramine's role in intractable diarrhea of infancy. (21) Total parenteral nutrition is not needed in the acute illness, but has an integral role in intractable or persistent diarrhea (Figs. 20.1, 20.2, 20.3). (22)

In the continued care of the patient with acute gastroenteritis, acquired disaccharide or monosaccharide intolerance must be watched for. Stools can be checked for reducing substances; remember that the validity of the test is dependent upon ingestion of the offending carbohydrate. (18,19) If intolerance is noted, either reduction of carbohydrate content or its exclusion must be enacted. Lactose should be the last to be reintroduced.

On the horizon is the feasibility of immunization against viral strains producing gastroenteritis. Reovirus-like agents in specific animal disease models share antigens with HRLVA, and, therefore, their administration may induce resistance. (See Table 20.1)

TABLE 20.1 Viral Agents and Gastroenteritis

Agent	Virus family
Rotavirus	Reoviruses
Enteric adenovirus	Adenoviruses
Norwalk virus	Caliciviruses
Astrovirus Hawaii virus Ditchling agent	27-nm viruses
Coxsackie virus	Picorna viruses

Modified from Yolken, R.H. (12)

REFERENCES

1. Flewett, T.H., Bruden, A.S., Davies, H., et al.: Relation between viruses from acute gastroenteritis of children and newborn calves. Lancet 2:61, 1974.

2. Hamilton, J.R., Gall, D.G., Kerzner, R., et al.: Recent development in viral gastroenteritis. Pediat Clin North Am 22:747, 1975.

3. Thornton, A. and Zuckerman, A.J.: The virus of acute diarrhea. Nature 254:557, 1975.

4. Kapikian, A.Z., Kim, H.W., Wyatt, R.G., et al.: Reovirus-like agent in stools: Association with infantile diarrhea and development of serologic tests. Science 185:1049, 1974.

5. Thornhill, T.S., Wyatt, R.G., Kalica, A.R., et al.: Detection by immune electron microscopy of 26-27 nm virus particles associated with two family outbreaks of gastroenteritis. J Infect Dis 132:20, 1977.

6. Middleton, P.J., Szymanski, M.T., Petric, M.: Viruses associated with acute gastroenteritis in young children. Am J Dis Child 131:733, 1977.

7. Middleton, P.J., Szymanski, M.T., Abbott, G.D., et al.: Orbivirus acute gastroenteritis of infancy. Lancet 1:1241, 1974.

8. Flewett, T.H., Bruden, A.S., Davies, H., et al.: Epidemic viral enteritis in a long-stay children's ward. Lancet 1:4, 1975.

9. Bortolussi, R., Szymanski, M., Hamilton, J.R., et al.: Studies on the etiology of acute infantile diarrhea. Pediatr Res 8:379, 1974.

10. Davidson, G.P., Bishop, R.F., Townley, R.R.W., et al.: Importance of a new virus in acute sporadic enteritis in children. Lancet 1:242, 1975.

11. Bishop, R.F., Davidson, G.P., Holmes, I.H., et al.: Virus particles in epithelial cells of duodenal mucosa from children with acute non-bacterial gastroenteritis. Lancet 2:1281, 1973.

12. Yolken, R.H.: Viral agents that cause diarrhea in children. Thirteenth Ross Roundtable, Columbus, Ohio, 1982, p. 8.

13. Schreiber, D.S., Blacklow, N.R., Trier, J.S.: The mucosal lesion of the proximal small intestine in acute infectious nonbacterial gastroenteritis. N Engl J Med 288:1318, 1973.

14. Barnes, G.L. and Townley, R.R.W.: Duodenal mucosal damage in 31 infants with gastroenteritis. Arch Dis Child 48:343, 1973.

15. Kerzner, B., Kelly, M.H., Gall, D.G., et al.: Transmissible gastroenteritis: Sodium transport and the intestinal epithelium during the course of viral enteritis. Gastroenterology 72:457, 1977.

16. Schreiber, D.S., Trier, J.S., Blacklow, N.R.: Recent advances in viral gastroenteritis. Gastroenterology 73: 174, 1977.

17. Blacklow, N.R., Dolin, R., Fedson, D.S., et al.: Acute infectious nonbacterial gastroenteritis: Etiology and pathogenesis. Ann Intern Med 76:993, 1972.

18. Rodriguez-de-Duret, H., Lugo-de-Rivera, C., Torres-Pinedo, R.: Studies on infant diarrhea. IV. Sugar transit and absorption in small intestine after a feeding. Gastroenterology 59:396, 1970.

19. Ironside, A.G.: Gastroenteritis of infancy. Br Med J 1: 284, 1973.

20. Today's Drugs: Drugs for diarrhea. Br Med J 2:606, 1969 (Editorial).

21. Tamer, M.A., Santora, T.R., Sandberg, D.H.: Cholestyramine therapy for intractable diarrhea. Pediatrics 53: 217, 1974.

22. Heird, W.C. and Winters, R.W.: Total parenteral nutrition: The state of the art. J Pediatr 86:21, 1975.

23. Finberg, L., Harper, P.D., Harrison, H.E., et al.: Oral rehydration for diarrhea. J Pediatr 101:497, 1982.

24. Nalin, D.R., Mata, L., Vargus, W., et al.: Comparison of sucrose and glucose in oral therapy of an infant diarrhea. Lancet 2:77, 1978.

Case 21

CHRONIC DIARRHEA IN A 12-YEAR-OLD BOY

HISTORY

A 12-year-old white male presented with a history of altered bowel habit pattern of almost 3 months' duration. His usual bowel habit pattern, once daily, had changed to 3-5 bowel movements daily and in the past 2 weeks to twice daily. The bowel movements were loose to watery in consistency, usually yellow in color, and frequently large in amount. There was associated gaseousness on occasions. There was no history of nausea, vomiting, fever, melena, hematochezia, skin lesions, arthralgia, dysuria, jaundice, or trauma. Medication included Lactinex granules and Konsyl, both apparently without effect. The prior history included a confirmed diagnosis of Down's syndrome (mongolism) with congenital heart disease. The family history included the father with peptic ulcer disease and bronchiectasis, mother with diverticulosis, brother and one sister with bronchial asthma. Developmental history included slight vaginal bleeding during the 1st trimester, delivery by repeat C-section, and maternal age 36 years. Birth weight was 7 lb 13 oz, and the developmental pattern included walking without support at 3 years of age. There was a complete hearing loss on the left side, partial on the right side, confirmed at approximately 6 years of age. The remainder of the developmental history, social and family history, and review of systems was essentially noncontributory. There was no history of recurrent infections.

EXAMINATION

He was in no apparent distress, with normal vital signs, weight 39.7 kg, height 141 cm, and head circumference 57.75 cm. The

163

remainder of the examination was unremarkable except for mild
brachycephaly, mongoloid slant of eyes, high-arched palate, and
presence of a hearing aid in the right ear. There was bilateral
clinodactyly and a transverse crease of the left palmar area, as
well as mild symmetrical decrease in muscle tone and presence
of hypoactive deep tendon reflexes bilaterally.

LABORATORY DATA

Hemoglobin:	12.9 gm%
Hematocrit:	39%
White blood cell count:	6,800/mm^3
PMN's:	54%
lymphocytes:	44%
monocytes:	1%
eosinophiles:	1%
Urinalysis:	negative
Serum:	
SGOT:	18 units
SGPT:	21 units
carotene:	116 μg%
folate:	0.8 ng/ml
creatinine:	0.5 mg%
total protein:	6.7 gm%
albumin:	4.5 gm%
Stool:	
smear:	rare RBC
hemoccult:	negative
reducing substances:	negative
culture:	Shigella
ova and parasites:	negative

QUESTIONS

1. Which strains of this agent are most commonly encountered
   in the United States?
   A. S. dysenteriae
   B. S. flexneri
   C. S. sonnei
   D. S. paradysenteriae
   E. S. typhimurium

Questions 2 and 3: Answer true (T) or false (F).

2. S. sonnei is the only strain which produces an exotoxin.

3. Infection by this agent affects particularly the small intestine, especially the jejunum.

4. The typical stool contains which of the following?
   A. White blood cells
   B. Meat fibers
   C. Red blood cells
   D. Charcot-Leyden crystals
   E. Mucus

5. Which of the following studies are diagnostic for this agent?
   A. Stool culture
   B. Sigmoidoscopy
   C. Serum agglutinins in paired sera
   D. Rectal biopsy
   E. Barium enema

Question 6: Answer true (T) or false (F).

6. This agent generally produces a disease which is self-limited.

7. Which of the following are an indication for initiation of antibiotic treatment of this agent?
   A. All patients
   B. Severely ill children
   C. Newborn infants
   D. School-age children
   E. Children of all ages with persistent blood in stools

ANSWERS AND COMMENTS

1. (B,C) The overwhelming majority of cases are associated with S. flexneri and S. sonnei. More recently, S. sonnei has been most prevalent. (1-5) S. dysenteriae and paradysenteriae are rarely encountered. S. typhimurium is acutally Salmonella typhimurium.

2. (F) Actually, only S. dysenteriae produces an exotoxin. Otherwise, Shigellae do not produce toxins. (1-5)

3. (F) Shigella is an example of an agent which produces disease by invasion. It is spread by its ingestion orally in contaminated food or liquids; (1-5) in addition, flies can transmit it. Shigellae are gram-negative rods, consisting of approximately 40 serotypes. (1-6) This agent is particularly prevalent during

the warmer months and in tropical areas. (1-5) After ingestion, Shigellae can multiply, thereby allowing as few as 200 organisms to cause disease. (1-5) These organisms can then pen-
etrate the epithelium and multiply within the intestinal wall. (1-
5) This infection selectively involves the colon, particularly the
sigmoid colon and rectum. An acute inflammatory reaction is
produced in the mucosa and submucosa, and ulcerations or even
crypt abscesses may result. (1-5)

4. (A, C, E) A fresh, typical stool will contain mucus, white
blood cells, particularly polymorphonuclear, and red blood
cells. (1-9) In addition, cellular debris may be present. The
above seem to result from the localization of infection to the intestinal wall by white blood cells, particularly polys, and fibrin
thrombi. (1-5)

5. (A, C) As mentioned in answer 4, the typical stool contains
white blood cells, red blood cells, and mucus. On culture, Shigellae can be distinguished from normal flora because it is nonlactose fermenting. This organism is very hardy. Some media,
such as SS agar, seem to be too inhibitory, while others seem
to be more favorable, including MacConkey's XLD, and Hectoen
enteric. (1-11) The positive results of one culture range from
only 50 to 70%, while three or more cultures will produce a
yield of 80 to 95%. (1, 5, 9) Inoculation of plates should be done
as quickly as possible. Sigmoidoscopic examination may show
minimal changes, e.g., erythema, or increased friability, superficial, asymmetrical ulcerations, or significant erythema.
(1-11) In addition, during this examination, culture of stool or,
even more so, swabbing of ulcerations may establish the diagnosis. Rectal biopsy will demonstrate varying inflammatory
changes, ulcerations, or even crypt abscesses. Radiological
examination also shows nondiagnostic changes and, most commonly, is normal. (1-5, 9)
    The specific diagnosis can also be established by measure-
ment of agglutinins in serum. However, acute and convalescent
sera must be drawn for agglutinins, in order to establish the diagnosis. A fourfold or more increase in agglutinins establishes
the diagnosis, although it is certainly delayed by this method.
(1, 5, 9)

6. (T) Shigellosis is basically a self-limited disease (1-2
weeks). By the time of examination, the patient is frequently
improving or well. (1-11) Therefore, treatment is more often
aimed at a bacterial cure than at a symptomatic or clinical cure.

7. (B,C) As alluded to in answer 6, Shigellosis is a self-limited disease. Thus, the overwhelming majority of patients will
not be helped symptomatically by the use of antibiotics. However, in all severely ill patients or in newborns and infants less
than 1 year of age, antibiotic treatment is indicated. The antibiotic of choice is ampicillin, 100 mg/kg/day, for 5 to 7 days.
(9-12) Cure rates of 75 to 90% are usual. (8-11) However, ac-
quisition of R-factors (genetic), producing antibiotic resistance,
is facilitated by antibiotic administration. In addition, ampicillin resistance of Shigellae is significant in certain regions, in
general. Alternative antibiotic choices include trimethoprim-
sulfamethoxazole, tetracycline, in children over 9 years of age,
and chloramphenicol. (6) A prolonged carrier state with antibiotics is not the situation, as in salmonellosis. (13,14) All cases
should be isolated until at least three consecutive stool cultures
are negative, irrespective of whether antibiotics have been administered. (1-5,9,12)
   Other medication, such as Lomotil, which changes intestinal
motility, may actually be contraindicated. A recent report has
suggested actual prolongation of illness. (9,11) The use of vaccine in children has not been adequately assessed. (15)
   In all cases, fluid, electrolyte, and acid-base balance must
be assessed, and balance assured. This can be accomplished
orally in most cases, using glucose or sucrose as the carbohydrate; intravenous fluids should be reserved particularly for the
severely ill and infants less than one year of age.
   For more information on Shigella and Salmonella, see Table
21.1.

TABLE 21.1   Main Groups of Shigella and Salmonella

Shigella	
Group (Serology)	Member(s)
A	S. dysenteriae (1-10)
B	S. flexneri (1-6)
C	S. boydii (1-15)
D	S. sonnei (1)

TABLE 21.1   Main Groups of Shigella and Salmonella (Cont'd)

Salmonella	
Group (serology)	Member(s)
A	S. paratyphi A
B	S. schottmulleri S. typhimurium
C_1	S. paratyphi C S. choleraesuis S. montevideo
C_2	S. newport
D	S. typhi S. enteritidis S. gallinarum
E	S. anatum

REFERENCES

1. Levine, M.M., Dupont, H.L., Formal, S.B., et al.: Pathogenesis of Shigellae dysenteriae I (Shiga) dysentery. J Infect Dis 127:261, 1973.

2. Haltalin, K.C., Kusmiesz, H.T., Hinton, L.V., et al.: Treatment of acute diarrhea in outpatients. Am J Dis Child 124:555, 1972.

3. Haltalin, K.C.: Neonatal Shigellosis. Am J Dis Child 114: 603, 1967.

4. Nelson, J.D. and Haltalin, K.C.: Accuracy of diagnosis of bacterial diarrheal disease by clinical features. J Pediatr 78:519, 1971.

5. Nelson, J.D., Kusmiesz, H.T., Haltalin, K.C.: Endemic Shigellosis: A study of fifty households. Am J Epidemiol 86:683, 1967.

6.   Report of the Committee on Infectious Diseases, American Academy of Pediatrics, 19th edition, Evanston, Illinois, 1982, p. 235, 238.

7.   Harris, J.C., Dupont, H.L., Hornick, R.B.: Fecal leukocytes in diarrheal illness. Ann Intern Med 76:697, 1972.

8.   Dupont, H.I., Hornick, R.B., Dawkins, A.T., et al.: The response of man to virulent Shigella flexneri 2a. J Infect Dis 119:296, 1969.

9.   Tong, M.J., Martin, D.G., Cunningham, J.J., et al.: Clinical and bacteriological evaluation of antibiotic treatment in Shigellosis. J Am Med Assoc 214:1841, 1970.

10. Haltalin, K.C., Nelson, J.D., Kusmiesz, H.T., et al.: Comparison of intramuscular and oral ampicillin therapy for Shigellosis. J Pediatr 73:617, 1968.

11. Weissman, J.B.: Infectious diarrhea: When should you start to worry? Resid Staff Physician, p. 117, November, 1977.

12. Davies, J.R., Farrant, W.N., Uttley, A.H.C.: Antibiotic resistance of Shigella sonnei. Lancet 2:1157, 1970.

13. Rosenstein, B.J.: Salmonellosis in infants and children: Epidemiologic and therapeutic considerations. J Pediatr 70:1, 1967.

14. Tynes, B.S. and Utz, J.P.: Factors influencing the cure of Salmonella carriers. Ann Intern Med 57:871, 1962.

15. Istrat, G., Meitert, T., Ciufeco, C.: Treatment of dysentery bacilli carriers with a live nonpathogenic antidysenteric vaccine. Arch Immunol Ther Exp (Warsz) 16:333, 1968.

Case 22

VOMITING AND LACK OF WEIGHT GAIN
IN A 10-MONTH-OLD BOY

HISTORY

A 10-month-old white male presented with a history of recurrent
vomiting and poor weight gain of 2 months' duration. At approximately 7-1/2 months of age, he had an upper respiratory tract
infection and ear infection with associated vomiting. His ear infection was treated with antibiotics and apparently resolved, but
his vomiting persisted until the time of this evaluation. The
vomiting occurred twice daily (average), was nonprojectile, occurred with meals and usually 1-1/2 to 2 hours after meals.
There was no history of associated abdominal pain, diarrhea,
constipation, hematemesis, bile within the vomitus, or of hematochezia. The patient generally would have as many as 3-4
bowel movements a day, soft to firm in consistency, and brown
in color. There were no known food allergies or history of
wheezing, nasal stuffiness, skin rashes, or recurrent purulent
infections. Gestational and developmental history was unremarkable. His initial diet consisted of breast milk until 6 to 7
weeks of age when he was started on rice cereal, Isomil, and
applesauce, which he tolerated well. At 2-1/2 months of age,
he was started on vegetables, once again with no difficulty. At
6-1/2 months of age, his weight was 16 lbs 11 oz. At 7 to 7-
1/2 months of age, whole milk (homogenized) was started. The
remainder of the past history, developmental history, family
history, and review of systems was unremarkable.

EXAMINATION

He was alert, with normal vital signs. Height was 71 cm, weight
7.5 kg, and head circumference was 54.5 cm. The remainder
of the examination was unremarkable.

LABORATORY DATA

Hemoglobin:	11.6 gm%
Hematocrit:	34.8%
White blood cell count:	7,500/mm^3
PMN's:	40%
lymphocytes:	42%
monocytes:	5%
eosinophiles:	13%
platelets:	433,000/mm^3
sedimentation rate:	10.8 seconds
Serum:	
creatinine:	0.6 mg%
total protein:	6.6 gm%
albumin:	4.6 gm%
IgG:	375 mg%
IgA:	39 mg%
IgM:	52 mg%
IgE:	152 units/ml
RAST:	positive: α-lactalbumin, β-lactoglobulin, bovine serum albumin, whole milk
Urinalysis:	normal
Stool:	
pH:	6.5
reducing substances:	0%
culture:	negative
ova and parasites:	negative
Upper GI series:	(Fig. 22.1)
Fiberoptic upper endoscopy:	negative
Small intestinal biopsy:	(Fig. 22.2)
Duodenal fluid:	
aerobic and anaerobic cultures and ova and parasites:	negative

QUESTIONS

Questions 1-11: Answer true (T) or false (F).

1. From the clinical history and examination data, the presumptive diagnosis is regional enteritis.

2. This disorder always occurs as an isolated gastrointestinal disorder.

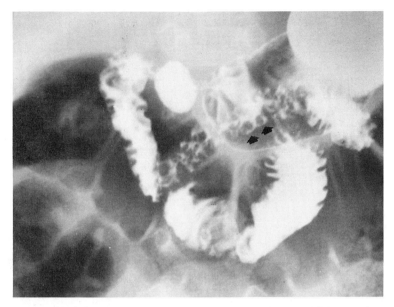

Figure 22.1 Barium swallow. Thickened mucosal folds with rounded, radiolucent lesions, coated with barium at the periphery (arrows), are seen in the distal duodenum and proximal jejunum.

3. This disorder can occur as a secondary condition, such as with celiac disease.

4. The most common protein component responsible for this disorder is beta-lactoglobulin.

5. There is no characteristic pathology in the small intestine, although prominent eosinophilia may be present.

6. Most children with this disorder do not have symptoms within the first 6 months of life.

7. An acute syndrome, vomiting, pallor, and possible shock-like state, or a chronic syndrome, vomiting, diarrhea, failure to thrive, can clinically characterize this condition.

8. The diagnosis of this disorder depends upon provocative skin testing with appropriate allergens (antigens).

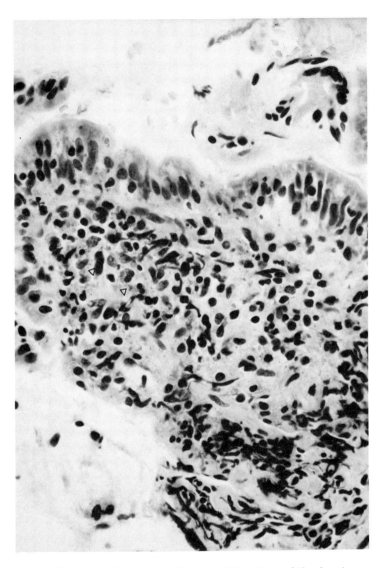

Figure 22.2 Duodenum. Cellular infiltration of the lamina propria is evident. These cells contain numerous granules, staining intensely with eosin (arrows) (H&E, X275).

9. The main entity in differential diagnosis is lactose intolerance.

10. The main treatment for this disorder is dietary elimination of the offending agent or agents.

11. A recent alternative treatment of this condition is oral disodium cromolyn glycate.

ANSWERS AND COMMENTS

1. (F) The presumptive diagnosis is cow's milk protein intolerance. Refer to answers 2 to 11.

2. (F) Intolerance to cow's milk protein may be associated with other allergic manifestations, such as eczema or asthma. (1-5)

3. (T) This condition can occur as a secondary phenomenon, such as with celiac disease. (1-5)

4. (T) Beta-lactoglobulin represents the major protein in cow's milk whey proteins, while it is lacking in human milk. (1-5) It has been the most commonly incriminated protein (allergen). (1-5) Other important protein components include β-lactalbumin and casein (milk). Cow's milk protein in toto contains three times more protein than human milk, but the same content of soluble protein (Table 22.1). The pathogenic response to these protein fractions gastrointestinally involves local intestinal sensitization at a time of impaired mucosal immune functional capability, e.g., early infancy, local infection (gastroenteritis). (1-12)

TABLE 22.1 Cow's Milk: Main Protein Components

Protein	g/m100 ml
caseins	2.5
β-lactoglobulin	0.3
α-lactalbumin	0.07
bovine serum albumin	0.03
immunoglobulins	0.06

5. (T) There is no characteristic pathology in the small intestine in cow's milk protein intolerance. However, in the majority of cases, the small intestinal mucosa is not normal. The small intestinal mucosa can range from normal to flat in appearance, most commonly showing partial villous atrophy (flattening). Eosinophilic infiltration of the lamina propria has been a variable finding, although some authors claim that this is a characteristic finding. (5-7) The eosinophilia can be the only finding, or it can be associated with variable villous changes. (5-7)

6. (F) Most children with this condition have symptomatology within the first six months of life. This presentation can be gastrointestinal in type, such as vomiting, diarrhea, blood in the stools (hematochezia or occult blood) or protein-loss, edema, or nongastrointestinal, such as urticaria or wheezing. (1-9) Thus, the spectrum of gastrointestinal manifestations includes enterocolitis and enteropathy with malabsorption in earlier childhood and eosinophilic gastroenteritis, more common in later childhood. (3,8,10)

7. (T) Children with predominantly gastrointestinal symptomatology may manifest an acute syndrome or a chronic syndrome. (1-9) The acute syndrome is characterized by the abrupt onset of vomiting, frequently followed by diarrhea, occasionally pallor, and rarely "shock." This complex can mimic an acute gastroenteritis. The chronic syndrome is one of gradual onset of vomiting and diarrhea with associated failure to thrive. Actual malabsorption with apparent steatorrhea may actually occur. (1-9) The frequency of steatorrhea, even by laboratory criteria, i.e., stool fat collection (3 day) has been the subject of controversy. (1,5,8) When evidence of steatorrhea is present, other laboratory studies also demonstrate abnormality, including d-xylose absorption (decreased), secondary disaccharidase deficiency (reducing substances in stool, increased breath hydrogen, H_2, with carbohydrate ingestion). Sigmoidoscopic examination may be normal or may disclose variable edema and/ or erythema, rarely significant friability and ulceration. (5,8) The rectal biopsy will be normal or reveal an inflammatory reaction in the lamina propria, including eosinophiles, polymorphonuclear leukocytes, and mononuclear cells, in particular. (5,8)

8. (F) Unfortunately, the diagnosis of cow's milk protein intolerance relies principally upon clinical studies, in particular elimination trials. In 1963, Goldman, et al., (11) described the following criteria, now generally accepted: (1) symptomatology subsides after milk elimination; (2) recurrence of symptomatology within 48 hours after milk challenge; (3) the same positive

reactions to three such challenges, i.e., similar onset, duration, and clinical features. However, a few authors, such as
Rey (9) suggest only one positive challenge is necessary for the
diagnosis. More recently, Powell (12) suggested the following
criteria for a positive response to challenges (enterocolitis
group): (1) diarrhea within 24 hours after administration of a
single challenge (100 ml milk or soy), (2) stools with WBC
(polys) and RBC after challenge, and (3) a change in the total
poly count (blood) postchallenge, 6-12 hours, (vs prechallenge)
of greater than 4,000/mm^3. Also, there is disagreement as to
whether cow's milk or the actual protein fractions should be
used for such challenges. (5,8-11)

In addition to the challenge method, other laboratory studies
have been performed in order to aid in the diagnosis of cow's
milk protein intolerance. Circulating antibodies to cow's milk
protein (precipitins, hemagglutinins) have been frequently measured. (1-3,8,13) Unfortunately, consistent correlation with clinical milk protein intolerance has not been confirmed. Antibodies
in feces, coproantibodies, are not correlative, either. (14) Provocative skin tests have been advocated as a diagnostic tool, but
variable positivity and, thereby, clinical correlation, have been
frequent, 50 to 100%. (3,8,15) Matthews and Soothill (16) studied complement activation after milk challenge in a small series, but larger, controlled series have been lacking. Quantitative immunoglobulin E levels have demonstrated significant overlap between normals and those with clinical disease. (3,8) The
radioallergosorbent test (RAST) which detects specific IgE antibodies to individual food proteins, such as milk, has not been
demonstrated to be reliable in diagnosis. (17) Preliminary lymphoblast transformation tests, carried out in the presence of
β-lactoglobulin, have been found to be a useful aid in diagnosis
due to their specificity. (18) Further studies will be necessary.

Small intestinal (jejunal) biopsy, as previously mentioned,
is not specific, but has been advocated by some authors as an
adjunct to the clinical milk challenge. This would involve biopsies before and after this milk challenge, thus demonstrating
normal and then abnormal small intestinal mucosa. (5-8)

9. (T) The most important differential diagnosis is lactose intolerance. Lactose intolerance can be excluded by the performance of a lactose tolerance test, involving the administration
of lactose, 2 grams per kilogram body weight or 50 grams per
meter^2 of body surface, and obtaining blood samples for glucose
determination at 0, 30, 60, 90, and 120 minutes. (8) To determine whether it is a primary or secondary phenomenon, small
intestinal (jejunal) biopsy must be performed and specific disaccharidase content in the mucosa determined. Even the usage of

the recently developed, noninvasive hydrogen (H_2) breath test
(collection of expired air and hydrogen measurement after carbohydrate, lactose administration) cannot distinguish primary
and secondary lactose intolerance. (8) Only morphological correlation with specific mucosal disaccharidase content may allow
this differentiation.

10. (T) The obvious cornerstone of treatment is elimination
of cow's milk from the diet as well as all foods containing cow's
milk. (3,8,19) Neglect of these restrictions results in therapeutic failure. Various milk substitutes, such as soy protein, goat's
milk, and elemental formulas, can be quite effective, although
some children may be intolerant to soy protein. (3,8,19) The
duration of the milk protein intolerance is usually temporary,
although the exact duration is usually unpredictable. However,
in general, after the age of 2 to 3 years, milk is tolerated without apparent untoward sequelae. (3,5,8)

11. (T) Disodium cromolyn glycate (Intal) was synthesized by
linking two chromone rings by an alkylene-hydroxy chain. (20)
This drug has the ability to interfere with allergy, in particular
type I reactions. (20) Despite its oral route, only 5 to 8% of the
administered dose is actually absorbed through the small intestinal mucosa. (20) Its excretion is via urine and bile. The apparent site of action of this drug is at the sensitized mast cell.
Its specific action is inhibition of antigen-induced (reagin) release of histamine, slow-acting substance (SRS-A), and other
factors from the mast cells. However, it does not inhibit fixation of antibodies or interfere with the antigen-antibody reaction,
but does suppress the response to this reaction. Preliminary
studies in patients with food allergy have been encouraging but
not consistent. (21-23) Further data, particularly studies in the
United States, will be necessary.

REFERENCES

1. Minford, A.M.B., MacDonald, A., Littlewood, J.M.: Food
   intolerance and food allergy in children: A review of 68
   cases. Arch Dis Child 57:742, 1982.

2. Goldstein, B., and Heiner, D.C.: Clinical and immunological perspectives in food sensitivity. J Allerg 46:270, 1970.

3. Goldman, A.S. and Heiner, D.C.: Clinical aspects of food
   sensitivity: Diagnosis and management of cow's milk sensitivity. Pediatr Clin North Am 24:133, 1977.

4. Gerrard, J.W., MacKenzie, J.W.A., Goluboff, N., et al.: Cow's milk allergy: Prevalence and manifestations in an unselected series of newborns. Acta Paediatr Scand 234 (suppl): S1-S21, 1973.

5. Freier, S.: Paediatric gastrointestinal allergy. Clin Allerg (suppl) 3:597, 1973.

6. Shiner, M., Ballard, J., Smith, M.E.: The small intestinal mucosa in cow's milk allergy. Lancet 1:136, 1975.

7. Kuituven, P., Rapola, J., Savilahti, E., et al.: Response of the jejunal mocosa to cow's milk in the malabsorption syndrome with cow's milk intolerance. Acta Paediat Scand 62:585, 1973.

8. Lebenthal, E.: Cow's milk protein allergy. Ped Clin North Am 22:827, 1975.

9. Rey, J.: The diagnostic criteria of cow's milk intolerance. Acta Paediat Scand 63:651, 1974.

10. Bock, S.A.: Food sensitivity. Am J Dis Child 134:973, 1980.

11. Goldman, A.S., Anderson, D.W., Sellers, W.A., et al.: Milk allergy: Oral challenge with milk and isolated milk proteins in allergic children. Pediatrics 32:425, 1963.

12. Powell, G.K.: Milk- and soy-induced enterocolitis of infancy: Clinical features and standardization of challenge. J Pediatr 93:553, 1978.

13. Peterson, R.D. and Good, R.A.: Antibodies to cow's milk protein: Their presence and significance. Pediatrics 31:209, 1963.

14. Kletter, B., Freier, S., Davies, A.M., et al.: The significance of coproantibodies to cow's milk protein. Acta Paediatr Scand 60:173, 1971.

15. Chua, Y.Y., Brenmer, K., Lakdawala, N., et al.: In vivo and in vitro correlates of food allergy. J Allerg Clin Immunol 58:299, 1976.

16. Matthews, T.S. and Soothill, J.F.: Complement activation after milk feeding in children with cow's milk allergy. Lancet 2:893, 1970.

17. Chua, Y.Y., Bremner, K., Llobet, J.L., et al.: Diagnosis of food allergy by the radioallergosorbent test. J Allerg Clin Immunol 58:477, 1976.

18. Scheinmann, P., Gendrel, D., Charlas, J., et al.: Value of lymphoblast transformation test in cow's milk protein intestinal intolerance. Clin Allerg 6:515, 1976.

19. Kuzemko, J.A. and Simpson, K.R.: Treatment of allergy to cow's milk. Lancet 1:338, 1975.

20. Cox, J.S.G.: Disodium cromoglycate - Mode of action and its possible relevance to the clinical use of the drug. Br J Dis Chest 65:189, 1971.

21. Nizami, R.M., Lewin, P.K., Baboo, M.T.: Oral cromolyn therapy in patients with food allergy: A preliminary report. Ann Allerg 39:102, 1977.

22. Dannaeus, A., Foucard, T., Johansson, S.G.O.: The effect of orally administered sodium cromoglycate on symptoms of food allergy. Clin Allerg 7:109, 1977.

23. Bierman, C.W., Furukawa, K.S.: Food Allergy. Pediatr Review 3:231, 1982.

Case 23

RECURRENT ABDOMINAL PAIN IN A 7-YEAR-OLD BOY

HISTORY

A 7-year-old white male presented with history of recurrent abdominal pain of 7 months' duration. The pain was located in the midabdomen without radiation, initially occurring once or twice monthly but increasing to daily for the last few weeks. The severity of the pain had increased, too. The pain would last minutes to hours and could recur during the same day. There was no relationship of the pain to time of day, bowel movements, position, and meals, but it was aggravated on occasion by excessive use of spices and possibly milk. He had associated pain during periods of increased stress. There was occasional associated nausea and infrequent vomiting. His bowel habit pattern was once daily but occasionally increased to 2-3 times daily without effect on the previously mentioned abdominal pain. There was no history of associated fever, constipation, dysuria, anorexia, weight loss, hematochezia, or melena; there was no history of associated trauma. The pertinent family history included the mother with a history of a nervous stomach and paternal aunt, as well as father with history of supposed hay fever. The pertinent social history included his present residence with his mother and 8-year-old brother, recent move about 6 months prior to this exam, and pressure for attainment of better grades in school by his mother. At home, he was expected to take care of his 8-year-old brother who had a history of hyperactivity, presently requiring usage of medication and counseling. His attendance at school also had suffered during this period of recurrent abdominal pain (absence from school for almost 6 weeks). The father had abandoned the family when the mother was pregnant with this patient. Subsequent divorce occurred, the mother raising the children.

EXAMINATION

He was alert and cooperative, weight 25.5 kg, height 118 cm, and normal vital signs. The remainder of the examination was unremarkable, including the abdomen and anorectal area.

LABORATORY DATA

Hemoglobin:	13.0 gm%
Hematocrit:	39.5%
White blood cell count:	$7,800/mm^3$
PMN's:	60%
lymphocytes:	34%
monocytes:	4%
eosinophiles:	2%
Sedimentation rate:	10 mm/hr
Serum:	
SGPT:	20 units
alkaline phosphatase:	150 IU
total protein:	6.8 gm%
albumin:	4.0 gm%
folate:	8 ng/ml
carotene:	170 μg%
serum amylase:	100 units
Urinalysis:	negative
Amylase (diastase):	2,400 units
Stool:	
reducing substances:	positive
occult blood:	negative
culture:	negative
ova and parasites:	negative
Upper gastrointestinal series:	negative

QUESTIONS

1. What is the probable diagnosis of this patient?
   A. Lactase deficiency
   B. Celiac disease
   C. Sucrase-isomaltase deficiency
   D. Giardiasis
   E. Whipple's disease

2. Lactase is characterized by which of the following statements?
   A. It is a brush border enzyme, hydrolyzing only lactose
   B. It splits lactose into the monosaccharides, glucose and fructose
   C. Its level can be altered by changing the amount or type of carbohydrate in the diet
   D. Its levels cannot be altered by changing the amount or type of carbohydrate in the diet
   E. Its splits lactose into the monosaccharides, glucose and galactose

3. Lactose intolerance is found in a high percentage of which ethnic groups?
   A. Scandinavians
   B. Greek Cypriots
   C. American Caucasians
   D. Ashkenazic Jews
   E. African Bantus

4. The usual clinical features of disaccharide (lactose) intolerance include which of the following?
   A. Watery diarrhea
   B. Abdominal cramps and borborygmi
   C. Fever
   D. Urticaria
   E. Nausea and vomiting

5. Which of the following laboratory studies are diagnostic of lactase deficiency?
   A. Clinical response to removal of the offending sugar from the diet
   B. Stool pH, reducing substances
   C. Blood glucose levels before and after oral administration of lactose
   D. Hydrogen excretion in breath after oral administration of lactose
   E. Small intestinal biopsy and enzyme (lactase) assay

6. The treatment consists of which of the following measures?
   A. Exclusion of lactose from the diet
   B. Oral antihistamines, e.g., Benadryl
   C. Oral anticholinergics, e.g., Probanthine
   D. Oral disodium cromoglycate
   E. Oral corticosteroids, e.g., Prednisone

ANSWERS AND COMMENTS

1. (A) The probable diagnosis is congenital (primary) lactase deficiency, albeit, an uncommon entity.
    The age of onset, lack of ingestion of sucrose- or gluten-containing foods, and the negative stool examinations would tend to rule out the remaining choices.

2. (A,D,E) Disaccharides are hydrolyzed by enzymes, disaccharidases, which are localized to the brush-border membrane of the intestinal villous cells lining the small intestine. (1) Their precise location is still unsettled, although their locus has been suggested to be as knob-like projections of the luminal surface of the microvilli. Their hydrolyzing ability is the result of their location, permitting the necessary binding and hydrolysis of disaccharides coming into contact with the intestinal cell surface. (1-3) Although there are two lactases (lysosome, brush-border), only one (brush-border) has digestive enzymatic properties. (1-3)
    Lactase levels rise during the perinatal period in full-term infants and, thereafter, can remain at a high level or decrease during childhood. (1-3) In some animals, the lactase level falls after weaning. (1-3) Although some controversy remains, lactase seems to be a disaccharidase that cannot be altered by a change in the type or quantity of lactose in the diet. (1-3) In weanling rats, lactase levels can be increased by oral lactose administration but only in large amounts. (1) Lactase activity is higher in the jejunum and proximal ileum than in the duodenum and distal ileum. (1-3)
    The actual hydrolysis of lactose into its monosaccharides, glucose and galactose, seems to occur at the surface of the intestinal microvilli, closer luminally to the membrane which controls intestinal transport and absorptive permeability. (1-6) The monosaccharides, except fructose, are transported actively across this membrane. The monosaccharides are apparently "trapped" in the glycocalyx or fuzzy coat covering the microvilli. Whether there are specific binding proteins for these monosaccharides remains unanswered. Fructose is apparently transported by facilitated diffusion. (1-6) Undigested disaccharides basically remain in the intestinal lumen and can act as an "osmotic force," resulting in an outpouring of fluid into the lumen. This increased fluid load then leads to the symptomatic pattern, as discussed in answer 4. In the colon, the undigested disaccharide, such as lactose, is fermented by bacterial enzymes, as discussed in answer 5. (1-6)
    Congenital lactase deficiency is apparently an "inborn" error of metabolism, being inherited and present from birth. Alpha-

glucosidase activities are not decreased. (7, 8) Dahlqvist (9) has suggested that congenital lactase deficiency is a structural mutation in which an abnormal protein without lactase activity is synthesized rather than the brush-border lactase.

3. (B,D,E) Low levels of lactase activity, as well as "milk intolerance," can occur in otherwise healthy individuals. Other disaccharidase activity, as well as intestinal mucosal integrity, is normal. The incidence of low lactase activity (intestinal) and/ or "milk intolerance" (lactose) is low in Western Europeans, Scandinavians, and American Caucasians, approximately 1 to 8% of the population. Conversely, lactose intolerance is quite prevalent in Greek Cypriots, Arabs, Ashkenazic Jews, and American Negroes, approximating 60 to 80%. (2,7,10-16) This increased prevalence of lactose intolerance is even more marked, 90% or greater, in African Bantus, Formosans, Filipinos, Thais, and Japanese. (2,7,10-16)

Interestingly, milk (lactose) intolerance is not common in apparently normal infants, even in populations where intestinal lactase levels are low. (10-16) With increasing age in childhood, the incidence of lactose intolerance increases. In American Negroes, only 40 to 50% clinically manifest lactose intolerance under the age of 10 years, while 60 to 80% of Thais, African Bantus, and Australian Aborigines will do so by this age. (10-16) Thus, the issue still remains whether ontogeny of this enzyme deficiency resulted from low lactase levels in beginning generations or whether milk consumption was low or nil during these generations. (2,7,10-16)

The consequences of these low lactase levels are variable. Obviously not all are bothered by milk consumption. Certainly many tolerate smaller amounts of milk, i.e., less than one quart daily. (8,13,17) Some will drink little, if any, milk after infancy, such as African Bantus, South Americans (e.g., Peruvians), and Asians, Thais, and Japanese. (10-16) Others will find that milk products, such as yogurt or cheese, a fermented form, will be well tolerated. (17) Thus, the common denominators are (1) the amount of milk consumed on any occasion and (2) individual responsiveness to this amount. (8,17)

4. (A,B,E) As described in answer 2, undigested lactose in the intestinal lumen acts as an osmotic force which results in an outpouring of fluid into the small intestine. The unabsorbed lactose holds the fluid in the lumen. The increased fluid load and resultant altered transit time produce abdominal distention/ bloating, abdominal discomfort (cramps), nausea, diarrhea, and, less so, vomiting. (1-4,7-17) In the colon, the undigested lactose undergoes fermentative degradation by bacterial

enzymes. The end products, carbon dioxide and hydrogen, may play a role in the bloating, flatulence, and diarrhea. (18-21)

5. (E) It is important to establish the lack of mucosal damage as well as a deficiency or lack of the disaccharidase, lactase in this patient, by direct assay. These aims can only be achieved by small intestinal biopsy (histology) and assay of enzyme activities, including sucrase, maltase, and lactase. (5-7, 22) However, the lack of histological abnormalities per se does not exclude the possibility of prior mucosal damage, now repaired, with a slow but incomplete return of lactase activity, taking up to 6 months in known cases. (7, 12, 22)

The other studies are very helpful in establishing an intolerance to one or more disaccharides, e.g., lactose, as a result of low or absent disaccharidase levels in the small intestinal mucosa, small intestinal transit alteration (increased rate), or a shortening (length) of the small intestine. (1, 3, 10, 22) The stool pH can be as low as 3.5 to 4.0. This lowered pH occurs when an undigested disaccharide, e.g., lactose, is fermented by bacterial enzymes in the colon, producing lactic acid as well as other short-chain fatty acids. In addition, reducing substances are present in the stools, being abnormal in amount if more than 0.5% (over 2+, using Clinitest tablets). (2, 7, 8, 10-16) An oral lactose absorption test can be performed to establish lactose intolerance. After an oral load of lactose, 2 gm/kg or 50 gm/m^2 surface area, as a 10% solution, blood glucose is measured at 30, 60, 90, and 120 minutes following administration. These levels are compared with the fasting level, normal being a rise of 30 mg/100 ml or more. (2, 7, 8, 10-16) Other factors, however, can influence the results, including gastric emptying time (delayed) and peripheral uptake of glucose (accelerated). (1, 2, 7, 8) The recent development of breath tests with oral administration of sugars has provided an accurate, noninvasive, easy method of establishing lactose intolerance. (20, 21) Hydrogen excretion in breath increases in lactose intolerance. Other orally administered agents, such as lactulose (transit), can be used to further distinguish lactase deficiency from lactose intolerance of other causes. (18, 19) Clinically, the response to removal of the offending sugar, the reproduction of the prior clinical pattern on administration of the sugar, and a good response to its removal once again further establish the diagnosis. Thus, lactase deficiency is suggested, lactose intolerance for whatever reason is established. (8, 17)

6. (A) Patients demonstrate a dramatic response to the exclusion of lactose from their diet. However, milk contains many important nutrients, and, therefore, attempts to prepare lactose-

free milk have existed for years. To avoid loss of minerals, vitamins, and the like, hydrolysis of lactose would be preferable to its removal. This hydrolysis can be accomplished enzymatically. One such preparation of lactase, Maxilact, has been used, but unfortunately, it involves the addition of a relatively large amount of foreign protein, as well as a significant cost factor. (9) Another method recently reported by Dahlqvist, et al. (9,23) has involved the incubation of milk, with a small amount of soluble lactase for a long time period. Commerically, Lact-aid® has been developed and used with good results and reasonable resultant taste.

Medication such as antihistamines, anticholinergics, corticosteroids, or sodium cromoglycate, are not of value for sugar intolerance and do not have any induction properties.

Finally, the vast majority of patients with apparent lactase deficiency shortly after birth seem to be able to tolerate small amounts and eventually normal amounts of lactose in later years. Therefore, this observation seems to shed doubt on the exist-

TABLE 23.1   Diagnostic Evaluation of Carbohydrate
Intolerance

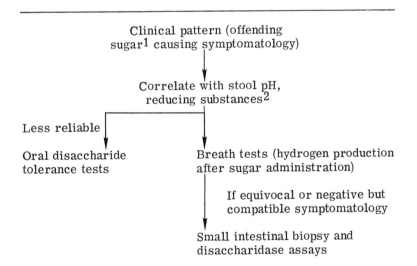

[1]Sugar = lactose, sucrose, glucose, fructose
[2]For sucrose, fructose: Acid hydrolysis (1N HCl) of stools before testing

ence, or certainly the magnitude, of congenital (primary) lactase deficiency. (9)

For further information on carbohydrate intolerance, see Table 23.1.

REFERENCES

1. Gray, G.M.: Carbohydrate digestion and absorption. Gastroenterology 58:96, 1970.

2. Launiala, K.: The mechanism of diarrhea in congenital disaccharide malabsorption. Acta Paediatr Scand 57:425,1968.

3. Gilat, T., Dolizky, F., Gelman-Malachi, E., et al.: Lactase in childhood - A nonadaptable enzyme. Scand J Gastroenterol 9:395, 1974.

4. Gracey, M. and Burke, V.: Sugar-induced diarrhea in children. Arch Dis Child 48:331, 1973.

5. Dahlqvist, A., Hammond, J.B., Crane, R.K., et al.: Assay of disaccharidase activities in peroral biopsies of the small intestinal mucosa. Acta Gastro-Enterol Belg 27:543, 1964.

6. Dahlqvist, A.: Assay of intestinal disaccharidases. Enzymol Biol Clin 11:52, 1970.

7. Bayless, T.M. and Christopher, N.L.: Disaccharidase deficiency. Am J Clin Nutr 22:181, 1969.

8. Bayless, T.M. and Huang, S.S.: Inadequate intestinal digestion of lactose. Am J Clin Nutr 22:250, 1969.

9. Dahlqvist, A.: The basic aspects of the chemical background of lactase deficiency. Postgrad Med J 53:57, 1977.

10. Asp, N-G. and Dahlqvist, A.: Intestinal β-galactosidases in adult low lactase activity and in congenital lactase deficiency. Enzyme 18:84, 1974.

11. Liebman, W.M.: Recurrent abdominal pain in children: Lactose and sucrose intolerance, a prospective study. Pediatrics 64:43, 1979.

12. Lifschitz, F.: Congenital lactase deficiency. J Pediatr 69:229, 1966.

13. Bolin, T.D., Davis, A.E., Seah, C.S., et al.: Lactose intolerance in Singapore. Gastroenterology 59:76, 1970.

14. Gilat, T., Kuhr, R., Gelman, E., et al.: Lactase deficiency in Jewish communities in Israel. Am J Dig Dis 15:895, 1970.

15. Sahi, T., Isokoski, M., Jussila, J., et al.: Lactose malabsorption in Finnish children of school age. Acta Paediatr Scand 61:11, 1972.

16. Cook, G.C., Asp, N-G., Dahlqvist, A.: Activities of brush-border lactase, acid β-galactosidase and hetero-β-galactosidase in the jejunum of the Zambian African. Gastroenterology 55:328, 1973.

17. Bayless, T.M., Paige, D.M., Ferry, G.D.: Lactose intolerance and milk-drinking habits. Gastroenterology 60:605, 1971.

18. Bond, J.H. and Levitt, M.D.: Quantitative measurement of lactose absorption. Gastroenterology 70:1058, 1976.

19. Lasser, R.B., Bond, J.H., Levitt, M.D.: The role of intestinal gas in functional abdominal pain. N Engl J Med 293:524, 1975.

20. Barr, R.G., Levine, M.D., Watkins, J.B.: Recurrent abdominal pain of childhood due to lactose intolerance: Prospective study. N Engl J Med 300:1449, 1979.

21. Barr, R.G., Watkins, J.B., Perman, J.A.: Mucosal function and breath hydrogen excretion: Comparative studies in clinical evaluation of children with nonspecific abdominal complaints. Pediatrics 68:526, 1981.

22. Nordstrom, C. and Dahlqvist, A.: Quantitative distribution of some enzymes along the villi and crypts of human small intestine. Scand J Gastroenterol 8:407, 1973.

23. Dahlqvist, A., Asp, N-G., Burvall, A., et al.: A new method for the preparation of lactose-free milk. Postgrad Med J 53:65, 1977.

Case 24

CHRONIC WATERY DIARRHEA IN A 3-YEAR-OLD GIRL

HISTORY

A 3-year-old white girl presented with watery diarrhea, 3 to 8 stools daily, since the neonatal period. She also had associated bloating and flatus without relationship to meals, food types, or time of day. There was no history of vomiting, fever, melena, hematochezia, rash, or jaundice. Growth and development were normal. Toilet training had not been completed. The remainder of the past, developmental, family, and social history was unremarkable, as was the review of systems.

EXAMINATION

She was alert and in no apparent distress, with normal vital signs, weight 14.1 kg, height 95 cm, and head circumference, 48 cm. The remainder of the examination, including the abdomen, was unremarkable.

LABORATORY DATA

Hemoglobin:	12.1 gm%
Hematocrit:	37%
White blood cell count:	$8,700/mm^3$
PMN's:	41%
lymphocytes:	52%
monocytes:	4%
eosinophiles:	3%
Sedimentation rate:	9 mm/hr
Urinalysis:	negative

189

Serum:
 total protein: 6.4 gm%
 albumin: 3.8 gm%
 folate: 5.2 ng/ml
 carotene: 108 μg%
 creatinine: 0.4 mg%
 calcium: 9.8 mg%
Stool:
 occult blood: negative
 reducing substances: negative (nonacidified);
 positive (acidified)
 culture: negative
 ova and parasites: negative

QUESTIONS

1. What is the most likely diagnosis of this patient?
   A. Duodenal ulcer
   B. Primary sucrose-isomaltase deficiency
   C. Celiac disease
   D. Regional enteritis
   E. Ulcerative colitis

Question 2: Answer true (T) or false (F).

2. This condition is inherited by dominant transmission.

3. As illustrated to some extent by this case, the usual clini-
   cal features include which of the following?
   A. Diarrhea
   B. Abdominal distention
   C. Vomiting
   D. Fever
   E. Variable failure to thrive

4. Diagnosis of this abnormality would be strongly suggested
   or confirmed by which of the following?
   A. Reducing substances in stools on known control diet
   B. Serum antibodies to disaccharide
   C. Oral sucrose tolerance test
   D. Small intestinal enzyme assay
   E. Secretin-pancreozymin stimulation test

5. Treatment of this condition includes which one of the following?
    A. Sucrose restriction in diet
    B. Antihistaminics
    C. Anticholinergics
    D. Sodium cromolyn
    E. Cimetidine

Question 6: Answer true (T) or false (F).

6. There is an excellent prognosis in this condition and the majority of patients will have improved tolerance for sucrose with increasing age.

ANSWERS AND COMMENTS

1. (B) The probable diagnosis of this patient is primary (congenital) sucrose-isomaltase deficiency (Table 24.1).
    The lack of pain relief by eating, nocturnal pain, vomiting, fever, hematochezia, more consistent and protracted diarrhea, and of weight loss would make the other choices less likely.

2. (F) Primary sucrase-isomaltase deficiency is probably the most common primary disaccharidase deficiency. (1-4) It is inherited by recessive transmission. There is always coexistent sucrase and isomaltase deficiency. (1-4) Recently, this deficiency has been explained as the absence of an inactive enzyme variant by a major (no-sense) structural gene mutation or by repression of regulatory mechanisms controlling the formation of the structural gene. (5) The first confirmation of deficient sucrase-isomaltase content in duodenal tissue was in 1962 by Anderson, et al. (3) although the first description of the clinical pattern associated with dietary sucrose ingestion was in 1961 by Weijers, et al. (7) and then others. (8-10) The estimated recessive inheritance in North Americans is 0.2%. (2,10)

3. (A,B,E) The most common symptom is diarrhea. (1-10) Diarrhea begins with the initiation of sucrose feedings in young infants, i.e., dextrin and starch (solid foods) such as fruits. (1-10) Bowel movements become loose or liquid, with a pungent odor. In addition, abdominal pain (crampy or colicky in nature and of variable location), variable distention and flatulence are frequent. (1-11) In the first few months of life, associated steatorrhea may be present, while in later infancy or the preschool period, difficulty in toilet training may be encountered. (1-10) Variable failure to thrive may be frequently present, too. How-

TABLE 24.1 Carbohydrate Assimilation

Diet	Luminal Enzyme	Luminal Digestive Product	Mucosal Enzyme	End Products
Amylopectin	Salivary and pancreatic alpha-amylase	Alpha-dextrins (1-6 alpha linkage)	Isomaltase	Glucose
Sucrose (30% of diet)		Sucrose	Sucrase	Glucose, fructose

Substrate (Dietary)		Intestinal Enzyme		Monosaccharide (End Product)
Starch (60%)(1,2)	Maltose, isomaltose	Salivary and pancreatic alpha-amylase		Glucose
Sucrose (30%)		Sucrase		Glucose, fructose
Lactose (10%)		Lactase		Glucose, galactose

(Modified from Gray, G. M.: Gastroenterology 58:96, 1970)

ever, the usual clinical picture is that of a healthy, normal-looking child whose height and weight are usually within normal limits. (1-11)

4. (A, C, D) The unhydrolyzed disaccharide sucrose produces a net secretion of water and electrolytes into the intestinal lumen, resulting in diarrhea, osmotic in type. (1-10) Therefore, sucrose will be present in the bowel movements. By testing the liquid portion of the feces with Clinitest tablets, first adding 1 N HCl and boiling for 30 to 60 seconds, reducing substances can be demonstrated without performing the more accurate paper chromatography. (1-10) Unabsorbed sucrose and isomaltose will be split into monosaccharides (glucose, fructose) by the colonic bacterial flora. Fermentation of these monosaccharides into lactic acid occurs, resulting in a lowering of fecal pH, usually to less than 5.5 (screening test). (1-10)

Another reliable test is the oral tolerance test (sucrose). (1-10) The lack of sucrose absorption is reflected in a flat glucose curve(0, 30, 60, 90, 120 minutes) after the feeding of sucrose (2 gm/kg), i. e. , less than 30-40 mg/100 ml rise above the basal level. (1-10) Diarrhea may also occur during the 6 to 12 hours after sucrose feeding, and reducing substances will be present in the feces. The small intestinal biopsy with enzyme (disaccharidase) assay can be diagnostic. The morphologic appearance is normal, while quantitative determination of sucrase reveals little or no activity. (13) Isomaltase activity is markedly reduced. (13) Lactase activity is normal to high normal.

In making decisions, one must remember that disaccharidase activity is normally higher in the jejunum and proximal ileum than in the rest of the small intestine. (12, 14) The other studies do not apply to this disorder.

Finally, the recent development of breath analysis offers an accurate, noninvasive technique for diagnosis of disaccharidase deficiencies. This technique involves the collection of expired breath before and 2 hours after feeding of a (lemon-flavored) sucrose solution. (12-17) Hydrogen in expired breath will be elevated in disaccharidase deficiencies, i.e., 25 ppm or more (12-17)

5. (A) Sucrose content in the diet must be eliminated or severely restricted, certainly initially. (11, 18-22) With time, most patients will tolerate a diet excluding only those foods with a high sucrose content, such as breakfast cereals, sugar (cane, beet, granulated, brown, powdered), and commercial baby foods. (18-22) One explanation for the increased tolerance has been normal growth and increased intestinal absorptive area. (18-22) In addition, jejunal sucrase activity has been increased by

194 / Case 24

certain dietary sugars, including fructose and sucrose. Furthermore, the levels were higher on high carbohydrate diets than on the low carbohydrate diets, i.e., a dose response. (18-22)

In rats, steroids (hydrocortisone) have produced an inducing effect on intestinal sucrase activity. (23) No controlled studies in children have been performed.

The other choices play no role in treatment of this condition.

6. (T) The prognosis in this abnormality is excellent. Despite continued reduced intestinal sucrase activity, dietary sucrose tolerance usually increases with age. (1-10, 20) However, dependent on dietary sucrose content, some degree of symptomatology can be expected for life. (1-10)

REFERENCES

1. Ament, M.E.: Malabsorption syndromes in infancy and childhood, J Pediatr 81:685, 867, 1972.

2. Davidson, M.M.D.: Disaccharide intolerance. Pediatr Clin North Am 14:93, 1967.

3. Anderson, C.M., Messer, M., Townley, R.R.W., et al.: Intestinal isomaltase deficiency in patients with hereditary sucrose and starch intolerance. Lancet 2:556, 1962.

4. Auricchio, S., Dahlqvist, A., Murget, G., et al.: Isomaltose intolerance causing decreasing ability to utilize starch. J Pediatr 62:165, 1963.

5. Gray, G.M., Conklin, K.A., Townley, R.R.W.: Sucrase-isomaltase deficiency. Absence of an inactive enzyme variant. N Engl J Med 294:750, 1976.

6. Sunshine, P. and Kretchmer, N.: Diarrhea and deficiency of intestinal disaccharidases. J Pediatr 63:844, 1963.

7. Weijers, H.A., Vandekamer, J.H., Dicke, W.K., et al.: Diarrhoea caused by deficiency of sugar-splitting enzymes. Acta Paediat Scand 50:55, 1961.

8. Weijers, H.A. and Vandekamer, J.H.: Aetiology and diagnoses of fermentative diarrhoeas. Acta Paediat Scand 52:329, 1963.

9. Anderson, C.M., Messer, M., Townley, R.R.W., et al.: Intestinal sucrase and isomaltase deficiency in two siblings. Pediatrics 31:1003, 1963.

10. Roy, C.C., Silverman, A., Cozzetto, F.J.: Pediatric Clinical Gastroenterology, 2nd Edition. The CV Mosby Co., St. Louis, 1975, p. 205.

11. Liebman, W.M.: Recurrent abdominal pain in children: Lactose and sucrose intolerance, a prospective study. Pediatrics 64:43, 1979.

12. Barr, R.G., Watkins, J.B., Perman, J.A.: Mucosal function and breath hydrogen excretion: Comparative studies in clinical evaluation of children with nonspecific abdominal complaints. Pediatrics 68:526, 1981.

13. Dahlqvist, A.: Method for assay of intestinal disaccharidases. Anal Biochem 7:18, 1964.

14. Auricchio, S., Rubino, A., Prader, A., et al.: Intestinal glycosidase activities in congenital malabsorption of disaccharides. J Pediatr 66:555, 1965.

15. Hepner, G.M.: Breath analysis: Gastroenterological applications. Gastroenterology 67:1250, 1974.

16. Barr, R.G., Perman, J.A., Schoeller, D.A., et al.: Breath tests in gastrointestinal disorders: New diagnostic opportunities. Pediatrics 62:393, 1978.

17. Perman, J.A., Barr, R.G., Watkins, J.B.: Sucrose malabsorption in children: Noninvasive diagnosis by interval breath hydrogen determination. J Pediatr 93:17, 1978.

18. Rosensweig, N.S. and Herman, R.H.: Dose response of jejunal sucrase and maltase activities to isocaloric high and low carbohydrate diets in man. Am J Clin Nutr 23:1373, 1970.

19. Greene, H.L., Stifel, F.B., Herman, R.H.: Dietary stimulation of sucrose in a patient with sucrase-isomaltase deficiency. Biochem Med 6:409, 1972.

196 / Case 24

20. Rosensweig, N.S. and Herman, R.H.: The dose response of jejunal disaccharidase activity to varying carbohydrate diets in man. Am J Clin Nutr 21:536, 1968.

21. Hardinge, M.G., Swarner, J.B., Crooks, H.: Carbohydrates in foods. J Am Diet Assoc 46:197, 1965.

22. Fomon, S.J.: Infant Nutrition, 2nd Edition. WB Saunders Co., Philadelphia, 1974.

23. Lebenthal, E., Sunshine, P., Kretchmer, N.: Effect of carbohydrate and corticosteroids on activity of alpha-glucosidases in intestine of the infant rat. J Clin Invest 51: 1244, 1972.

Case 25

CHRONIC DIARRHEA IN A 2-YEAR-OLD GIRL

HISTORY

A 2-year-old white female presented with an altered bowel habit
pattern, variable increase in number and bulk of bowel movements, for a duration of almost one year. The prior bowel habit
pattern had been once daily, soft to firm in nature, brown in
color, and had increased to 2-4 bowel movements daily, larger
in amount, bulky in nature, infrequently floating on top of the
toilet bowl water, but with increased odor. The patient's appetite had decreased slightly, and there had been no weight gain
between 1 and 2 years of age. Her activity continued to remain
good. There was no associated history of nausea, vomiting, fever, constipation, melena, hematochezia, skin lesions, arthralgia, dysuria, or jaundice. The family history included the father with variable bowel habit pattern, thin in habitus, but no
other specific conditions. The remainder of the past history,
developmental history, family history, social history, and review of systems was noncontributory.

EXAMINATION

She was alert, active, and in no distress, with normal vital
signs, weight 9.0 kg, height 88 cm, and head circumference
47.5 cm. The remainder of the examination was unremarkable
except for the abdomen, which was slightly distended, with no
shifting dullness, fluid wave, masses, or palpable liver, spleen,
and kidneys.

LABORATORY DATA

Hemoglobin:	13.2 gm%
Hematocrit:	40%
White blood cell count:	10,000/mm^3
PMN's:	41%
lymphocytes:	56%
monocytes:	2%
eosinophiles:	1%
Platelet count:	250,000/mm^3
Sedimentation rate:	3 mm/hr
Urinalysis:	negative
Serum:	
total protein:	6.6 gm%
albumin:	4.3 gm%
SGOT:	19 units
alkaline phosphatase:	170 IU
carotene:	5 μg%
folate:	2 ng/ml
IgG:	800 mg%
IgM:	80 mg%
IgA:	48 mg%
calcium:	9.4 mg%
creatinine:	0.6 mg%
T$_4$:	4.4 μg%
Stool:	
occult blood:	negative
reducing substances:	negative
culture:	negative
ova and parasites:	negative
Chest films:	negative
Barium enema:	negative
Upper GI - small bowel series:	thickening of mucosal folds in distal duodenum, jejunum, and proximal ileum
Bone age:	12 months (chronological age, 2 years)
Small intestine biopsy (histology):	(Fig. 25.1)
culture (aerobic, anaerobic):	negative
ova and parasites:	negative
thin layer chromatography:	negative
Sweat:	
sodium:	32 meq/L
chloride:	24 meq/L

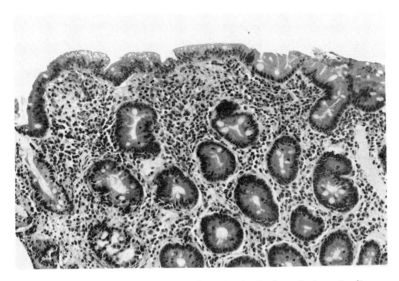

Figure 25.1 Jejunum. Foci of acute (polys) and chronic (lymphocytes, plasma cells) inflammatory cells are present throughout the lamina propria. The superficial epithelial layer is preserved in few areas, while others demonstrate absence or a variable loss. The villus-to-crypt ratio is <2:1; villi are atrophic (H&E X 125).

QUESTIONS

1. Celiac disease is one of the most common causes of malabsorption in infants and children. Which one of the following is the other most common cause?
    A. Zollinger-Ellison syndrome
    B. Giardiasis
    C. Shwachman-Diamond syndrome
    D. Cystic fibrosis
    E. Crohn's disease

2. The possible pathogenetic mechanisms in celiac disease include which of the following?
    A. Hypergastrinemia
    B. Hypoperfusion
    C. Peptidase deficiency
    D. Infectious (viral)
    E. Immunological disorder

Question 3: Answer true (T) or false (F).

3. As in the present case, abnormal fecal fat excretion (steatorrhea) is invariably present (95-100%).

4. The histological features of celiac disease include which of the following?
   A. Shortening of villi
   B. Increased cellularity of lamina propria, predominantly polys
   C. Increased cellularity of lamina propria, predominantly plasma cells
   D. Lacteal dilatation in lamina propria
   E. Granuloma formation in submucosa

5. Treatment may include which of the following?
   A. Gluten-free diet
   B. Milk-free diet
   C. Antacids
   D. Anticholinergics
   E. Corticosteroids

6. Common complications of this condition include which of the following?
   A. Crisis
   B. Peptic ulcer
   C. Pancreatitis
   D. Inflammatory bowel disease (Crohn's disease)
   E. Malignancy

ANSWERS AND COMMENTS

1. (D) Celiac disease and cystic fibrosis constitute the most common causes of malabsorption in infants and children. (1-5) Celiac disease is a disorder of the small intestine, producing clinical evidence of malabsorption, characterized by structural (histological) abnormality of the mucosa, reversed by gluten withdrawal. (1-5) The incidence of this condition is significantly higher in Europe than in the United States, i.e., as frequent as 1:300 to 1:500 in Western Ireland. (1,4) More than one member of a family may be affected, e.g., small intestinal mucosal abnormalities in first-degree relatives, 2 to 15%. (6) In addition, a link has been found genetically, i.e., histocompatibility antigens, most notably HLA-B8 and HLA-DW3. (7,8) The likely explanation for this finding rests with the immune response (Ir) genes which have been linked to the histocompatibility loci

in man, as well as animals. (7,8) Yet, 20 to 30% of patients
with celiac disease do not have the HLA-B8 antigen and more do
not have the HLA-DW3 antigen. (7,8) Other HL-A antigens have
been associated with celiac disease, too, e.g., HLA-B1 antigen.
(7) Therefore, other factors, such as environmental and genetic, play a role in the development of celiac disease.

2.   (C,E) In the 1950s, Dicke initially, others later, observed
the association of gluten in the diet with the resultant enteropathy, celiac disease. (1.4) The consumption of gluten (wheat
protein) or one of two ethanol extract fractions, gliadin, produces this condition, while their strict dietary elimination results in remission. (1,4) Acidic peptide products of gliadin,
such as fraction IX or alpha gliadin, have been particularly implicated. (1,4)
    Two major proposals have been frequently mentioned as the
cause(s) of the intestinal lesion upon exposure to gluten or toxic
peptides. (1,4) In general, these two are intestinal peptidase
deficiency and an immunological disorder. (1,4) The former
proposal is based on the lack of an intestinal peptidase, necessary for the detoxification of gluten. (1,4) Although peptidase
deficiency is present, mucosal injury is also present. This deficiency is more likely secondary to the intestinal lesion because
healed mucosa has normal peptidase concentration, suggesting
a nonprimary nature. (1,4)
    The second proposal has been receiving increased attention,
especially because of recent studies with in vitro organ cultures
(intestinal mucosa bathing in special medium). Biopsy specimens from the small intestinal mucosa of normals, patients
with gluten enteropathy, and from patients with other intestinal
disorders have been studied by this technique. Immunoglobulin
synthesis, IgA and IgM antibody with antigluten specificity, was
found to be increased only in patients with gluten enteropathy.
(9,10) In addition, IgA-antigen complexes have been found in
the small intestinal mucosa of patients with gluten enteropathy
after gluten challenge. (9,10) No effect with gluten challenge
(protein) was noted in specimens of patients in remission.
Therefore, these results suggest that gluten protein must first
produce an internal change in tissue integrity of susceptible individuals, e.g., activation of an endogenous effector(s), before
toxicity occurs. (9,10) This hypothesis has been strengthened
further by the production of mucosal changes in the presence of
gluten protein only when cultured with the mucosa of a patient
with active disease. (9,10)
    Other aspects of the immune status in gluten enteropathy
have been extensively studied. Atrophy of the spleen has been
confirmed in several reports. (11) Up to a third of patients may

be affected. The cause remains undefined. An increased risk
of blood-borne infections is a possibility. Humoral (B-cell) investigations have been numerous. (1,12-14) Serum IgG levels
have been generally high, while serum IgM levels have usually
been low. Elevated, as well as low or normal, serum IgE levels have been reported. (12) Two percent of patients have associated isolated IgA deficiency. (13) Conversely, elevated levels
of IgG, IgA, and IgM are usually found in intestinal secretions.
(15) Immunocytes (IgA, IgG, IgM) in the intestinal mucosa are
increased in number; and increased synthesis of IgA and IgM
has been noted in organ culture experiments. (16,17) Cell-mediated (T-cell) studies have been numerous, too. Reduced numbers and function of circulating T-cells have been reported,
using rosetting technique and lymphocyte PHA (phytohemagglutinin) responsiveness, respectively. (18) However, clinical evidence of T-cell deficiency has not been observed, e.g., viral/
fungal infections. (18)

In an attempt to synthesize a unifying concept Grüttner and
Stern (19) suggested that intraluminal partial hydrolysis of gliadin leads to a fraction that binds to the small intestinal mucosa,
possibly corresponding to specific glycoprotein receptors (configuration). Then the molecular fraction binds or stimulates the
gut-associated lymphoid structures, this association possibly
facilitated by the HL-A antigens. Sensitization results, a local
reaction causing the mucosal injury. As a result of the mucosal
insult, immunological events occur, e.g., immune complexes.
Obviously, further investigation will be necessary to confirm,
or not, this hypothesis.

The other choices (answers) have not been demonstrated to
be present in gluten enteropathy.

3. (F) Steatorrhea (excessive fecal fat excretion) is absent in
10 to 30% of children with confirmed celiac disease and is apparently related more to extent than severity of the intestinal mucosal lesion. (1,2,4,5) Usually the 3-day stool fat collection between nonabsorbable markers in untreated celiacs reveals fat
excretion over 10 to 15% (normal, 5% or less. (1,2,4,5)

Other laboratory studies, including d-xylose absorption, have
frequently been performed in the evaluation of possible celiac
disease. Both urinary excretion (5 hours) and blood levels (0,
30, 60, 90, and 120 minutes) should be measured after an oral
dose of d-xylose, 0.5 gm/kg body weight or 14.5 gm/M^2, as a
10% aqueous solution. A rise of less than 30 mg/100 ml indicates mucosal abnormality. Some authors, particularly Rolles,
et al. (20) have reported the complete separation of untreated
celiacs from controls by use of only the fasting and 1-hour blood
levels. Based on this abnormal value, small intestinal biopsy

has or has not been performed. Serum total protein and albumin levels have been decreased in only 50 to 70% of untreated celiacs. (1-5) In addition, nitrogen losses in stools are abnormally high in only 50%. (1-5) The cause(s) of the protein abnormalities appears to be abnormal exudation through damaged mucosa, increased cell exfoliation, and diminished amino acid uptake by the damaged mucosa. (1,4)

Altered pancreatic functional status, specifically reduced volume, bicarbonate, and enzyme output, is probably related to impaired release of secretin and cholecystokinin-pancreozymin (CCK-PZ) from damaged small intestinal mucosa. Altered release and/or synthesis of endogenous CCK-PZ also results in decreased bile delivery and impaired fat absorption. (21) Low serum iron and folate levels and, less so, vitamin B_{12} have been found, as have low prothrombin levels. (1-5)

Radiologic studies may be helpful. Bone age may be retarded in long-standing, untreated celiacs. Osteoporosis and osteomalacia are not infrequent. (1,4,5) Rickets per se is not frequent. (1,4,5) The "classical signs" of celiac disease on small bowel series include dilatation (jejunum especially), segmentation (large barium clumps within dilated loops), and hypersecretion (flocculation). (1,4,5) In addition, transit time may be slow, and diffuse thickening of the mucosal folds may be visualized. (1,4,5)

4. (A,C) The histological features of celiac disease have been well described. The small intestinal tissue is obtained by peroral small biopsy, using one of several types of biopsy capsules, e.g., Crosby-Kugler. Initially, there is an accelerated rate of enterocyte loss (shedding). (1,4) This results in a compensatory increase in the proliferative zone of the intestinal crypts. (1-5) The mucosal architecture will then be altered when the compensatory effort is inadequate. (1-5) Subtotal or total atrophy of villi occurs, specifically shortening and clubbing. The crypts become elongated, increased in diameter and tortuous. (1-5) This produces an alteration in the normal villus-to-crypt ratio (over 2:1). In addition, there is increased cellularity of the lamina propria, predominantly plasma cells, less so lymphocytes. (1-5) Increased collagen may be noted in the subepithelial part of the lamina propria. (1-5) These changes are particularly prominent in the proximal jejunum. (1-5)

Disaccharidase assay of the involved mucosa has revealed decreased levels, particularly lactase. (21) In addition, decreased alkaline phosphatase, peptide hydrolase, and other enzymes, have also been found. (22) Increased lymphocytic infiltration (T-cell) of the mucosal layer with gluten challenge may aid in the diagnosis when noted.

The other answers, granuloma formation, particularly suggestive of granulomatous bowel disease, and lacteal dilatation,
suggestive of lymphatic obstruction or disorder, e.g., intestinal lymphangiectasia, are incorrect.

5. (A, B, E) The obvious form of treatment is a gluten-free
diet (Table 25.1). The initial response is usually dramatic and
reasonably rapid, usually within days. The stools become less
frequent and more formed, and the appetite and disposition improve. (23-25) Catch-up growth (height, weight) is noted within
months. Normal mucosal architecture is usually achieved within 3 to 6 months. (24,25) Conversely, celiac disease is a permanent condition, and reintroduction of gluten to the diet will be
followed by recurrence of mucosal abnormalities. (22-25) Yet,
many authors maintain children on a gluten-free diet for at least
2 years and then reintroduce gluten. "Tolerance" to gluten is
truly a matter of trial and error, requiring careful, continued
observation in order to assure adequate appetite, activity, and
growth and development. (25, 26) These clinical assessments
should be substantiated periodically by repeat laboratory tests
and repeat peroral intestinal biopsy. If symptomatology reap-
pears or there is a lack of clinical response after 6 months while
on a gluten-free diet, repeat evaluation, including intestinal biopsy, is in order. A diagnosis other than celiac disease is likely. (23-27)

Because the disaccharidases of the small intestinal mucosa
are frequently reduced in celiac disease, particularly lactase,
the corresponding substrates (sugars) should be restricted in
the diet, mainly lactose. (24) Usually this dietary restriction
is maintained for a minimum of 8 weeks. (24) In infants, a special formula can be used, e.g., Pregestimil, Vivonex, or even
Nutramigen (sucrose). (24)

Corticosteroids have produced variable responsiveness, including improved appetite, activity, growth, and decreased stools.
(28, 29) Their use has been primarily in more severely affected
children and in infrequent crises, and consists of prednisone,
40-60 mg/M^2 surface area/24 hr, orally; or in crisis, intravenous hydrocortisone, 10 mg/kg/24 hr. The steroids are continued for 4 to 8 weeks before progressive weaning. (28, 29)

Antacids and anticholinergics do not have a place in the usual
management.

6. (A, E) Celiac crisis is fortunately uncommon since it is a
life-threatening complication. It may be precipitated by prolonged fasting or intercurrent infection. (28, 29) Dehydration
and metabolic acidosis occur due to the protracted diarrhea and
vomiting. Treatment includes nasogastric suction, intravenous

TABLE 25.1 Gluten-Free Diet

Foods Avoided

---

1. All breads and cereals containing wheat flour, bread flour, all-purpose flour, barley, cracked wheat, bran, farina, cracker meal, bread crumbs, and pretzels
2. All cakes, cookies, pies, donuts, ice cream cones, prepared puddings and mixes (cake, cookie mixes), and commercial ice cream
3. Commercial candies containing cereal products
4. Fish or meat patties/loaves from bread/cracker crumbs or wheat flour and croquettes
5. Meat products with wheat, such as cold cuts, sausages, and frankfurters
6. Noodles, dumplings, spaghetti, macaroni
7. Commercial salad dressings
8. Sauces/gravies with wheat flour
9. Creamed soups, unless without wheat and all canned soups
10. Coffee, instant (wheat), Postum, malted drinks, ale, and beer

---

fluid therapy, colloid administration if shock or undue hypoproteinemia is present, and usually parenteral corticosteroid administration. Refer to answer 5.

In celiac disease in adults especially, malignancy may develop. Lymphoma of the small intestine is most common, but carcinoma of the gastrointestinal tract, such as the esophagus, may develop. (30-32) Strict adherence to a gluten-free diet does decrease this incidence. (30-32)

The other answers have not been consistently associated with celiac disease.

For a summary of malabsorption studies, see Table 25.2

TABLE 25.2 Malabsorption: Selective Studies

Initial Studies (Screening)

---

complete blood count
sedimentation rate
serum carotene
serum folate (folic acid)
serum total protein, albumin

urinalysis

stool suspension (pH, reducing substances, Sudan III stain, culture, ova, cysts, parasites)

Intermediate Studies

---

upper gastrointestinal - small bowel series
d-xylose (5hr-urine; blood, 0,1,2 hr)
quantitative stool fat (72hr collection)
sweat test
quantitative immunoglobulins

Special Studies

Breath tests
    CO_2 (C^{14}, C^{13})   fat, protein, bile acid
    hydrogen   carbohydrate
                           (lactose, sucrose, glucose)

small intestinal biopsy (histology, disaccharidase assay)

duodenal aspiration (aerobic/anaerobic culture, bile acids, pancreatic enzymes, enterokinase)

secretin-pancreozymin stimulation test (pancreas)

Cr^{51} albumin or I^{131} PVP excretion study (stool) (G.I. protein loss)

REFERENCES

1. Kowlessar, O.D. and Phillips, L.D.: Celiac disease. Med Clin North Am 54:647, 1970.

2. Young, W.E. and Pringle, E.M.: 110 children with celiac disease, 1950-1969. Arch Dis Child 46:421, 1971.

3. Anderson, C.M., Gracey, M., Burke, V.: Celiac disease: Some still controversial aspects. Arch Dis Child 47:292, 1972.

4. McNeish, A.S. and Anderson, C.M.: The disorder in childhood. Clin Gastroenterol 3:127, 1974.

5. Meeuwisse, G.W.: Diagnostic criteria in coeliac disease. Acta Paediatr Scand 59:461, 1970.

6. Asquith, P.: Family studies in coeliac disease. In: Cardiac Disease: Proceedings of the Second International Coeliac Symposium. Hekkens, J.M. and Pena, A.S. (Eds.). Leiden, Stenfert, Kroese, 1974, p. 332.

7. Stokes, P.L., Asquith, P., Holmes, G.K.T., et al.: Histocompatibility antigens associated with adult coeliac disease. Lancet 2:162, 1972.

8. Scott, B.B., Swinburne, M.L., Rajah, S.M., et al.: HL-A8 and the immune response to gluten. Lancet 2:374, 1974.

9. Ferguson, A., MacDonald, T.T., McClure, J.P., et al.: Cell-mediated immunity to gliadin within the small intestinal mucosa in coeliac disease. Lancet 1:895, 1975.

10. Falchuk, Z.M., Gebhard, R.L., Sessoms, C., et al.: An in vitro model of gluten-sensitive enteropathy: Effect of gliadin on intestinal cells of patients with gluten-sensitive enteropathy in organ culture. J Clin Invest 53:487, 1974.

11. Ferguson, A., Maxwell, J.D., Hutton, M.M.: Splenic function in adult coeliac disease. Scot Med J 14:261, 1969.

12. Asquith, P., Thompson, R.A., Cooke, W.T.: Serum immunoglobulins in adult coeliac disease. Lancet 2:129, 1969.

13. MacWhinney, H. and Tomkin, G.H.: Gluten enteropathy associated with selective IgA deficiency. Lancet 2:121, 1971.

208 / Case 25

14. Browth, I.L., Ferguson, A., Carswell, F., et al.: Auto-antibodies in children with coeliac disease. Clin Exp Immunol 13:313, 1973.

15. Savilahti, E.: Intestinal immunoglobulins in children with coeliac disease. Gut 13:958, 1972.

16. Blecher, T.E., Brzechwa-Adjukiewicz, A., McCarthy, C.F., et al.: Serum immunoglobulins and lymphocyte transformation studies in coeliac disease. Gut 10:57, 1969.

17. Pettingale, K.W.: Immunoglobulin and specific antibody responses to antigenic stimulation in adult coeliac disease. Clin Sci 38:16, 1970.

18. O'Donoghue, D.P., Lancaster-Smith, M., Kumar, P.J.: Depletion of thymus-dependent lymphocytes in adult coeliac disease. Gut 16:392, 1975.

19. Gruttner, R., Stern, M.: Celiac disease. Monat Kinderleif 128:109, 1980.

20. Rolles, C.J., Nutter, S., Kendall, M.J., et al.: One-hour blood-xylose screening test for celiac disease in infants and young children. Lancet 2:1043, 1973.

21. Colombato, L.O., Parodi. H., Cantor, D.: Biliary function studies in patients with celiac sprue. Am J Dig Dis 22:96, 1977.

22. Pena, A.S., Truelove, S.C., Whitehead, R.: Disaccharidase activity and jejunal morphology in celiac disease. Q J Med 41:451, 1972.

23. Hamilton, J.R., Lynch, M.J., Reilly, B.J.: Active celiac disease in childhood. Q J Med 38:135, 1969.

24. Roy, C.C., Silverman, A., Cozzetto, F.J.: Pediatric Clinical Gastroenterology, 2nd Edition. The CV Mosby Co., St. Louis, 1975, p. 226.

25. Sheldon, W.: Prognosis in early adult life of celiac children treated with a gluten-free diet. Br Med J 2:401, 1969.

26. Hamilton, J.R. and McNeill, L.K.: Childhood celiac disease: Response of treated patients to a small uniform daily dose of wheat gluten. J Pediatr 81:885, 1972.

27. Rossi, E., Moser, H.: Genetic abnormalities of pancreatic and intestinal function. In: Textbook of Gastroenterology and Nutrition in Infancy. E. Lebenthal (Ed). Raven Press, New York, 1981, p. 876.

28. Lloyd-Still, J.D., Grand, R.J., Khaw, T., et al.: The use of corticosteroids in celiac crisis. J Pediatr 81:1074, 1972.

29. Heiner, D.C. and Liebman, W.: Celiac syndrome. In: Pediatric Therapy. Shirkey, H.C. (Ed). The CV Mosby Co., St. Louis, 1975, p. 639.

30. Barry, R.E. and Read, A.E.: Celiac disease and malignancy. Q J Med 42:665, 1973.

31. Harris, O.D., Cooke, W.T., Thompson, H., et al.: Malignancy in adult coeliac disease and idiopathic steatorrhea. Am J Med 42:899, 1967.

32. Ferguson, R., Asquith, P., Cooke, W.T.: The jejunal cellular infiltrate in coeliac disease complicated by lymphoma. Gut 15:834, 1974.

Case 26

CHRONIC SWELLING OF THE TRUNK AND LOWER EXTREMITIES IN A 15-YEAR-OLD BOY

HISTORY

A 15-year-old white male presented with a 2-month history of progressive swelling of the lower extremities, scrotum, and abdomen. There was an associated altered bowel habit pattern, an increase to 3-4 bowel movements daily, looser in nature, and brown in color as compared to his normal pattern of once daily, firm, and brown in color. There was no associated history of fever, anorexia, nausea, vomiting, constipation, melena, hematochezia, weight loss, skin lesions, jaundice, arthralgia, dysuria, dyspnea, chest pain, ocular difficulty, or trauma. No medication was being taken during this period of time. Activity and appetite remained unchanged. There was no history of exposure to unusual food, drug, or plant, or of a trip outside of area of residence during the preceding 1-2 years. The remainder of the past history, developmental history, family history, social history, and review of systems was noncontributory. Preliminary studies by his private physician included normal complete CBC, urinalysis, chest X-ray, EKG, and chemistries, including total protein 4.2 gm/100 ml, albumin 2.1 gm/100 ml.

EXAMINATION

He was alert, cooperative, and in no distress, with normal vital signs, weight 68 kg, and height 173 cm. The remainder of the examination was unremarkable except for apparent abdominal distention, shifting dullness, and a definite fluid wave in the abdomen, and scrotal, pretibial, and pedal edema pitting in type.

LABORATORY DATA

Hemoglobin:	12.5 gm%
Hematocrit:	38%
White blood cell count:	7,500/mm^3
PMN's:	78%
lymphocytes:	7%
monocytes:	10%
eosinophiles:	3%
basophils:	2%
Sedimentation rate:	13 mm/hr
Urinalysis:	negative
Serum:	
SGPT:	18 units
SGOT:	20 units
alkaline phosphatase:	147 IU
prothrombin time:	11.7 seconds
partial thromboplastin time:	32 seconds
creatinine:	0.4 mg%
carotene:	32 μg%
folate:	4 ng/ml
total protein:	4.6 gm%
albumin:	2.1 gm%
calcium:	8.4 mg%
cholesterol:	110 mg%
triglyceride:	68 mg%
sodium:	138 meq/L
potassium:	9.1 meq/L
chloride:	102 meq/L
bicarbonate:	24 meq/L
Stool:	
quantitative fat (72 hr):	11% (per 24 hr)
Cr^{51} albumin isotope scan:	9.4% (72 hr value) ($<$ 2%)
Upper GI - small bowel series:	edema, thickening of mucosal folds of duodenum, jejunum, proximal ileum
Barium enema:	negative
Percutaneous lymphangiography:	no specific abnormality
Small intestinal biopsy:	(Fig. 26.1)
cultures (aerobic, anaerobic):	negative
ova and parasites:	negative

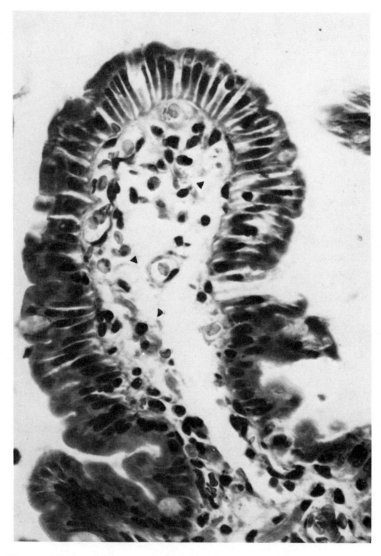

Figure 26.1   Jejunum.   Normal villous architecture with large, dilated lacteals (arrows) in the lamina propria (H&E, X 125.)

QUESTIONS

1. The probable diagnosis in this patient is
   A. constrictive pericarditis
   B. intestinal lymphangiectasia
   C. Menetrier's disease
   D. celiac disease
   E. ulcerative colitis

2. Excessive loss of enteric proteins is due to which basic pathological pathways?
   A. Decreased bone marrow production
   B. Excessive urinary excretion
   C. Lymphatic blockage
   D. Decreased hepatic synthesis
   E. Abnormal mucosal permeability

3. The clinical entities associated with enteric protein loss may include which of the following?
   A. Constrictive pericarditis
   B. Acute pancreatitis
   C. Crohn's disease
   D. Whipple's disease
   E. Celiac disease

4. The clinical picture usually includes
   A. diarrhea
   B. fever
   C. anasarca
   D. failure to thrive
   E. vomiting

5. Laboratory findings in this disorder usually include
   A. low serum albumin level
   B. low immunoglobulin levels
   C. lymphopenia
   D. low serum calcium
   E. steatorrhea

6. Radiographic findings in this disorder may include
   A. intestinal fold enlargement
   B. normal small intestinal pattern
   C. double-bubble sign
   D. significant dilatation
   E. linear ulcerations

7. Quantitation of enteric protein loss can be accomplished by which of the following methods?
   A. ^{51}Cr-albumin
   B. Radioiodinated serum albumin (RISA)
   C. Fe^{59}-iron dextran (Imferon)
   D. I^{131} polyvinylpyrrolidone ($I^{131}PVP$)
   E. Radioactive selenomethionine (^{75}Se)

Question 8: Answer true (T) or false (F).

8. Small intestinal biopsy may be specific for this condition.

9. The management of these cases may include
   A. localized surgical resection
   B. cimetidine
   C. oral disodium cromoglycate
   D. medium-chain triglycerides
   E. pancreatic enzyme supplementation (Viokase, Cotazym)

Question 10: Answer true (T) or false (F).

10. With appropriate management, the condition gradually disappears in essentially all cases.

ANSWERS AND COMMENTS

1. (B) Intestinal lymphangiectasia is the probable diagnosis. The radiographic findings, cardiac studies, and small intestinal biopsy virtually eliminate the other possibilities.

2. (C, E) There are two basic pathological mechanisms for enteric protein loss: (1) lymphatic blockage and (2) abnormal intestinal mucosal permeability to protein. (1-6) Refer to answer 3.

3. (A, C, D, E) As previously stated in answer 2, there are two basic mechanisms for enteric protein loss. Disease entities involving lymphatic blockage include intestinal lymphangiectasia, Crohn's disease, intestinal malrotation, Whipple's disease, neoplasm, and constrictive pericarditis, or congestive heart failure. (1-7) Disease entities involving altered intestinal permeability to protein include celiac disease (nontropical sprue), tropical sprue, various gastrointestinal infections, hypertrophic gastritis (Menetrier's disease), and radiation enteritis. (1-7) In the vast majority of cases, associated malnutrition and malabsorption are involved, resulting in a compromise of the ability of the liver to synthesize protein compensatingly. (1-7)

4. (A,C,D,E) In this disorder, the symptomatic pattern can be quite variable. The predominant manifestation is nongastrointestinal, i.e., edema, localized or generalized. This reflects the lowered plasma oncotic pressure due to low serum albumin levels. (1-7) This edema may even be asymmetrical. Chylous ascites may be present. Failure to thrive and abdominal distention are prominent features, too. Gastrointestinal symptomatology may be mild, at times severe, including diarrhea, vomiting, and abdominal discomfort or pain. (1-7) In addition, recurrent infections, tetany (calcium), and evidence of anemia or fat-soluble vitamin loss may be features. (1-7) The anemia may be secondary to iron loss, folic acid or vitamin B_{12} malabsorption, or severe protein loss. (1-7)

5. (A,B,C,D,E) The main laboratory features are low serum albumin level, low serum immunoglobulin levels, lymphopenia, lymphocytes in stool smears, and frequently, low serum calcium level and anemia, hemoglobin (8-10 gm/100 ml). Quantitative stool fat determinations are usually significantly abnormal (over 5 to 7% of the daily total fat intake). (1-9)
   The immunoglobulin and albumin deficiencies reflect the increased rate of protein loss into the intestinal lumen. Lymphopenia is due to the loss of lymphocytes into the gastrointestinal tract. However, the rate of immunoglobulin synthesis and antibody response to antigenic stimulation are essentially normal. (1-8) Conversely, delayed hypersensitivity reactions are minimal or nonexistent, resulting in anergy and impaired homograft rejection. (1-8)
   Refer to answer 7 for further discussion of enteric protein loss and kinetics of plasma protein metabolism (Fig. 26.2).

6. (A,B) Radiographic examination of the small intestine may be normal in 10 to 20%. (1-9) When abnormal, the radiographic findings include (1) intestinal fold enlargement, (2) minimal dilatation of the small intestine, (3) dilution of barium, and (4) coarsening of the mucosal pattern. (1-9) Obviously, these findings are suggestive but not pathognomonic of this disorder and must be correlated with the clinical and laboratory findings.

7. (A,C,D) The techniques for demonstration of enteric protein loss may be the only means of identifying the abnormality of the intestinal tract. When serum proteins are lost into the gastrointestinal tract, catabolism occurs and results in the formation of constituent amino acids which are subsequently reabsorbed. (10-12) When the synthetic capacity is exceeded, hypoproteinemia occurs.

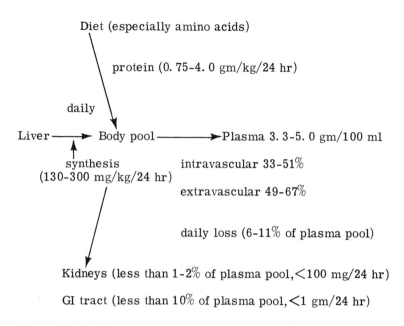

Diet (especially amino acids)

protein (0. 75-4. 0 gm/kg/24 hr)

daily

Liver ──→ Body pool ──────→ Plasma 3. 3-5. 0 gm/100 ml

synthesis   intravascular 33-51%
(130-300 mg/kg/24 hr)
                        extravascular 49-67%

                        daily loss (6-11% of plasma pool)

Kidneys (less than 1-2% of plasma pool, <100 mg/24 hr)

GI tract (less than 10% of plasma pool, <1 gm/24 hr)

Figure 26.2 Albumin metabolism in childhood. Modified from
Rothschild, M.A., et al.: N Engl J Med 286:748, 1972.

Gastrointestinal protein loss has generally been determined
by measuring the fecal excretion of a radioactive label previously administered intravenously. To be maximally effective, the
label should be attached to the protein without altering the nature
of the protein, should not be absorbed, and should not be excreted into the gastrointestinal tract except bound to protein.
(10-12) None of the currently available radioactive-labeled macromolecules fulfill all of these requirements. Radioiodinated
serum proteins, such as albumin (RISA), can be used to determine protein size, protein catabolic rate, and protein synthetic
rate but not enteric protein loss, per se. For example, reduced
circulating pools of quantitative immunoglobulins and albumin
are present, while the synthetic rate is normal or slightly increased. (10-12) For the determination of gastrointestinal protein loss itself, other labeled macromolecules were developed.
One was iodinated polyvinylpyrrolidone (PVP), a large polymer
apparently not metabolized. This agent was administered intravenously, and the percentage of this dosage determined in feces

over the subsequent 4 days. The normal excretion is 0 to 1.5% of the intravenously administered dose of radioactivity. (10-12) Unfortunately, variable amounts are absorbed, and it differs from serum proteins in size, structure, and charge. Another commonly used agent has been ^{51}Cr-labeled proteins, including ^{51}Cr-transferrin and ^{51}Cr-albumin. The latter has been most widely used. This label is not significantly secreted into or absorbed from the gastrointestinal tract. Less than 2% of intravenously administered ^{51}Cr-albumin is excreted in feces over a 4-day period of collection. Limitations of this technique include the relatively long survival of ^{51}Cr-albumin, the differential transit time of radioactivity, and the elution of the chromium from the albumin and association of the label with other proteins. Other agents have included ^{59}Fe-labeled iron dextran, ^{95}Nb-labeled albumin, and ^{67}Cu-labeled ceruloplasmin. The former is poorly absorbed and has little or no urinary excretion. However, its limitations include rapid clearance from the plasma. (10-12)

Thus, the size of the protein pool and rate of protein catabolism and synthesis can be measured by ^{125}I-protein (albumin) and rate of the gastrointestinal protein loss quantitated by ^{51}Cr-labeled protein clearance. The magnitude of disease and efficacy of treatment can be evaluated by repeated testing with ^{51}Cr-labeled serum proteins, e.g., albumin. (10-12)

A simpler technique for assessment of gastrointestinal protein loss has been more recently introduced, specifically, fecal alpha-1-antitrypsin (A-AT) measurement. (13) Fecal A-AT clearance has been easy, requiring no radioisotopes, and further controlled data in children with various disorders are being accumulated. (13)

8. (T) The small intestinal biopsy can be quite specific. Light microscopic studies will reveal normal villous architecture. However, there will be significant dilatation of the lymphatics of the lamina propria and submucosa, i.e., lacteals, many filled with lipid-filled macrophages (lipophages), and some villous distortion. As previously mentioned, villous and crypt epithelial cells appear normal. (5, 7)

Electron microscopic studies of the intestinal epithelial cells have generally been normal. At the base of absorptive cells at the villous tips, membrane-bound lipid droplets have been noted. The droplets have a trilaminar unit structure. Lymphatics have revealed a prominent basal lamina of flattened endothelial cells. There have been no open gaps, as well as altered tight cell junctions, noted in this condition, while in normals there are open gaps at cell junctions. (14, 15) Adjacent to endothelial nuclei are a large number of fibrils. Cellular components of the lamina propria appear normal. (14)

9. (A,D) Treatment of these patients is somewhat difficult. Diuretics are usually ineffective or only transiently effective. Medium-chain fatty acids (MCT), C6 to C10 length, may be quite effective in returning total serum proteins to normal and in causing edema to disappear. MCT are absorbed directly into the portal venous system rather than by the intestinal lacteals. This causes a reduction in lymphatic flow and diminishes the protein-rich lymph loss into the intestinal lumen. Thus, MCT are substituted for long-chain triglcerides (LCT), e.g., MCT oil or as part of elemental formulas/liquids, such as Vivonex®, Precision Isotonic®. Water-soluble vitamins and calcium supplements are necessary if levels are excessively low. For infections, antibiotics are used. (16-18)

If the involved segment is localized, surgical resection can be performed. Surgical treatment for more extensive lesions has been generally unsatisfactory, for example, peritoneal anastomosis of a saphenous vein. (5,7) Refer to answer 10.

10. (F) Relapses and remissions may occur in this condition. The previously mentioned dietary changes can bring about dramatic results in some cases, while in other cases, MCT seem to have little or no effect in changing the course. As previously mentioned, surgical treatment may or may not be "curative." (5-7) Furthermore, none of the laboratory, radiological, or morphological findings can predict those patients who will or will not respond to treatment, or the type of treatment to use.

REFERENCES

1. Herskovic, T., Winawer, S.J., Goldsmith, R., et al.: Hypoproteinemia in intestinal lymphangiectasia. Pediatrics 40:345, 1967.

2. Shimkin, P.M., Waldmann, T.A., Krugman, R.L.: Intestinal lymphangiectasia. Am J Roentgenol Rad Ther Nucl Med 110:827, 1970.

3. Strober, W., Wochner, R.D., Carbone, P.P., et al.: Intestinal lymphangiectasia: A protein-losing enteropathy with hypogammaglobulinemia, lymphocytopenia and impaired homograft rejection. J Clin Invest 46:1643, 1967.

4. Mistilis, S.P., Skyring, A.P., Stephen, D.D.: Intestinal lymphangiectasia: Mechanism of enteric loss of plasma-protein and fat. Lancet 1:77, 1965.

5. Schussheim, A.: Protein-losing enteropathies in children. Am J Gastroenterol 58:124, 1972.

6. Vardy, P.M., Lebenthal, E., Schuachman, H.: Intestinal lymphangiectasia. Pediatrics 55:842, 1975.

7. Nugent, F.W., Ross, J.R., Huexthal, L.M.: Intestinal lymphangiectasia. Gastroenterology 47:536, 1964.

8. McGuigan, J.E., Purkerson, M.L., Trudeau, W.L., et al.: Studies of immunologic defects associated with intestinal lymphangiectasia. With some observations on dietary control of chylous ascites. Ann Int Med 68:398, 1968.

9. Waldman, T.A.: Protein-losing enteropathy. Progress in gastroenterology. Gastroenterology 50:422, 1966.

10. Jarnum, S.: The ^{131}I-polyvinylpyrrolidine (^{131}I-PVP) test in gastrointestinal protein loss. Scand J Clin Lab Invest 13:447, 1961.

11. Waldmann, T.A.: Gastrointestinal protein loss demonstrated by [51] α-labelled albumin. Lancet 2:121, 1961.

12. Kerr, R.M., Dubois, J.J., Holt, P.: Use of ^{125}I and ^{51}Cr-labeled albumin for the measurement of gastrointestinal and total albumin catabolism. J Clin Invest 46:2064, 1967.

13. Bernier, J.J., Desmazures, C.H., Florent, C.H., et al.: Diagnosis of protein-losing enteropathy by gastrointestinal clearance of alpha-1-antitrypsin. Lancet 2: 1978.

14. Dobbins, W.O., III: Electron microscopic study of the intestinal mucosa in intestinal lymphangiectasia. Gastroenterology 51:1004, 1966.

15. Bujanover, Y., Liebman, W.M., Goodman, J.R., et al.: Primary intestinal lymphangiectasia: A radiological and ultrastructural study. Digestion 21:107, 1981.

16. Jeffries, G.H., Chapman, A., Sleisenger, M.H.: Low-fat diet in intestinal lymphangiectasia: Its effect on albumin metabolism. N Engl J Med 270:761, 1964.

17. Holt, P.: Dietary treatment of protein loss in intestinal lymphangiectasia. Pediatrics 34:629, 1964.

18. Gracey, M., Burke, V., Anderson, C.M.: Medium-chain triglycerides in pediatric practice. Arch Dis Child 45:445, 1970.

Case 27

RECURRENT ABDOMINAL PAIN IN A 17-YEAR-OLD BOY

HISTORY

A 17-year-old white male presented with a history of recurrent abdominal pain of 4-5 weeks' duration, initially generalized in location, now predominantly localized to the right lower quadrant. The pain would occur about 20 minutes after meals, could recur during the same day, and lasted 1/2 to 2 hours. On occasions, the pain would occur before meals. The pain was not associated with position, time of day, food types, and/or bowel movements. There was infrequent associated nausea, but no history of fever, vomiting, constipation, melena, hematochezia, skin lesions, ocular difficulty, or anorexia. The family history included a maternal aunt with peptic ulcer disease.

Medication included Donnatal tablets without apparent effect. The developmental history, family, social history, and review of systems were unremarkable.

EXAMINATION

He was alert, cooperative, active, and in no apparent distress, with normal vital signs. Height was 173 cm, weight 62.5 kg. The remainder of the examination was rather unremarkable except for mild tenderness in the right lower quadrant of the abdomen, without rebound tenderness, distention, masses, or palpable liver, spleen, and kidneys. Active bowel sounds were present with no bruits.

LABORATORY DATA

Hemoglobin:	13.0 gm%
Hematocrit:	40%
White blood cell count:	13,100/mm^3
PMN's:	72%
lymphocytes:	20%
monocytes:	7%
eosinophiles:	1%
Sedimentation rate:	23 mm/hr
Urinalysis:	negative
Urine amylase:	2,800 units
Serum:	
SGPT:	21 units
alkaline phosphatase:	145 IU
carotene:	120 μg%
folate:	16 ng/ml
total protein:	6.9 gm%
albumin:	4.4 gm%
amylase:	110 units
ANA:	negative
Stool:	
hemoccult:	negative
reducing substances:	negative
culture:	negative
ova and parasites:	negative
Barium enema:	negative
Upper GI - small bowel series:	negative

QUESTIONS

1. The most likely diagnosis in this patient is which of the following?
   A. Regional enteritis
   B. Ulcerative colitis
   C. Amebic colitis
   D. Yersinia infection
   E. Acute appendicitis

Question 2: Answer true (T) or false (F).

2. This disorder is rare in children less than 5 years of age.

3. The responsible agent can be characterized as which one of the following?
   A. Anaerobic, nonhemolytic, gram-positive rod
   B. Aerobic, hemolytic, gram-positive coccus
   C. Aerobic, hemolytic, gram-negative rod
   D. Anaerobic, nonhemolytic, gram-negative rod
   E. Aerobic, nonhemolytic, gram-negative rod

4. In older children, the condition may include which of the following?
   A. Persistent abdominal pain and fever
   B. Acute diarrhea
   C. Peripheral edema
   D. Recurrent diarrhea
   E. Acute right lower quadrant pain

5. Clinicopathologic findings may include which of the following?
   A. Mesenteric lymphadenitis
   B. Appendicitis, with or without ulcerations
   C. Terminal ileitis
   D. Edematous pancreatitis
   E. Diffuse esophagitis

6. Diagnosis can be made by which of the following studies?
   A. Stool cultures, including special media
   B. Serology (agglutinins)
   C. Histology of lymph node(s)
   D. Serum orosomucoid concentration
   E. Immunoelectrophoresis

7. Treatment of this condition includes which of the following?
   A. Chloramphenicol
   B. Nystatin
   C. Metronidazole
   D. Ampicillin
   E. Tetracycline

8. Complications of this disease include which of the following?
   A. Anterior uveitis
   B. Arthritis
   C. Myocarditis
   D. Spondylitis
   E. Erythema nodosum

ANSWERS AND COMMENTS

1. (D) Yersinia infection is the probable diagnosis. The clinical pattern and course, as well as the negative stool examinations for ova and parasites, barium enema, and small bowel series, would make the other choices less likely. (1-5)

2. (F) In most series, the majority of infections with Y. enterocolitica occur in the first 3 to 5 years of life. (1-4) Over 80% of Yersinia strains in laboratories have been isolated from the stools of children less than 10 years of age. (1-4)

3. (E) Yersinia enterocolitica is a nonhemolytic, aerobically growing, gram-negative rod, which resembles nonlactose fermenting Escherichia coli. It was formerly called Pasteurella X, Pasteurella pseudotuberculosis, and Bacterium enterocoliticum. (1-4) There are 34 serotypes of Y. enterocolitica and 5 serotypes of Y. pseudotuberculosis. The latter has been associated with an acute, appendicitis-like illness, diarrhea, sepis, and erythema nodosum. (5) Transmission can occur by food, water, infected persons, and pets. (1-5)

4. (A,B,D,E) This organism produces variable clinical symptomatology. The probable incubation period is 7 to 10 days. (1-4) The clinical picture can be that of (1) acute gastroenteritis, including diarrhea, with or without fever, vomiting, and variable dehydration; (2) blood in stools (20-25%), recurrent or chronic diarrhea; (3) persistent abdominal pain in any location with or without fever, vomiting, anorexia, weight loss; (4) acute right lower quadrant pain with or without fever, vomiting, anorexia, and (5) asymptomatic carriers (5-15%). (1-8)

5. (A,B,C) The gross and microscopic gastrointestinal pathological findings have included (1) terminal ileitis (acute, chronic) almost always without granulomas and with or without ulceration(s), usually superficial; (2) acute, subacute appendicitis with or without variably sized ulceration(s); (3) mesenteric lymphadenitis (acute, chronic), frequently with large pyroninophilic cells; (4) diffuse gastroenteritis (acute), with or without ulcerations, mucosal necrosis, pseudomembrane formation; (5) colitis (acute, chronic), right-sided especially, with or without associated enteritis, usually without ulceration. (1,3,8)

6. (A,B) The stool specimens usually contain many white blood cells (polys) and red blood cells (RBC). Routine screening of stool specimens for Y. enterocolitica have generally revealed a low rate of so-called asymptomatic carriers. (1,2,6)

The organism can be identified by conventional culture methodology. However, it is slow-growing, easily overlooked, and its identification can be facilitated by notifying laboratory personnel of its possible presence. Thus, prolonged incubation at 30°C on routine media or culturing on special media will augment its recognition. (1,2,8-9) Serological techniques have provided additional identification. The principal quantitation has been that of agglutination titers (agglutinins), against various serotypes (O-antigen, OH-antigen). A serological diagnosis, however, requires examination of specimens during the illness and 10 to 14 days later. (10)

Although lymph node (mesenteric especially) histology may disclose significant abnormalities, such as large pyroninophilic cells, diffuse hyperplasia, inflammatory reaction, germinal center activity, and interfollicular pulp mitoses, these changes are not specific and are at best "suggestive." (1,2,8,11) However, Yersinia itself may be identified in the lymph nodes.

Serum orosomucoid concentrations (lysozyme) may be helpful in determining infection in general or activity of disease. However, elevated levels have been found in a number of conditions, such as Yersinia infections and Crohn's disease. The magnitude of elevation is not specific, either.

Immunoelectrophoresis or quantitative immunoglobulin determinations also are nonspecific. Moreover, the results are usually normal. Tests of cell-mediated immunity are usually normal, too, except in cases with complications, such as peritonitis. (4,5) Standard laboratory studies, such as complete blood count, sedimentation rate, total protein and albumin levels, are frequently normal or nonspecifically abnormal.

7. (A,E) Most cases are usually self-limited and therefore do not require antibiotic treatment. Yersinia is usually sensitive to aminoglycosides, tetracycline, and chloramphenicol. The dosage of tetracycline is 20-40 mg/kg/day for 10 to 14 days, and of chloramphenicol, 25-50 mg/kg/day for 10 to 14 days. Clinical symptomatology usually disappears within 2 to 4 weeks. (5,15)

8. (B,C,E) As previously mentioned, the infection is usually self-limited, lasting 1-2 weeks. However, recurrent chronic diarrhea may occur and last several months or longer. Myocarditis, arthritis, erythema nodosum, severe gastrointestinal hemorrhage, and perforation with peritonitis have all been associated with Yersinia infections of the gastrointestinal tract. (1-8,12-15) These complications have been rare, however.

REFERENCES

1. Mollaret, H.H.: L'inflection humaine a "Yersinia entero-
    colitica." Pathol Biol 14:981, 1966.

2. Winblad, S., Nilehn, B., Sternby, N.J.: Yersinia enter-
    ocolitica (Pasteurella X) in human enteric infections. Br
    Med J 2:1363, 1966.

3. Bradford, W.D., Noce, P.S., Gutman, L.T.: Pathologic
    features of enteric infection with Yersinia enterocolitica.
    Arch Pathol 98:17, 1974.

4. DeLorme, J., Laverdiere, M., Martineau, B., et al.:
    Yersiniosis in children. Can Med Assoc J 110:281, 1972.

5. Report of the Committee on Infectious Diseases, American
    Academy of Pediatrics, 19th edition, Evanston, Illinois,
    1982, p. 288.

6. Marks, M.I., Pai, C.H., Lafleur, L., et al.: Yersinia
    enterocolitica gastroenteritis: A prospective study of clin-
    ical, bacteriologic, and epidemiologic features. J Pedi-
    atr 96:26, 1980.

7. Gurry, J.F.: Acute terminal ileitis and Yersinia infection.
    Br Med J 2:264, 1974.

8. Nilehn, B. and Sjostrom, B.: Studies on Yersinia entero-
    colitica. Occurrence in various groups of acute abdominal
    disease. Arch Pathol Microbiol Scand 71:612, 1967.

9. Doraiswamy, N.V., Currie, A.B.M., Gray, J., et al.:
    Terminal ileitis: Yersinia enterocolitica isolated from
    faeces. Br Med J 1:23, 1977.

10. Winblad, S.: Studies on serological typing of Yersinia en-
    terocolitica. Acta Pathol Microbiol Scand (suppl) 187:115,
    1967.

11. Jansson, E., Wallgren, G.R., Ahvonen, P.: Yersinia
    enterocolitica as a cause of acute mesenteric lymphaden-
    itis. Acta Paediat Scand 57:448, 1968.

12. Ahronen, P., Sievers, K., Aho, L.: Arthritis associated
    with Yersinia enterocolitica infection. Acta Rheum Scand
    15:232, 1969.

13. Winblad, S.: Erythema nodosum associated with infection with Yersinia enterocolitica. Scand J Infect Dis 1:11, 1969.

14. Nilehn, B.: Studies on Yersinia enterocolitica with special reference to bacterial diagnosis and occurrence in human acute enteric disease. Acta Pathol Microbiol Scand (suppl) 206:177, 1969.

15. Van Trappen, G., Ponette, E., Geboes, K., et al.: Yersinia enteritis and enterocolitis. Gastroenterology 72:220, 1977.

Case 28

RECURRENT ABDOMINAL PAIN, ABDOMINAL DISTENTION, NAUSEA, AND VOMITING IN A 10-YEAR-OLD GIRL

HISTORY

A 10-year-old white female presented with a history of recurrent abdominal pain, associated abdominal protuberance, and nausea with vomiting, usually bilious in type, of 16 months' duration. The pain was generally sudden in onset, lasting hours or longer, midabdominal and epigastric in location, unrelated to meals, food types, time of day, position, and/or bowel movements. With the onset of the abdominal pain, protuberance also occurred. In addition, the patient's appetite and activity would be decreased during these episodes. Four such episodes had occurred during this 16-month period. There was no associated history of fever, diarrhea, definite constipation, melena, hematochezia, jaundice, skin lesions, and/or trauma. Patient's bowel habit pattern was generally once daily, firm to soft in nature. Her prior appetite, activity, and development had been within normal limits. Family history included a father with a history of peptic ulcer disease. Otherwise, the remainder of the family history, social history, and review of systems was unremarkable.

EXAMINATION

She was alert and in moderate abdominal distress, pulse 110 per minute, respiration 30 per minute and nonlabored, oral temperature 37.5°C, height 135 cm, weight 32 kg. The remainder of the examination was unremarkable except for moderate abdominal distention without masses, shifting dullness, fluid wave, or palpable liver, spleen, and kidneys. The abdominal distention seemed to be generalized in nature. There was associated mild tenderness to direct palpation but no rebound tenderness. Increased bowel sounds were present with no bruits.

LABORATORY DATA

Hemoglobin:	11.9 gm%
Hematocrit:	36%
White blood cell count:	11,300/mm^3
PMN's:	58%
lymphocytes:	34%
monocytes:	4%
eosinophiles:	4%
Sedimentation rate:	24 mm/hr
Urinalysis:	negative
Urine amylase:	3,400 units/24 hr
Serum:	
sodium:	138 meq/L
potassium:	4.2 meq/L
chloride:	102 meq/L
bicarbonate:	24 meq/L
creatinine:	0.6 mg%
total bilirubin:	0.5 mg%
direct bilirubin:	0.4 mg%
SGOT:	21 KU
alkaline phosphatase:	140 IU
amylase:	111 units
Esophageal manometry:	mean LES pressure 13 mmHg normal relaxation no definite primary peristaltic contractions in body of esophagus

QUESTIONS

1. In general, the condition in this patient is characterized by which of the following?
   A. Episodes of apparent intestinal obstruction
   B. Episodes of hematemesis
   C. Malabsorption
   D. Jaundice
   E. Constipation

2. Which organs may be affected by this condition?
   A. Esophagus
   B. Stomach
   C. Small intestine
   D. Colon
   E. Liver

3. Typical clinical features in this condition include which of the following?
   A. Constipation
   B. Diarrhea
   C. Abdominal pain
   D. Melena
   E. Hyperphagia

4. Radiological features of this condition include which of the following?
   A. Increased intestinal mucosal fold thickness
   B. Stenosis of small intestine, particularly the distal ileum
   C. Dilation of small intestine
   D. Delayed intestinal transit time
   E. Increased intestinal transit time

5. Motility studies of the gastrointestinal tract may reveal which of the following?
   A. Lack of contractile activity in the body of the esophagus
   B. Insensitivity of the body of the esophagus to cholinergic stimulants
   C. Elevation of lower esophageal sphincter pressure
   D. Lack of contractile activity of segments of small intestine at rest
   E. All of the above

6. Histological examination of the small intestine usually reveals which of the following?
   A. Villous shortening
   B. Cellular infiltration of the lamina propria
   C. Elongated crypts
   D. Lacteal dilation
   E. Normal architecture

7. Management of this condition includes which of the following?
   A. Nasogastric or small intestinal intubation suction
   B. Cholinergic medication, e.g., Bethanechol
   C. Antibiotics
   D. Intravenous hyperalimentation
   E. Surgical resection

Question 8: Answer true (T) or false (F).

8. The prognosis in this condition is excellent with few or no recurrences or progression.

ANSWERS AND COMMENTS

1. (A, C, D) The apparent disorder in this patient is chronic, idiopathic intestinal pseudo-obstruction (IIP). IIP describes a syndrome characterized by recurrent symptomatology of mechanical intestinal obstruction without evidence of a mechanical obstruction lesion. (1-5) In addition, this distinct entity may have episodes of malabsorption, malnutrition, and/or constipation/obstipation over the years. (1-5) Most cases become symptomatic during the first decade of life. (1-6)

2. (A, B, C, D) IIP more typically involves the esophagus, small intestine, and colon. (1-5) The esophageal involvement may actually mimic achalasia. Involvement of the stomach has been recently reported and described in some detail. Refer to answer 5. However, the stomach is usually spared; the small intestine is more often affected than the large intestine. (6, 7)

3. (A, B, C) The common clinical features consist of constipation or obstipation, abdominal pain, predominantly colicky or crampy, nausea and/or vomiting, variable appetite, even anorexia, and diarrhea. The diarrhea is probably secondary to small intestinal stasis and subsequent bacterial overgrowth. (4, 5) The growth pattern is also affected, the height and weight demonstrating a rapid and significant slowing or even a plateau effect.

4. (C, D) The radiological features more commonly seen include (1) lack of peristalsis in the distal half to two-thirds of the esophagus; (2) significant dilation of the small intestine, the duodenum and jejunum in particular, the distal half of the ileum frequently being spared; (3) hypomotility of the small intestine in general; (4) delayed transit time, commonly 12 to 24 hours or longer; (5) significant colonic dilation. (1-5)

In addition, gastroesophageal reflux may be present, and, not infrequently, a stricture of the distal esophagus may be detected after several years. (1-5)

5. (A, B, C) More recent studies of mechanical and electrical activity of the gastrointestinal tract have provided some answers as to the functional defect(s) resulting in the clinical pattern of

this interesting, yet uncommon disorder. (8-13) Esophageal manometry has revealed normal peristalsis in the upper few centimeters, while the rest of the esophagus demonstrated minimal simultaneous rises in pressure with swallowing. A lack of contractile activity is present in the distal half to two-thirds of the esophagus. (1-5) The lower esophageal sphincter showed normal relaxation, and mean pressure has been within normal limits, i.e., 15 to 30 mmHg. (1-5)

Gastric fundic pressure has recently been measured at rest and after balloon distention. Gastric fundic relaxation was impaired at rest, and there was a more rapid increase in pressure upon distention. (14,15) Contraction waves per se have appeared normal.

Laboratory studies frequently reveal the presence of anemia, hypoalbuminemia, and steatorrhea (fecal fat, 72 hr). (1-7) Small intestinal cultures (aerobic, anaerobic) confirm the presence of bacterial overgrowth (fecal microflora), while breath tests with bile acid or carbohydrate will demonstrate abnormal breath carbon dioxide and hydrogen, respectively. (6,7)

Small intestinal studies have been confined predominantly to the duodenum and jejunum. Resting contractile activity has been noted to be essentially normal. After injections of cholinergic agents, such as Bethanechol (muscarinic) or Edrophonium (anticholinesterase), marked contractile activity occurred. (14, 15) Conversely, electrical activity, principally control waves and response activity ("spikes"), has not been normal at rest; specifically there was reduced and irregular electrical control activity. (14,15) In preliminary studies, if control activity is absent, electrical stimulation will not restore it. (16,17)

Colonic studies have been principally confined to the left colon, particularly sigmoid. (1,2,14-16) Electrical activity, control waves and response activity were present at rest and after drug administration, such as morphine, respectively. (14,15) This suggests that acetylcholine release is present and that colonic muscle can respond accordingly. (14,15)

In addition to the previously mentioned studies, preliminary in vitro work has been performed on muscle strips of the intestine, specifically longitudinal and circular jejunum. (14,15) In comparison to similar muscle strips from normals, only quantitative differences have been noted in comparing the relative effects of transmural stimulation of intrinsic cholinergic and non-adrenergic inhibitory nerves and of drugs, such as acetylcholine, physostigmine, serotonin, catecholamines, and ATP. (14,15) Electrical control activity was absent except during the migration of the myoelectrical complex, characterized by response potentials being superimposed on every control potential, appearing proximally and spreading distally. (14,15) Sarna, et al.,

(14, 15) concluded that hyperpolarization of intestinal smooth muscle may explain this absence of electrical control activity.

6. (E) The lack of histologic abnormalities in peroral biopsies and essentially all autopsy material, in conjunction with the clinical and radiological pattern, is almost diagnostic of this abnormality and important in differentiation from other conditions, such as scleroderma. (14, 16) However, one case has been reported in which the number of axons and neurons in the intestinal wall were reduced, and another case was reported in which smooth muscle degeneration was found in the jejunal wall. (16, 17) In neonates presenting with Hirschsprung's disease-like symptomatology, decrease in argyrophil neurons has been observed. (16-18) In other cases, atrophy and degeneration of smooth muscle has been reported. (16-18)

7. (A, C, D, E) Episodes of intestinal obstruction must be managed by either nasogastric or small intestinal intubation, e.g., Cantor tube and suction. Intravenous fluid therapy is also instituted to maintain or re-establish fluid and electrolyte balance. Intravenous (peripheral, central) hyperalimentation is used to correct significant malnutrition and provide more extensive "intestinal rest." (1-5, 14, 17) A home program of total parenteral nutrition (TPN) has become a reality. (18)

Treatment of bacterial overgrowth secondary to small intestinal stasis will improve the malabsorption syndrome but not the pseudo-obstructive phenomena. Broad-spectrum antibiotics, such as tetracycline, are used for this purpose. Obviously, their effect lasts only as long as the treatment does. Cholestyramine has not been evaluated.

Small intestinal resection has been used frequently in this condition when absolutely necessary. Unfortunately, this treatment does not prevent recurrences and, in addition, adds further problems, specifically shortening of the small intestine of variable extent with resultant absorptive deficits and nutritive consequences. (1-5, 17)

Cholinergic therapy has generally been of no value. Recently, temporary, partial improvement with subcutaneous neostigmine was reported. (14) However, most authors do not suggest cholinergic use.

Finally, the use of stimulants, such as prostaglandins, specifically the F group (F2a), may be a future hope. These could produce electrical control and response activity, although not of normal quality. (19) Whether this will be effective in small intestinal transit remains for future studies.

234 / Case 28

8. (F) This is a progressive condition. Prolonged remissions
have been noted, but with time, episodes of intestinal obstruction and resultant malabsorption become more frequent and severe. Ultimately, an early demise is to be expected. The long-
est reported survival has been only 34 years. (1-5,16,17)

REFERENCES

1. Maldonado, J.E., Gregg, J.A., Green, P.A.: Chronic
   idiopathic intestinal pseudo-obstruction. Am J Med 49:
   203, 1970.

2. Moss, A.A., Goldberg, H.I., Brotman, M.: Idiopathic
   intestinal pseudo-obstruction. Am J Roentgenol Radium
   Ther Nucl Med 115:312, 1972.

3. Schuffler, M.D. and Pope, E.I., II.: Esophageal motor
   dysfunction in idiopathic intestinal pseudo-obstruction.
   Gastroenterology 70:677, 1966.

4. Pearson, A.J., Brzechwa-Ajdukiewicz, A., McCarthy,
   C.F.: Intestinal pseudo-obstruction with bacterial overgrowth in the small intestine. Am J Dig Dis 12:200, 1969.

5. Naish, J.M., Capper, W.M., Brown, N.J.: Intestinal
   pseudo-obstruction with steatorrhea. Gut 1:62, 1960.

6. Anuras, S., Christensen, J.: Recurrent or chronic intestinal pseudo-obstruction. Clin Gastroenterol 10:177, 1981.

7. Hanks, J.B., Meyers, W.C., Andersen, D.K., et al.:
   Chronic primary intestinal pseudo-obstruction. Surgery
   89:175, 1981.

8. Duthie, H.L.: Electrical activity of gastrointestinal
   smooth muscle. Gut 15:669, 1974.

9. Bennett, A., and Stockley, H.L.: The intrinsic innervation of the human alimentary tract and its relation to function. Gut 16:433, 1975.

10. Sarna, S.K. and Daniel, E.E.: Electrical stimulation of
    small intestinal electrical control activity. Gastroenter-
    ology 69:660, 1975.

11. Carlson, G.M., Bedi, B.S., Code, C.F.: Mechanism of propagation of intestinal interdigestive myoelectric complex. Am J Physiol 222:1027, 1972.

12. Sarna, S.K., Daniel, E.E., Waterfall, W.E.: Myogenic and neural control systems for esophageal motility. Gastroenterology 73:1345, 1977.

13. Sujmers, R.W., Helm, J., Christensen, J.: Intestinal propulsion in dog: Its relation to food intake and the migratory myoelectric complex. Gastroenterology 70:753, 1976.

14. Lewis, T.D., Daniel, E.E., Sarna, S.K., et al.: Idiopathic intestinal pseudo-obstruction. Report of a case with intraluminal studies of mechanical and electrical activity, and response to drugs. Gastroenterology 74:107, 1978.

15. Sarna, S.K., Daniel, E.E., Waterfall, W.E., et al.: Postoperative gastrointestinal electrical and mechanical activities in a patient with idiopathic intestinal pseudo-obstruction. Gastroenterology 74:112, 1978.

16. Schuffler, M.C., Pope, C.E., II., Lowe, M.C., et al.: Idiopathic intestinal pseudo-obstruction in a 15-year-old girl: Pathologic and family studies. Gastroenterology 70: 935, 1976.

17. Philippon, E. and Goujon, G.: Pseudo—obstruction intestinale chronique idiopathique. Arch Fr Mal App Dig 61: 145, 1972.

18. Silverman, A., Roy, C.C.: Pediatric Clinical Gastroenterology, 3rd edition. The CV Mosby Company, St. Louis, 1983, p. 123.

19. Luderer, J.R., Demers, L.M., Bonnem, E.M., et al.: Elevated prostaglandin E in idiopathic intestinal pseudo-obstruction. N Engl J Med 295:1179, 1976.

Case 29

RIGHT LOWER QUADRANT PAIN, WEIGHT LOSS, AND FEVER IN A 14-1/2-YEAR-OLD BOY

HISTORY

A 14-1/2-year-old white male presented with a history of recurrent abdominal pain, right lower quadrant in location, of almost 3 months' duration. There was no radiation of the pain from the right lower quadrant. It occurred almost daily, without relationship to meals, food types, time of day, or position. The patient denied a relationship of the pain with bowel movements. Bowel movements were 1 or 2 daily, brown in color and firm in consistency. There was associated fever almost daily, weight loss of over 14 lbs, occasional nausea and vomiting, but no history of diarrhea, hematochezia, melena, skin lesions, arthralgia, jaundice, ocular difficulty, hematemesis, or dysuria. The patient's activity and appetite had decreased during this period of time. Medication had included Tylenol for the fever, Vibramycin (a tetracycline), ferrous sulfate, and vitamins without apparent effect. Pertinent prior history included a maternal first cousin with similar clinical course approximately 2 weeks prior to the onset of the patient's history but resolving within 2 to 3 weeks. The remainder of the past history, family history, developmental history, social history, and review of systems was unremarkable.

EXAMINATION

He was alert, thin, slightly pale, and in no apparent distress, with normal vital signs including temperature, weight 42.8 kg and height 159 cm. The remainder of the examination was unremarkable except for mild tenderness to palpation in the right lower quadrant of the abdomen, without rebound tenderness, masses, distention or palpable liver, spleen and kidneys.

LABORATORY DATA

Hemoglobin:	9.1 gm%
Hematocrit:	28.8%
White blood cell count:	6,700/mm^3
PMN's:	60%
lymphocytes:	38%
monocytes:	1%
eosinophiles:	1%
Sedimentation rate:	61 mm/hr
Urinalysis:	negative
Serum:	
SGOT:	19 units
SGPT:	20 units
total bilirubin:	0.9 mg%
direct bilirubin:	0.6 mg%
total protein:	5.9 gm%
albumin:	3.1 gm%
carotene:	90 μg%
folate:	8 ng/ml
vitamin B$_{12}$:	420 ng/ml
iron:	110 μg%
iron-binding capacity:	300%
calcium:	8.9 mg%
phosphorus:	2.8 mg%
cholesterol:	170 mg%
glucose:	84 mg%
creatinine:	0.6 mg%
PBI:	5.6 μg%
IgG:	1,420 mg%
IgA:	109 mg%
IgM:	10 mg%
ANA:	negative
Schilling test:	
without intrinsic factor:	1.9%
with intrinsic factor:	2.0%
Proctosigmoidoscopy:	normal findings
rectal biopsy:	normal findings
Stool:	
culture:	negative
ova and parasites:	negative
hemoccult:	negative
Barium enema:	negative except for minimal irregularity of the terminal ileum
Upper GI - small bowel series:	(Fig. 29.1)

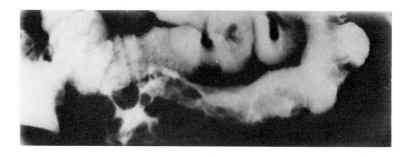

Figure 29.1   Barium swallow. Mucosal thickening with cobblestone appearance is shown in the terminal ileum.

QUESTIONS

1.   The most likely diagnosis is:
     A. duodenal ulcer
     B. acute pancreatitis
     C. regional enteritis
     D. amebiasis
     E. ulcerative colitis

2.   Which age group (years) in children is most commonly af-
     fected by this condition?
     A. 0-1
     B. 1-2
     C. 2-5
     D. 5-10
     E. 10-15

3.   Which of the following are implicated most commonly in the
     etiology of this disease?
     A. Autonomic imbalance
     B. Vascular insufficiency
     C. Infection (transmissible agent)
     D. Immunological dysfunction
     E. Psychosomatic factors

4. The predominant symptom of this condition is
   A. fever
   B. nausea, vomiting
   C. abdominal pain
   D. rectal bleeding
   E. weight loss

5. In this case, distal small intestinal involvement only, the
   differential diagnosis includes
   A. eosinophilic enteritis
   B. Y. enterocolitica
   C. M. tuberculae
   D. E. histolytica
   E. lymphoma

6. Characteristic microscopic features of this condition include
   A. disruption of superficial epithelium
   B. eosinophilic infiltration of lamina propria
   C. absence of ganglion cells
   D. noncaseating granuloma
   E. ulceration extending into submucosa

7. Usual uncomplicated treatment of this condition may consist
   of which of the following?
   A. Cimetidine
   B. Salicylazosulfapyridine (Azulfidine)
   C. Corticosteroids
   D. Azathioprine
   E. Surgery

8. Associated complications in Crohn's disease include
   A. obstruction (intestinal)
   B. massive hemorrhage
   C. arthritis (migratory)
   D. duodenal ulceration
   E. growth retardation

9. Prognosis of Crohn's disease is characterized by
   A. high incidence of cure (disease resolution)
   B. high incidence of progression of disease
   C. cancer risk greater than ulcerative colitis
   D. cancer risk less than ulcerative colitis
   E. postsurgical recurrence

ANSWERS AND COMMENTS

1. (C) The most likely diagnosis is regional enteritis because of a compatible history (abdominal pain, low-grade fever, diarrhea), negative proctoscopy, positive rectal biopsy (granuloma), abnormal terminal ileum noted on the small bowel series, negative barium enema examination, and negative stool examinations for ova and parasites. Thus, the diagnoses of duodenal ulcer (A), amebiasis (D), and ulcerative colitis (E) have been effectively eliminated. Although the chest radiograph and tuberculin skin test were negative, intestinal tuberculosis cannot be eliminated. However, the clinical course makes it less likely.

2. (E) Twenty to thirty years ago, Crohn's disease was thought to be confined to the distal small intestine. Today, Crohn's disease is accepted as potentially involving the digestive tract from the oral cavity to the anus. However, the ileocecal area is still the most frequently involved segment, 60-85%. (1-9) Recently, Bergman and Krause (10) in Sweden, reported an incidence of 5 new cases per 100,000 population, while Brahme, et al. (11) reported an incidence of 6 per 100,000. Most studies have reported a peak age distribution of 15 to 25 years (ileum and colon). (1-11) In the pediatric population, the most common age group affected is 10 to 15 years. (1-12) Twenty percent of the cases are within the pediatric population. (2,4,9,10,12) Annual incidence rates of Crohn's disease have included 3 to 4.0 per 100,000. (12,13) The earlier the onset, the more severe is the disease's course.

Fluctuation in incidence is not only present between countries, but also between regions within countries. (1,2,6,10,11) Increased incidence is present among Jews and whites versus nonwhites. In addition, familial involvement, including monozygotic twins, has been reported. (1,6) In the United States, the average annual incidence has varied between 0.8 to 3.1 per 100,000. (1,6)

3. (C,D) The precise etiology of Crohn's disease remains unknown. A number of theories have been proposed in order to explain this granulomatous reaction. Two, in particular, have been prominently mentioned: (1) infectious (transmissible) agent, and (2) immunological dysfunction.

With reference to an infectious agent, the histologic similarity between Crohn's disease and tuberculosis spurred interest in finding this and/or other agents. (1,6,12) Direct culture of intestinal tissue for bacterial agents, as well as serological studies and subsequent animal inoculation studies, were and have repeatedly been negative. (1,4,6) However, fecal coliform counts, antibody titers to colon microorganisms, and electron microscopic identification of intramural bacteria have been reported. (1,3,4,6) The separation of primary etiology versus secondary phenomena due to stasis and/or disrupted epithelial barrier was and is not possible. Investigation for possible fungi or parasites has also been unrewarding. Recently, transmission to experimental animals and virological correlation have resulted in extensive investigation of potential agents. In both mice and rabbits, transmission studies have suggested that Crohn's disease is associated with a transmissible agent, less than 220 nm in diameter. (14) In addition, in tissues of such patients, a viral agent, small and RNA in type, has been isolated. Further studies are being pursued to relate human and experimental animal models.

Abnormal bacterial agents have not been routinely identified, although cell wall-defective forms of pseudomonas (L-forms) and clostridium difficile have been implicated. Unfortunately, consistent findings have not been confirmed. (12,14) Recent bacteriological investigation has focused on normal bacterial flora. (17) In addition, as previously mentioned, viral agents may play an important role. (1,9) Positive Kveim reactions have also been reported in Crohn's disease. The potential link between sarcoidosis and Crohn's disease is under continued investigation. (1,6,9) An abnormal immunological reaction (local or generalized) to such agents remains a possibility.

As with ulcerative colitis, current views of the immunological role in Crohn's disease center on (1) abnormal response to an infectious agent, (2) allergic reaction to an exogenous antigen, and (3) autoimmune phenomenon. (1,9,15,16)

In Crohn's disease, dietary antibodies, e.g., cow's milk, have been uncommonly detected. (13) Skin testing with purified antigens has also been unrewarding. (1,9,15) Peripheral and/or tissue eosinophilia have not been identified. (1,2,9) Serum IgE levels have not been informative, either. (1,2,15) Specific IgE antibodies to dietary antigens (allergens), e.g., radioallergosorbent test (RAST) studies, have not been adequately evaluated. However, interest continues due to recent reports of the efficacy of cromolyn sodium (immediate hypersensitivity effect). (12,18) The association of autoimmune disorders with Crohn's disease has been infrequently reported. (9,15,16) In as many as 25% of patients, antibody reacting with reticulin has been demonstrated.

Serum immunoglobulin levels have not shown consistent abnormalities compared to normals, except for a statistically increased incidence of secretory IgA. (9,15,16) Increased catabolism of IgM has been reported, too. Serum complement levels, particularly total hemolytic complement, C_3 or C_4, have not produced consistent results as an index of an immune complex process. Small immune complexes of IgG have been clinically correlated with disease activity in some cases, however. (20) Finally, circulating complexes may be involved in the extraintestinal manifestations, but further studies to demonstrate these complexes and/or complement in the involved tissues remain to be accomplished.

Cell-mediated immunity has also been extensively studied. In controlled studies, consistent evidence of either anergy or the presence of normal delayed hypersensitivity to dinitro chlorobenzene (DNCB) has been found. Conflicting results have been reported in lymphocyte transformation studies in response to plant mitogens, such as phytohemagglutinin (PHA), concanavalin A (Con A), and pokeweed. (19) Most have shown normal response, while a few have demonstrated reduced responsiveness. (15,18)

The response in a mixed lymphocyte reaction has been normal or reduced. (9,15) The number of T and B cells has been reported as normal or reduced. (13,19) Using antigens from feces and intestinal mucosa, for example, in vitro leukocyte migration inhibition and/or lymphocyte transformation, has been found to be normal or abnormal in comparison to controls. (18) Korsmeyer, et al. (21) have reported lymphocytotoxic activity in sera of Crohn's disease patients, more for normal lymphocytes than for those of patients with inflammatory bowel disease. Strickland, et al. (22) then demonstrated a cold reactive lymphocytotoxin, responsible for this cytotoxicity. Further correlative studies are needed.

Histocompatibility antigen profiles have been studied. The results have been discouraging, although HLA-B27 and HLA-B8 have been more frequent in occasional reports. (12,18)

Autonomic imbalance (A) and vascular insufficiency (B) have not been primarily implicated in Crohn's disease. Psychosomatic factors (E) have been implicated in disease exacerbation rather than in primary causation.

4. (C) Crampy abdominal pain is the predominant symptom in Crohn's disease. (1,2,6,8,9) The pain is usually more severe than in ulcerative colitis. It is usually periumbilical in location, but can frequently be in the right lower quadrant. (1,2,6, 8.9) Defecation may be associated with the pain, producing temporary relief after completion. The pain may be triggered by meals, with no particular association with types of foods (lactose?).

The other answers also are frequently present in Crohn's disease. Looser, more frequent stools are common (45 to 80%). Rectal bleeding is less frequent than in ulcerative colitis (15 to

35%). As in ulcerative colitis, the patient may be awakened from sleep by the urge to defecate, particularly with colonic involvement. Appetite is usually decreased during the active phase of disease. Resultant weight loss occurs, too. Nausea and vomiting also occur during active disease, but less often. Delayed sexual maturation may be present in older patients. Fever occurs in up to 70%. Extraintestinal manifestations occur in many patients, e.g., 1 to 10% (skin) or up to 30 to 35% (joint symptomatology). (1-5,12)

5. (B,C,E) If the inflammatory process involves the small and large intestine, inflammatory bowel disease, particularly Crohn's disease, is rather likely. However, with colonic involvement only, ulcerative colitis, as well as other conditions, such as amebiasis (E. histolytica), must be ruled out. With small intestinal involvement only, other granulomatous conditions must be considered, including tuberculosis, histoplasmosis, sarcoidosis, yersinosis, and, rarely, amebiasis (questionable). Other possibilities include lymphoma, adenocarcinoma, and, lastly, chronic granulomatous disease.

6. (D,E) Macroscopically, the intestinal wall is thickened, and the lumen is narrowed. Longitudinal and transverse ulcerations, deep in nature, may be present. Mucosa between crevices or fissures leads to the cobblestone appearance of the involved intestine. (1-11) The lesions tend to be discontinuous (normal intervening areas), producing so-called skip areas. (1-11) Associated lymph nodes are enlarged, and the mesentery may be thickened. (1-11)

Microscopically, a granulomatous reaction may be present with associated edema and fibrosis of all bowel layers. (1-11, 23) The most suggestive feature is the presence of noncaseating granulomas with multinucleated giant cells and epithelioid cells. (1-11,20,21) These are present in 50% or more of cases. (1-11, 23) Another helpful feature is the presence of ulceration extending into the submucosa and muscularis. Lymphoid elements and inflammation may be present in the submucosa.

7. (B,C,E) The treatment of Crohn's disease, especially during its active phase, embraces many components. Nutritional care is one important aspect of management. Smaller, more frequent meals may be helpful. High-protein content and addition of vitamins, especially fat-soluble and B_{12}, trace metals (elements), iron and folic acid (folate), are necessary. In some cases, an elemental diet may be necessary in order to supply adequate calories, protein, carbohydrate, and fat, as medium-chain triglycerides (MCT), either at regular feeding times or by

continuous tube drip. If obstruction is evident, nasogastric or
intestinal suction will be necessary, and the patient will take
nothing by mouth. During this same time, intravenous therapy
should be administered. In those patients with more significant
malnutrition, hyperalimentation, parenteral or central, may be
quite helpful and necessary in improving the nutritional status
in debilitated patients, as well as in providing "bowel rest."
(24-26) Remission can be induced in as many as 80%. (12-25)
In addition, in some patients, reduced disaccharidase activity
is present, and a lactose-free diet may provide relief. As previously mentioned, MCT may be helpful since some patients
have bile acid and/or hydroxy fatty acid diarrhea due to ileal
involvement. (3,9,23)

Antidiarrheal agents have occasionally been helpful in control of stools, e.g., propantheline bromide (probanthine), loperamide (Imodium). Cholestyramine is indicated and provides
relief in those patients with mild to moderate loss of bile salts
into the colon (4-12 gm/day).

Salicylazosulfapyridine (Azulfidine) has been demonstrated
to be effective in suppressing inflammation, although its precise
mode of action is unknown. Refer to discussion, ulcerative colitis. Usually the initial dose is 1.5 to 2.0 gm daily. In 3 to 5
days, the dosage is increased to 4 to 6 gm/day (loading dose).
After 2 to 3 weeks, the dosage is reduced to maintenance level,
2.0 gm/day. This drug is not likely to be particularly effective
in patients with more extensive bowel involvement. However, it
does seem to be effective in providing and maintaining remission
during the initial active stage and may be effective in preventing
relapses. (1-3,8,9,17)

Corticosteroids also may be necessary in the treatment of
this condition. If illness is severe, intravenous use of corticosteroids, e.g., hydrocortisone, 300 mg/24 hr, should be considered. The alternative use of ACTH, 40-60 mg/12 hr, does
not offer any significant advantage. (24) With satisfactory initial
response, oral therapy, i.e., prednisone, 2 mg/kg, can be initiated and should be continued for 4 to 6 weeks before progressive tapering. Once a daily dosage of 10 mg is achieved, an alternate day regimen can be contemplated, e.g., 20 mg every
other day. Subsequently, prednisone can be tapered and then
discontinued after a satisfactory asymptomatic duration. A significant number will have a relapse and require reinitiation of
steroid therapy. Azulfidine is frequently administered concom-
itantly. Steroid therapy has been effective in achieving remission after the initial active stage but questionably effective in
maintaining remission. (1,3,8,9,27)

In anal involvement, steroid administration can be by retention enema; 15% of the drug is absorbed by this method. The initial dose is 100 mg hydrocortisone twice daily for at least 2 to 3 weeks before reduction to once daily. (1)

Azathioprine (D), an immunosuppressive agent, has been used as primary treatment but in controlled trials has been found to be less effective than either Azulfidine or corticosteroids. (28) However, this drug has permitted a reduction of necessary steroid dosage. (25) The usual dosage has been 2 mg/kg/24 hr. (12, 25, 28) Recently, 6-mercaptopurine (6-MP) 1.5 mg/kg/24 hr, proved effective in patients with colitis and ileocolitis rather than enteritis only. (29) Few studies, however, are available.

Antibiotics, broad-spectrum, e.g., ampicillin, have not been consistently beneficial, although helpful in those patients with stricture and bacterial overgrowth. Metronidazole (Flagyl), 1.0 to 1.5 mg/kg/24 hr, has also been beneficial in some patients, and a recent cooperative study in Sweden demonstrated superior efficacy to sulfasalazine. (12, 30, 31) Further studies are needed.

Cholestyramine, an anion-binding resin, is indicated in patients with more significant bile salt loss into the colon with a secondary choleretic effect (diarrhea). This agent must be gradually instituted, eventually reaching a dose of 4 to 12 gm/24 hr. If stenosis is present, this agent should not be administered.

Surgery is utilized in a different manner than in ulcerative colitis. Some surgeons favor early radical procedures. However, there is a tendency for disease relapse, so intensive medical treatment has been advocated initially. When surgery is indicated, resection must be restricted. Surgery is indicated for patients with severe symptomatology, continued poor health, significant growth retardation, or with complications, such as free perforation, uncontrollable massive bleeding, rarely toxic dilatation, and perianal problems, e.g., fistulization. (1-11, 32-35) As previously mentioned, surgery, i.e., resection, is the procedure of choice. Surgery may be necessary in as many as 70% of patients within 5 to 10 years. (1-5, 12, 32-35) Recurrence after surgery is high, 30 to 70%. (1, 3, 4, 6-9, 32, 35) Conversely, some patients have responded quite favorably, particularly with reference to growth, sexual maturation, and more normalized activity. (1, 3, 4, 6-9, 32-35)

Cimetidine (A) is an H_2-receptor antagonist (gastric acid secretion inhibitor).

8. (A, C, E) Crohn's disease generally follows a chronic pattern, although acute exacerbations are not infrequent. Free

perforation and uncontrolled massive hemorrhage are infrequent. (1-11,20,32-36) More frequent complications, however, include obstruction, intestinal stasis, internal fistulization, e.g., ileosigmoid, and abscess formation. (1-11,20,32-35) Malabsorption can result from the chronic inflammatory process with associated structural alterations. More recently, an increased risk of cancer formation has been reported in both small and large intestinal Crohn's disease, i.e., twentyfold. (35)

Nearly 50 to 80% of patients will have significant growth retardation, weight more commonly than height. (1-11,20,35-38) Delayed sexual maturation is also frequent, i.e., 30 to 50%. (1, 3,6-9,12,36) Conversely, 10 to 20% of patients will have few symptoms and will be "healthy." (1-5,12,36) In addition to these complications, migratory polyarthritis can occur in as many as 25%. Refer to description of ulcerative colitis.

Other complications include oxalate (excessive colonic reabsorption) and uric acid stones, hepatobiliary disease, i.e., pericholangitis, cholelithiasis, and amyloidosis. Skin manifestations occur less commonly than in ulcerative colitis although they are the same in type, e.g., erythema nodosum. Refer to discussion of ulcerative colitis. (1-11,23-32)

9. (B,C,D) Mortality is relatively low, while morbidity is relatively high. (36) In most cases, the disease is progressive and complications are frequent. Poor health is the result. With small intestinal involvement, subsequent colonic involvement is not infrequent. With colonic extension, subsequent small intestinal extension is significantly less common. (1-11,32-39)

As mentioned in answer 8, cancer risk is increased in Crohn's disease but is less common than in ulcerative colitis. (37) Adenocarcinoma is the most common type of cancer in these cases.

As mentioned in answer 7, surgery should be judiciously employed. Postsurgical recurrence is high. (1-11,32,34,35)

For a summarized comparison of ulcerative colitis and Crohn's disease, see Table 29.1.

TABLE 29.1   Inflammatory Bowel Disease

Symptom/Feature	Ulcerative Colitis	Crohn's Disease
pain	less frequent	frequent
rectal bleeding (gross)	frequent	less frequent
diarrhea		
appetite loss	frequent to less frequent	frequent
weight loss	frequent	frequent (more severe than u.c.)
growth retardation	frequent to less frequent	frequent
extraintestinal involvement (hepatic, skin, joints)	frequent	frequent
ileum	infrequent	frequent
colon	frequent	less frequent
rectum	frequent	infrequent
anus	uncommon	infrequent
radiological	symmetrical; distal or universal; superficial ulcerations; haustral loss; no skip areas	asymmetrical; segmental in distribution; right-sided colonic involvement, small intestine; longitudinal fissures, thumb printing; string sign
histological	diffuse mucosal inflammation; crypt abscesses; rarely granulomas (?)	focal transmural inflammation; granulomas frequent

TABLE 29.1 Inflammatory Bowel Disease (Cont'd)

Symptom/Feature	Ulcerative Colitis	Crohn's Disease
treatment response		
Azulfidine/steroids (medical)	frequent	infrequent
surgery	frequent	infrequent to less frequent
prognosis/complications		
remission	frequent	probably infrequent to less frequent
relapse (following medical treatment or surgery)	uncommon to infrequent	less frequent
cancer development	infrequent	uncommon

Key: Frequent = 50% or more; less frequent = 20 to 50%; infrequent = 5 to 20%; uncommon = 5% or less

REFERENCES

1. Ament, M. E.: Inflammatory disease of the colon: Ulcerative colitis and Crohn's colitis. J Pediatr 86:322, 1975.

2. Ehrenpreis, T.H., Gierup, J., Lagercrantz, R.: Chronic regional enterocolitis (Mb Crohn) in children and adolescents. Acta Paediat Scand 60:209, 1971.

3. Grand, R.J. and Homer, D.R.: Approaches to inflammatory bowel disease in childhood and adolescence. Pediat Clin North Am 22:835, 1975.

4. Guttman, F.M.: Granulomatous enterocolitis in childhood and adolescence. J Pediatr Surg 9:115, 1974.

5. Law, D.H.: Regional enteritis. Gastroenterology 56:1086, 1969.

6. Winkelman, E.I.: Regional enteritis in adolescence. Pediatr Clin North Am 14:141, 1967.

7. Shofield, P.F.: Some aspects of Crohn's disease. Dis Colon Rectum 10:262, 1967.

8. Truelove, S.C. and Pena, A.S.: Course and prognosis of Crohn's disease. Gut 17:192, 1976.

9. Daum, E., Boley, S.J., Cohen, M.I.: Inflammatory bowel disease in the adolescent patient. Pediatr Clin North Am 20:933, 1973.

10. Bergman, L. and Krause, U.: The incidence of Crohn's disease in central Sweden. Scand J Gastroenterol 10:725, 1975.

11. Brahme, E., Lindstrom, C., Wenckert, A.: Crohn's disease in a defined population. An epidemiological study of incidence, prevalence, mortality and secular trends in the city of Malmo, Sweden. Gastroenterology 69:342, 1975.

12. Silverman, A., Roy, C.C.: Pediatric Clinical Gastroenterology, 3rd edition. The CV Mosby Company, St. Louis, 1983, pp. 349,370.

13. Mendeloff, A.I.: The epidemiology of inflammatory bowel disease. Clin Gastroenterol 9:259, 1980.

14. Beeken, W.L., Mitchell, D.N., Cove, D.R.: Evidence for a transmissible agent in Crohn's disease. Clin Gastroenterol 5:289, 1976.

15. Whorwell, P.J. and Wright, R.: Immunological aspects of inflammatory bowel disease. Clin Gastroenterol 5:303, 1976.

16. Bolton, P.M., James, S.L., Newcombe, R.G., et al.: The immune competence of patients with inflammatory bowel disease. Gut 15:213, 1974.

17. West, B., Lendrum, R., Hill, M.J., et al.: Effects of
     sulphasalazine (salazopyrin) on focal flora in patients with
     inflammatory bowel disease. Gut 15:960, 1974.

18. Sachar, I.B., Auslander, M.O., Walfish, J.S.: Aetiolog-
     ical theories of inflammatory bowel disease. Clin Gastro-
     enterol 9:231, 1980.

19. Aas, J., Huizenga, K.A., Newcomer, A.D., et al.: In-
     flammatory bowel disease: Lymphocytic responses to non-
     specific stimulation in vitro. Scand J Gastroenterol 7:299,
     1972.

20. Jewell, D.P. and MacLennan, I.C.M.: Immune complexes
     in inflammatory bowel disease. Clin Exp Immunol 14:219,
     1973.

21. Korsmeyer, S., Strickland, R.G., Wilson, I.D., et al.:
     Serum lymphocytotoxic and lymphocytophilic antibody ac-
     tivity in inflammatory bowel disease. Gastroenterology
     67:578, 1974.

22. Strickland, R.G., Friedler, F.M., Henderson, C.A., et
     al.: Serum lymphocytotoxins in inflammatory bowel dis-
     ease: Studies of frequency and specificity for lymphocyte
     subpopulations. Clin Exp Immunol 21:384, 1975.

23. Aluwihare, A.P.R.: The electron microscope and Crohn's
     disease. Clin Gastroenterol 1:279, 1972.

24. Vogel, C.M., Corwin, T.R., Baue, A.E.: Intravenous
     hyperalimentation in the treatment of inflammatory dis-
     eases of the bowel. Arch Surg 108:460, 1974.

25. Gryboski, J., Hillemeier, C.: Inflammatory bowel dis-
     ease in children. Med Clin North Am 64:1185, 1980.

26. Conen, M.I., Boley, S.E., Winslow, P.R., et al.: The
     role of parenteral alimentation in the primary management
     of regional enteritis in children and adolescents. Pediatr
     Res 7:336/108, 1973.

27. Cooke, W.T. and Fielding, J.F.: Corticosteroid or cor-
     ticotrophin therapy in Crohn's disease. Gut 11:921, 1970.

28. Willoughby, J.N.T., Kumar, P.J., Beckett, J., et al.:
     Controlled trial of azathioprine in Crohn's disease. Lancet
     2:944, 1971.

29. Present, D.H., Korelitz, B.I., Wisch, N., et al.: Treatment of Crohn's disease with 6-mercaptopurine. N Engl J Med 302:981, 1980.

30. Ursing, B., Alm, T., Barany, F., et al.: A comparative study of metronidazole and sulfasalazine for active Crohn's disease: The cooperative Crohn's disease study in Sweden. II. Result. Gastroenterology 83:550, 1982.

31. Ursing, B. and Kamme, C.: Metronidazole for Crohn's disease. Lancet 1:775, 1975.

32. DeDombal, F.T., Burton, I.L., Clamp, S.E., et al.: Short-term course and prognosis of Crohn's disease. Gut 15:435, 1974.

33. McCaffery, T.D., Nasr, K., Lawrence, A.M., et al.: Severe growth retardation in children with inflammatory bowel disease. Pediatrics 45:386, 1970.

34. Ventteerden, J.A., Sigler, R.M., Lynn, H.B.: Regional enteritis in children: Surgical aspects. Mayo Clin Proc 42:100, 1967.

35. DeDombal, F.T.: The results of surgical treatment for Crohn's disease. Br J Surg 59:826, 1972.

36. Banks, D., Zetzel, L., Richter, H.S.: Morbidity and mortality in regional enteritis. Am J Dig Dis 14:367, 1969.

37. Weedon, D.D., Shorter, R.G., Ilstrup, D.M., et al.: Crohn's disease and cancer. N Engl J Med 21:1099, 1973.

38. Jorgensen, T.G., Vang, O., Pederson, G.: Thirty-three patients with acute terminal ileitis operated on for suspected appendicitis and followed up after 5 to 22 years. Nord Med 82:1415, 1969.

Case 30

PERIUMBILICAL PAIN, VOMITING, AND
FEVER IN A 2-YEAR-OLD BOY

HISTORY

A 2-year-old white male presented with the sudden onset (11 hr)
of mid-abdominal pain, migrating to the right lower quadrant.
Nausea and subsequent vomiting occurred. The rectal temperature ranged from 99.6 to 101.2°F. His appetite and activity
had decreased. He had had no bowel movement. There was no
associated history of hematemesis, diarrhea, melena, hematochezia, rash, jaundice, dysuria, or trauma. The remainder of
the past, developmental, family, and social history, as well as
review of systems, was unremarkable.

EXAMINATION

He was in apparent distress, rectal temperature 100.6°F.
Weight was 12.4 kg, height 88 cm, and head circumference 45.6
cm. The remainder of the examination was unremarkable, except for moderate generalized abdominal tenderness, no rebound
tenderness or masses, and hypoactive bowel sounds. The anorectal examination revealed referred tenderness to the umbilical
region with right and left rectal wall palpation.

LABORATORY DATA

Hemoglobin:	11.7 gm%
Hematocrit:	35%
White blood cell count:	13,200/mm^3
PMN's:	62%
lymphocytes:	32%

monocytes:	5%
eosinophiles:	1%
Sedimentation rate:	24 mm/hr
Urinalysis:	1-3 WBC/HPF
Plain films of abdomen:	multiple bowel loops; no free air
Stool:	
occult blood:	negative

QUESTIONS

Questions 1-15: Answer true (T) or false (F).

1. The most likely diagnosis is acute appendicitis.

2. Acute appendicitis is the most common condition requiring abdominal surgery during childhood.

3. Acute appendicitis is common during the first 2 years of life.

4. Fecaliths are found in almost 50% of cases.

5. Important predisposing factors include parasites, fecaliths, and lymphoid hyperplasia.

6. The usual clinical triad consists of abdominal pain, fever, and tenderness, localized to the right lower quadrant.

7. Vomiting occurs in the majority of patients, while diarrhea never occurs.

8. The main physical finding is localized right lower quadrant tenderness.

9. A reliable physical finding is the presence of rebound tenderness.

10. Laboratory studies are not specific in diagnosis of acute appendicitis.

11. Radiographically, air in the appendix without air throughout the intestinal tract is strongly suggestive of appendicitis.

12. Free peritoneal air is usually present in patients with a ruptured appendix.

13. Potential complications in this disorder include peritonitis, intra-abdominal abscess, appendiceal mucocele, and pyogenic abscess of the liver.

14. The treatment of choice is surgery.

15. The major reason for complications in this condition is delay in diagnosis.

ANSWERS AND COMMENTS

1. (T) The clinical pattern (pain pattern and location, vomiting) is quite compatible with this diagnosis. Refer to answers 2 through 15.

2. (T) Acute appendicitis is the most common condition requiring abdominal surgery during childhood. (1-5) Next in frequency is inguinal hernia. (1-5)

3. (F) Acute appendicitis has been and is apparently uncommon in the first 2 years of life. (1-6) However, appendicitis with perforation does occur not infrequently in the neonatal period, frequently in association with other conditions, such as Hirschsprung's disease. (1-4)

4. (F) Fecaliths are present in 10 to 25% of cases. (1-4) These fecaliths apparently produce obstruction with probable secondary bacterial invasion. When a fecalith is present in children with abdominal pain, as many as 50% will have appendiceal perforation. (1,7-10) Refer to answer 5.

5. (T) Important predisposing factors include parasites, fecaliths (answer 4), and lymphoid hyperplasia. (1-6) Other less common but probably predisposing factors include enteric infections, viral, bacterial, and fungal, extraintestinal infections, such as viral upper respiratory and pneumonia. (1-11) The role of pinworms remains controversial, although they are found in 3-10% of cases. (1-6)

6. (T) The "typical" clinical triad of abdominal pain, fever, and localized tenderness, right lower quadrant, indicates acute appendicitis until proven otherwise. (1-11) The right lower quadrant pain is usually preceded by cramplike epigastric or umbilical pain for 6 to 8 hours. (1-11) However, a pelvic appendix usually produces little abdominal pain, instead manifesting fecal as well as urinary symptomatology, while a retrocecal appendix

frequently produces variable pain. In addition, there may be a history of indigestion or flatulence for 1-5 days before the acute attack. Nausea generally precedes the vomiting and anorexia is common. (1-6) The previously mentioned fever is usually low-grade, 100-101°F. Constipation develops, although diarrhea may be present in a small percentage, 5 to 15%. (1-6) Diarrhea is quite common in those children with perforated appendices. (1-10)

7. (F) Refer to answer 6. Vomiting, with or without nausea, occurs in the majority of patients; vomiting, when it occurs, follows the pain. Diarrhea does occur in a small percentage of patients, 5 to 15%. (1-6) Refer to answer 6.

8. (T) The most important criterion in confirming a diagnosis of acute appendicitis is the presence of localized tenderness, right lower quadrant, in particular. This point tenderness is in the right iliac fossa, overlying the so-called McBurney's area (point). Guarding will be maximal where the tenderness is maximal; percussion can be used to detect tenderness or where it is maximal. Percussion in other parts of the abdomen may elicit pain referred to the right lower quadrant. In addition, external rotation of the flexed right thigh and leg will stretch the internal obturator muscle, producing pain if there is an adjacent inflamed appendix (obturator sign). (1-11) With the patient on his right side, stretching of the iliopsoas muscle may produce pain in the right iliac fossa (psoas sign), too. (1-11)
If a perforation has occurred, abdominal examination may disclose a mass if walled-off. Generalized tenderness and guarding may be present if there is a free perforation. (1-10) The child will usually lie still, the right lower extremity being drawn up.

9. (F) Rebound tenderness in the right iliac fossa is routinely assessed, but is generally an unreliable sign, especially in younger children and infants. (1-10) Pain/tenderness and muscle spasm may be elicited over the entire abdominal wall in infants.
In a small percentage of cases (1-10%), a palpable mass is noted, males greater than females. (11)

10. (T) In most patients, the white blood cell count is between 9,000 and 12,000 cells per mm^3, seldom higher than 15,000, with an increase in the percentage of polymorphonuclear leukocytes. (1,2,11) If the white blood cell count is over 15 to 18,000, perforation is suggested. (1-4,7-10) Conversely, a low white blood cell count with an increased percentage of

polymorphonuclear leukocytes may be present with an abscess or even with generalized peritonitis. Urinalysis is usually normal or demonstrates ketonuria; on occasions, white and/or red blood cells may be present if the inflamed appendix is adjacent to the bladder.

Other studies, such as the sedimentation rate (normal or mildly elevated), are also nonspecific in nature. Cultures, in particular of blood, are usually negative. (1-4)

11. (T) Air in the appendix without air throughout the intestine is highly suggestive of acute appendicitis. (1,2,4) Chest X-rays must be done in order to rule out intrathoracic conditions. Abdominal films may demonstrate the previously described finding, the presence or not of free air, or, in 10 to 25% of cases, the presence of a round or oval calcified fecalith. (1,7-10) Additionally, sentinel loops (small-bowel loops with air in the right lower quadrant), fluid levels in the right colon, or abdominal wall edema, and scoliosis (curvature of the spine toward the right) may be present.

Barium enema examination has been helpful in improving diagnostic accuracy in difficult cases, e.g., children with other diseases, such as diabetes mellitus, neoplasms, preschool children, mentally retarded children. (12,13) More recent experience in children in early appendicitis has suggested its use as an adjunct, especially if positive, i.e., nonfilling of the appendix with pericecal inflammation, while if negative, should not be the major determinant of surgery or not. (12, 14)

12. (F) Free air in the peritoneum is seldom seen with a ruptured appendix. (1,7-10) Signs of paralytic ileus or partial obstruction of the small intestine are frequently present on plain films of the abdomen. (1,7-10) Refer to answer 11.

13. (T) In the United States, 25 to 50% of children with appendicitis have a ruptured organ before surgery can be performed. This incidence is even higher in children less than 2 years of age. (1-10) After the initial perforation, there is temporary relief of pain, followed by the onset of fever, diffuse abdominal pain and tenderness, then rigidity (peritonitis). There may be a localization of the inflammatory process in the pelvic area and later fistulization (rectum, vagina). In addition, infection may spread to the subdiaphragmatic area, liver, or other foci (abscess). Pleural effusion may also occur. In most cases, a mass may be palpable; abdominal wall redness or edema is less common. If the infection invades the portal system, pyelphlebitis can result, terminating in the development of liver abscesses. Other potential complications include appendiceal mucocele

secondary to obstruction of the appendiceal lumen and mucus accumulation and small intestinal obstruction secondary to inflammatory adhesions. (1-10)

14.   (T) As the diagnosis is being made, the patient is placed on intravenous fluid therapy, nothing by mouth, and clinical observations, as well as repeat complete blood counts, urinalysis, abdominal X-rays, and intravenous pyelography, are performed as indicated. When the diagnosis is "certain," appendectomy should be performed as soon as possible. A nasogastric tube is passed, the stomach emptied, correction of any fluid and electrolyte deficit initiated, and the operating room readied. Recent studies have suggested the benefit of antibiotic administration or metronidazole (Flagyl) prior to or just after surgery in unruptured appendicitis. (15, 16)

   If perforation has occurred, the type of complication dictates treatment. A localized abscess requires incision and drainage as well as removal of the appendix. Antibiotic therapy is initiated, broad spectrum in nature, our choice being ampicillin, 200 mg/kg/day and gentamicin, 5-10 mg/kg/day. Intravenous fluid therapy, nothing by mouth, nasogastric tube passage, and analgesia, narcotics or substitute, are administered, too. With generalized peritonitis, once the patient is stabilized, surgery is performed, in particular, appendectomy and suctioning of peritoneal purulent contents. (1-10) Powers, et al. (16) have suggested initial antibiotic treatment with delayed operative intervention because of reduced complications, e.g., peritonitis, obstruction (adhesions).

15.   (T) Delay in diagnosis is the major reason for complications; therefore, if the diagnosis is considered probable, surgery is advocated. By necessity, this approach will lead to operations disclosing normal appendices, the generally accepted incidence being 15 to 25%. (1-6,12,17,18) This is obviously a difficult problem to resolve satisfactorily: the possibility of rupture versus the finding of a normal appendix. There is no clear-cut answer other than to assess each patient carefully, maintain a high index of suspicion, and recommend surgery if highly suspected. The overall mortality rate is 0.5 to 1.9%. (12,17)

REFERENCES

1.   MacIntyre, R.: Acute appendicitis. J Abdom Surg 11:125, 1969.

2. Grosfeld, J.L., Weinberger, M., Clatworthy, H.W.: Acute appendicitis in the first 2 years of life. J Pediatr Surg 8: 285, 1973.

3. Lansden, F.T.: Acute appendicitis in children. Am J Surg 106:938, 1963.

4. Smith, P.H.: The diagnosis of appendicitis. Postgrad Med J 41:2, 1965.

5. Brickman, T.D. and Leon, W.: Acute appendicitis in childhood. Surgery 60:1083, 1966.

6. Parsons, J.M., Miscall, B.G., McSherry, C.K.: Appendicitis in the newborn infant. Surgery 69:841, 1970.

7. Ackerman, N.B.: The continuing problems of perforated appendicitis. Surg Gynecol Obstet 139:29, 1974.

8. Holgersen, L.A. and Stanley-Brown, E.G.: Acute appendicitis with perforation. Am J Dis Child 122:288, 1971.

9. Shandling, B., Ein, S.H., Simpson, J.S., et al.: Perforating appendicitis with antibiotics. J Pediatr Surg 9: 79, 1974.

10. Foek, G., Gastrin, U., Josephson, S.: Appendiceal peritonitis in children. Acta Chir Scand 135:534, 1969.

11. Jordan, J.S., Kovalcik, P.J., Schwab, C.W.: Appendicitis with a palpable mass. Ann Surg 193:227, 1981.

12. Liebman, W.M. and St. Geme, J.W., Jr.: Enteroviral pseudoappendicitis. Am J Dis Child 120:7, 1970.

13. Hatch, E.I., Naffis, D., Chandler, N.W.: Pitfalls in the use of barium enema in early appendicitis in children. J Pediatr Surg 16:309, 1981.

14. Fee, H.J., Jones, P.C., Kadel, B., et al.: Radiologic diagnosis of appendicitis. Arch Surg 112:742, 1977.

15. Welch, C.E., Malt, R.A.: Abdominal surgery (first of three parts). N Engl J Med 308:629, 1983.

16. Powers, R.J., Andrassy, R.J., Brennan, L.B., et al.: Alternate approach to the management of acute perforated appendicitis in children. Surg Gynecol Obstet 152:473, 1981.

17. Salzberg, A.M. and White, N.K.: Current mortality for appendicitis in infants and children. Am J Surg 115:651, 1968.

18. Blair, G.L. and Gaisford, W.: Acute appendicitis in children under 6 years. J Pediatr Surg 4:445, 1969.

Case 31

ALTERNATING CONSTIPATION AND DIARRHEA
IN A 13-MONTH-OLD BOY

HISTORY

A 13-month-old white male presented with a history of altered
bowel habit pattern of 3 months' duration. The frequency of bowel movements varied from 0 to 4-5 bowel movements daily,
loose to soft in nature. In addition, there was probable associated increased flatus passage on occasions. There was no history of fever, vomiting, abdominal pain, melena, hematochezia,
skin lesions, anorexia, jaundice, or dysuria. Appetite and activity remained good. Growth pattern, height and weight remained within normal limits. There was no relationship of the
bowel movements with meals, time of day, or food types. The
parents had eliminated milk products on their own, but this produced no effect. The remainder of the past history, developmental history, family history, social history, and review of
systems was noncontributory. Medications have included Lactinex granules without apparent effect.

EXAMINATION

He was alert, active, and in no distress, with normal vital signs.
Height was 76 cm, weight 11.3 kg, and head circumference 46.5
cm. The remainder of the examination was negative, including
the abdomen and anorectal area.

LABORATORY DATA

Hemoglobin: 12.0 gm%
Hematocrit: 36%

White blood cell count:	7,200/mm^3
PMN's:	44%
lymphocytes:	54%
monocytes:	1%
eosinophiles:	1%
Platelets:	275,000/mm^3
Sedimentation rate:	7 mm/hr
Urinalysis:	negative
Serum:	
sodium:	139 meq/L
potassium:	4.1 meq/L
chloride:	102 meq/L
bicarbonate:	22 meq/L
total protein:	6.2 gm%
albumin:	4.5 gm%
calcium:	9.4 mg%
glucose:	90 mg%
creatinine:	0.5 mg%
SGOT:	18 units
alkaline phosphatase:	180 IU
carotene:	115 μg%
folate:	9.0 ng/ml
Stool:	
occult blood:	negative
reducing substances:	negative
culture:	negative
ova parasites:	negative
Barium enema:	negative
Upper GI - small bowel series:	negative

QUESTIONS

1. Which is the most likely diagnosis of this patient?
    A. Duodenal ulcer
    B. Irritable colon syndrome
    C. Celiac disease
    D. Ulcerative colitis
    E. Regional enteritis

2. Which of the following are the usual clinical features of this condition?
    A. Recurrent dysphagia
    B. Slow growth and development
    C. Chronic diarrhea
    D. Recurrent vomiting
    E. Recurrent abdominal pain ("colic")

Question 3: Answer true (T) or false (F).

3.   There is a marked female preponderance in this condition.

4.   Which factor(s) have been most implicated in its etiology?
     A. Altered transit time (slowed)
     B. Altered transit time (accelerated)
     C. Exaggerated response to stress
     D. Hormonal imbalance
     E. Allergy

5.   Which of the following studies would usually be indicated in
     the evaluation of such patients?
     A. Complete blood count, urinalysis
     B. Stool pH, reducing substances, and culture
     C. Sigmoidoscopy
     D. Fiberoptic endoscopy
     E. Intravenous pyelography

6.   Which of the following measures have been frequently help-
     ful in the treatment of this condition?
     A. Antispasmodics
     B. Antacids
     C. Antihistaminics
     D. Sedatives, tranquilizers
     E. Supportive counseling

ANSWERS AND COMMENTS

1.   (B) The irritable colon syndrome (ICS) is the most likely
diagnosis of this patient.
     The pattern of pain, specifically without relationship to loca-
tion, time of day, meals and food types, or to bowel movements,
as well as the lack of nausea and vomiting, fever, hematochezia,
anorexia, weight loss, and reduced activity, make the possibilities less likely of duodenal ulcer disease, celiac disease, and
inflammatory bowel disease.

2.   (C, E) The key feature suggesting this condition, and, in
fact, the usual clinical feature, is the presence of a well child.
Thus, growth and development are normal. The main symptom
of this well child is chronic diarrhea. The diarrhea usually consists of less than 6 to 7 bowel movements daily. The bowel
movements are usually described as being mushy or loose, with
variable odor, mainly brown in color, and not floating on top of
the water in the toilet bowel. Mucus is frequently noted in the

stools, and undigested food may also be present at times. Blood
(red streaks) is infrequent. Melena and occult blood positive
stools rarely occur. The diarrhea may be precipitated by stress
or any type of infection. The pattern of diarrhea may be continuous, recurrent, or limited to a few weeks or months. In early
infancy, this pattern seems to clear spontaneously by 3-1/2 to
4 years of age. (1-5) Recurrent abdominal pain (RAP), colicky
in nature, frequently occurs. Its localization may be difficult to
ascertain, most commonly being in the periumbilical region.
There is usually no relationship to time of day, meals, specific
foods, or to bowel movements. Its duration is quite variable,
usually not interfering significantly with patient activity. Nausea, vomiting, fever, anorexia, pyrosis, and dysphagia essentially do not occur.

3.   (F)   There is only a slight male preponderance in this condition. The usual age of onset in infancy is 8 to 18 months of
age, although the age range can be 3 months to 30 months. (1-5)

4.   (B,C)   The exact cause (or causes) of ICS in unknown. Many
associated conditions have been mentioned in conjunction with
ICS, including food allergy, constipation, aerophagia, "teething," Mittelschmerz, and abdominal "migraine." However, the
main etiological factors mentioned have been stress (emotions)
and altered transit time (accelerated). (1-13)
   The former has been implicated on the basis of extensive interviews and observations (patient, family) in patients with ICS;
and the resultant effect of various stimuli, such as familial interactions, peer relationships, play activity, has been an exaggerated response or summation, expressed in somatic symptomatology, including diarrhea and abdominal pain. (1-13) Whether
a generalized disturbance or imbalance of the autonomic nervous
system is involved remains unsettled, despite reports of exaggerated responses to stimulation, e.g., pupillary response to
cholinergic drugs. (6,7,10) Altered transit time is frequently
present, usually 40 to 50% less than age-matched controls, determined by use of a marker system, such as carmine. (8) Mass
movements, particularly of the left colon, propel fecal material
to the rectosigmoid area. Lower colonic segment tone and pressure have been found to be elevated in some patients subjected
to anorectal manometry. This increase could provide a resistance to material moving down, reducing subsequent desiccation
due to fluid absorption. (12,13) Additionally, recent studies of
basal electrical rhythm by transducers have revealed increased
slow wave frequency in ICS. (13) Therefore, altered motor activity (increased) is a component; moreover, some authors have
demonstrated this increase in potential reactivity even when all
symptoms are in remission. (12-14)

No evidence of malabsorption, e.g., fat, nitrogen, bile acids, reducing substances, parasitic infestation, allergic diathesis, or abnormal electroencephalography have consistently been found in ICS. Finally, a family history of the same or other functional bowel disorders has been found in 20 to 35% of cases. (1-5,11-13) However, a true genetic or ethnic predisposition has not been found.

5. (A,B) It is advisable to restrict the number of studies performed during the initial evaluation unless the history, examination, and/or clinical course suggest otherwise. As previously mentioned, a well child with only chronic diarrhea and normal growth and development suggests this entity. There are no absolute diagnostic studies for confirmation of this condition. Radiological examinations, including barium enema, are nonspecific. The demonstration of an area of spasm in the splenic flexure-proximal descending colon during barium enema examination is not a specific finding. (12,13)

Proctosigmoidoscopic examination usually is of no significant aid. One series emphasized findings, such as patches of hyperemia, dilatation of the rectal lumen, and pallor, as reflecting exaggerated responses to stress, but most authors would agree that these findings are quite common in asymptomatic normals. (9,12,13) Fiberoptic upper endoscopy is obviously of little value unless pathology is expected in the esophagus, stomach, or proximal duodenum. Fiberoptic lower endoscopy will infrequently demonstrate an abnormality in such cases in preschool children, while being more helpful in older children, e.g., inflammatory bowel disease, parasite infestation. (12,13) Therefore, a complete blood count, urinalysis, sedimentation rate, and stool examinations for occult blood, reducing substances and/or pH, and culture are usually sufficient, when normal, to reassure the parents and physician that significant organic disease is not likely. When the history is atypical, appropriate radiological and laboratory studies are indicated.

6. (E) This is one of the more taxing problems in pediatric practice, requiring time, patience, and understanding. The physician must be willing to spend time to explain his findings convincingly to the parents, to provide support and guidance as to dietary and activity management, and to be available in the future for further aid. The physician's thoroughness in initial and subsequent evaluations further reduces anxiety. With reference to diet, between-meal snacks should be avoided. Chilled foods and drinks (trigger mass movements) should be limited or avoided. Adequate caloric intake, however, must be maintained.

An adequate intake of undigestible bulk has been the most important single factor to the well-being of adult patients with ICS. (15,16) Bulk-providers, e.g., unprocessed wheat bran, psyllium seed derivatives, e.g., Metamucil®, Effersyllium®, were more effective than placebos in double-blind therapeutic trials. (15) The wet weight of colonic contents is increased, and intraluminal pressure from muscular activity is reduced. (15,16)

The usage of various drugs should be discouraged since they generally do not help, confuse the clinical picture, and, additionally, create unwanted dependence. However, occasional symptomatic relief of severe pain is warranted, e.g., analgesics, such as acetaminophen, 4-6 mg/kg every 4 hours. (12,13) Extreme anxiety may necessitate temporary use of tranquilizers, such as chlorpromazine, 0.5 mg/kg per dose 3 times daily. (13) The therapeutic purpose of antispasmodic/anticholinergic agents is to reduce contraction frequency and force and can be effective on occasions, especially if there is no gaseous distention. Antacids and antihistaminic preparations have produced inconsistent results. In summary, a patient, understanding, and available physician to provide guidance and support to the family is the key to successful treatment.

In ICS of infancy, the prognosis is excellent, with spontaneous disappearance occurring in essentially all patients by 3-1/2 to 4 years of age. In older children and adolescents, ICS tends to be more chronic and intermittent, with 30 to 60% lasting into adulthood, regardless of treatment or type. (2,17)

REFERENCES

1. Davidson, M. and Wasserman, R.: The irritable colon of childhood. J Pediatr 69:1027, 1966.

2. Apley, J.: The Child with Abdominal Pain, 2nd Edition. Blackwell Scientific Publications, Oxford, 1975.

3. Apley, J.: Psychosomatic illness in children: A modern synthesis. Br Med J 2:756, 1973.

4. Kirsner, J.B. and Palmer, W.C.: The irritable colon. Gastroenterology 34:491, 1958.

5. Lumsden, K., Chaudhary, N., Truelove, S.C.: The irritable colon syndrome. Q J Med 31:123, 1962.

6. Kopel, E., Kim, I., Barbero, G.H.: Comparison of rectosigmoid motility in normal children, children with recurrent abdominal pain, and children with ulcerative colitis. Pediatrics 39:4, 1967.

7. Rubin, L.S., Barbero, G.J., Sibinga, M.S. : Pupillary reactivity in children with recurrent abdominal pain. Psychosomatic Med 29:111, 1967.

8. Dimson, S.B.: Transit time related to clinical findings in children with recurrent abdominal pain. Pediatrics 47: 666, 1971.

9. Stone, R.T. and Barbero, G.J.: Recurrent abdominal pain in childhood. Pediatrics 45:732, 1970.

10. Apley, J., Haslam, D.R., Tulloc, C.G.: Pupillary reaction in children with recurrent abdominal pain. Arch Dis Child 46:337, 1971.

11. Stone, R.T.: Abdominal pain in childhood. Clin Med 80: 27, 1973.

12. Roy, C.C., Silverman, A., Cozzetto, F.J.: Pediatric Clinical Gastroenterology, 2nd Edition. The CV Mosby Co., St. Louis, 1975, p. 195.

13. Liebman, W.M. and Thaler, M.M. : Pediatric considerations of abdominal pain and the acute abdomen. In: Gastrointestinal Disease. Sleisenger, M.H. and Fordtran, J.S. (Eds). WB Saunders Co. , Philadelphia, 1978, p. 411.

14. Taylor, I., Parby, C., Hammond, P.: Is there a myoelectrical abnormality in the irritable colon syndrome? Gt 19:391, 1978.

15. Ritchie, J.: Pain in IBS. Pract Gastroenterol 3:16, 1979.

16. Heaton, K.W. (ed): Dietary fiber: Current developments of importance to health. Technomic Publishing Company, Inc., Westport, Connecticut, 1979, p. 1.

17. Christensen, M.E. and Mortensen, O.: Long-term prognosis in children with recurrent abdominal pain. Arch Dis Child 50:110, 1975.

Case 32

BLOOD IN STOOLS IN A 2-YEAR-OLD GIRL

HISTORY

A 2-year-old white female presented with a history of recurrent
blood, occult more than gross, in the bowel movements since 6
months of age. Evaluation at that time, by another physician,
revealed the presence of anemia, macrocytic and megaloblastic
in type. Urine and plasma amino acid screen was normal at that
time while both serum folate and vitamin B_{12} levels were low.
Bone marrow examination was unremarkable at that time, too.
Treatment was begun with folate and vitamin B_{12}. However,
there was no response to this regimen, and a one-unit transfusion of whole blood was administered. The hemoglobin level
was raised from 7.0 gm/100 ml to 9.0 gm/100 ml. In addition,
since birth the patient has had isolated episodes of vomiting or
atypical segmental rashes while receiving several types of formula and baby foods. In addition, she has had vague abdominal
cramping, related and unrelated to meals or to various formulas or foods, with no episodes of vomiting, diarrhea, fever, or
melena. Her growth pattern has continuously been within normal limits for age. The patient's present diet consisted of Pregestimil, rice, and applesauce. Past history, developmental
history, family history, and review of systems were unremarkable.

EXAMINATION

She was alert and active. Weight was 13.2 kg and height 92 cm.
Head circumference was 49.5 cm. Examination revealed only
a grade I-II/VI systolic murmur heard along the lower left sternal border, disappearing with deep inspiration and with no lateral radiation. The rest of the examination, including the abdomen, was unremarkable.

LABORATORY DATA

Hemoglobin:	12.4 gm%
Hematocrit:	37%
White blood cell count:	8,300/mm^3
PMN's:	45%
lymphocytes:	50%
monocytes:	4%
eosinophils:	1%
reticulocyte count:	0.7%
Hb electrophoresis:	normal pattern
Platelet count:	504,000/mm^3
Serum:	
iron:	77 μg/100 ml
iron-binding capacity:	267 μg/100 ml
folate:	12 ng/ml
IgG:	635 mg/100 ml
IgA:	66 mg/100 ml
IgM:	57 mg/100 ml
Urinalysis:	normal
Sweat test:	
sodium:	11 meq/L
chloride:	16 meq/L
Pertechnetate ^{99m} isotope scan:	negative
Upper GI series:	negative
Barium enema:	(Fig. 32.1)
Proctosigmoidoscopy:	minimal erythema
Rectal biopsy:	focal collection of lympho-cytes

QUESTIONS

1. Which one of the following is the most likely diagnosis?
   A. Peptic ulcer disease
   B. Regional enteritis
   C. Benign lymphoid hyperplasia of colon
   D. Ulcerative colitis
   E. Familial polyposis coli

Questions 2-4: Answer true (T) or false (F).

2. Collections of lymphocytes in the mucosa and submucosa of the gastrointestinal tract are an abnormal finding, primary or secondary.

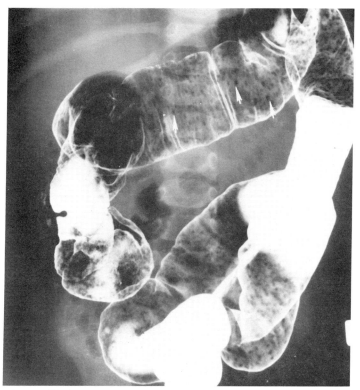

Figure 32.1 Barium enema. Multiple, small radiolucent, round nodules throughout the colon are noted. None of these demonstrate central umbilication (arrows).

3. Lymphoid hyperplasia may occur in the small or large intestine.

4. When present in the colon only, lymphoid hyperplasia is usually confined to the ascending colon.

5. The clinical pattern in lymphoid hyperplasia of the colon usually includes which of the following?
   A. Fever
   B. Abdominal pain
   C. Vomiting
   D. Diarrhea
   E. Rectal bleeding

6. The peak age incidence of this disorder is
   A. 1-3 months
   B. 6-12 months
   C. 1-3 years
   D. 3-6 years
   E. 6-12 years

7. Treatment may include which of the following?
   A. No treatment
   B. Acetaminophen
   C. Azulfidine
   D. Corticosteroids
   E. Surgery

ANSWERS AND COMMENTS

1. (C) Benign lymphoid hyperplasia is the most likely diagnosis. The lack of fever, abdominal pain, diarrhea, weight loss, and significant hematochezia would tend to eliminate the other choices.

2. (F) Collections of lymphocytes in the mucosa and submucosa may be a normal finding in the gastrointestinal tract. (1.2) If less than 5 mm in diameter, they may be visible and are termed follicular hyperplasia. (1-6) The follicles consist of mature lymphocytes and reticulum cells. (1-6) If greater than 5 mm in diameter, they will appear as nodular (nodular hyperplasia). (1-6) In the ileum, submucosal nodules (Peyer's patches) will result.

3. (T) Lymphoid hyperplasia of the small as well as of the large intestine may occur in a number of conditions, including immunoglobulin deficiencies, particularly, selective IgA deficiency and pernicious anemia. (1-8) Association with giardiasis has been reported; however, its true significance remains unresolved, since hypogammaglobulinemia, particularly IgA, has almost always been present. (1-8) The immunological component (B cell, not T cell) has been predominantly associated with small intestinal involvement. (1-8) When polypoid in nature, lymphoid polyps have been reported in association with adenomatous polyps, as well as Gardner's and Cronkhite-Canada syndromes. (6,9)

4. (F) When limited to the colon, the condition may be limited to the rectum or may be diffuse throughout the colon. Thus, any segment of the colon may be affected. The condition may be

follicular, nodular, or polypoid in configuration. (1-6) The ascending colon per se is rarely, if ever, affected. (1-12)

5.   (B,D,E) The clinical pattern may be one of no symptomatology, rectal bleeding, looser and more frequent bowel movements, and/or nonspecific, vague abdominal discomfort. Most commonly, minimal rectal bleeding, bright red, without anemia, has been associated. (1-13) The polypoid form has infrequently been linked with intussusception. (1-12) Other associated symptomatology has included constipation and anorectal discomfort. (1-6) There are no specific laboratory studies. (1,2,6)

Radiologically, lymphoid hyperplasia is characterized by small, relatively symmetrical, umbilicated lesions. A small amount of barium may be present in the center of the lesion, i.e., polyps (umbilication). The latter has not been observed in adenomatous or juvenile polyposis. (1-6)

Endoscopy (sigmoidoscopy, colonoscopy) does allow direct inspection, as well as potential tissue inspection, by biopsy. Unfortunately, bleeding from lymphoid hyperplasia has rarely been confirmed at direct inspection. (6,14)

6.   (C) The general age range is 6 months to 12 years, while the peak incidence is 1 to 3 years. (1,2,6) Other ages have not been affected.

7.   (A,D) Due to the obvious difficulty in differentiation from polypoid lesions themselves, prior treatment has included radiation, surgery, i.e., subtotal or total colectomy, as well as corticosteroid administration. (1-6) However, if the diagnosis of lymphoid hyperplasia is confirmed, no treatment is necessary, as spontaneous regression usually results. (1-12)

If severe abdominal pain or significant rectal bleeding persists, then some authors have suggested use of corticosteroids, i.e., prednisone, 1-2 mg/kg/day, for 2 to 4 weeks. Surgery would be reserved for obstructive symptomatology only, a rare occurrence. (1-12)

REFERENCES

1.   Poley, J.R. and Smith, E.I.: Benign lymphatic hyperplasia of the rectum. So Med J 65:420, 1972.

2.   Capitanio, M.A. and Kirkpatrick, J.A.: Lymphoid hyperplasia of the colon in children. Radiology 94:323, 1970.

3. Collins, J.O., Falk, M., Guibone, R.: Benign lymphoid polyposis of the colon: A case report. Pediatrics 38:897, 1966.

4. Franken, E.A., Jr.: Lymphoid hyperplasia of the colon. Radiology 94:320, 1970.

5. Ferran, J.L., Betoulieres, P., Bonnet, H., et al.: L-hyperplasie lymphoide du colon. Presentation de deux observations. Arch Franc Pediat 32:405, 1975.

6. Liebman, W.M. and Rosental, E-D.: Benign lymphoid hyperplasia of the colon. A case report and review. West J Med 127:416, 1977.

7. Hermans, P.E.: Nodular lymphoid hyperplasia of the small intestine and hypogammaglobulinemia: Theoretical and practical considerations. Fed Proc 26:1601, 1967.

8. Gryboski, J.D., Self, T.W., Clement, A., et al.: Selective immunoglobulin A deficiency and intestinal nodular lymphoid hyperplasia: Correction of diarrhea with antibiotics and plasma. Pediatrics 42:833, 1968.

9. Sheahan, D.G., Martin, F., Baginsky, S., et al.: Multiple lymphomatous polyposis of the gastrointestinal tract. Cancer 28:408, 1971.

10. Shaw, E.B. and Hennigar, G.R.: Intestinal lymphoid polyposis. Am J Clin Pathol 61:417, 1974.

11. Louw, J.H.: Polypoid lesions of the large bowel in children with particular reference to benign lymphoid polyposis. J Pediatr Surg 3:195, 1968.

12. Robinson, M.J., Podron, S., Rywlin, A.M.: Enterocolitis lymphofollicularis. Arch Pathol 196:311, 1973.

13. Schifter, P., Szakáll, S.Z., Várbiró, M., et al.: Intestinal lymphoid hyperplasia causing pseudopolyposis and intussusception. Orv Hetil 121:2331, 1980.

14. Euler, A.R., Seibert, J.J.: The role of sigmoidoscopy, radiographs, and colonoscopy in the diagnostic evaluation of pediatric age patients with suspected juvenile polyps. J Pediatr Surg 16:500, 1981.

Case 33

DIARRHEA AND BLOOD IN A 10-YEAR-OLD BOY

HISTORY

A 10-year-old white male presented with a 3-week history of increased bowel movements, as many as 5 to 6 loose bowel movements daily, with associated gross blood, bright red, on top of the bowel movements and mixed with the bowel movements. There was associated lower abdominal pain, cramping in nature, left-sided more than right-sided, occurring a few minutes before the bowel movements and relieved by the bowel movements. The patient had awakened from sleep on occasions in order to have a bowel movement. There had been a mild decrease in appetite with a loss of 1-1/2 lbs during these 3 weeks. There had been no associated history of nausea, vomiting, fever, melena, dysuria, skin lesions, arthralgia, ocular difficulty, or trauma. Medication had included Tegopen and Prostaphlin (almost 2 weeks for a supposed infectious gastroenteritis; staph in one stool culture). The pertinent family history included the mother with a history of inflammatory bowel disease, type unknown, currently being treated with antibiotics, and a sister and father with history of bronchial asthma. The pertinent prior history included the patient's growth pattern, height and weight being at approximately the 3rd percentile throughout his life, and a history of constipation for the last 2 years prior to the onset of the present clinical pattern. Review of the past history, developmental history, family history, social history, and review of systems was noncontributory.

EXAMINATION

He was alert, cooperative, and in no apparent distress, with normal vital signs, weight 22 kg, and height 124 cm. The

273

remainder of the examination was unremarkable except for mild tenderness in the lower abdomen, left greater than right.

LABORATORY DATA

Hemoglobin:	11.8 gm%
Hematocrit:	35%
White blood cell count:	11,000/mm^3
PMN's:	64%
lymphocytes:	32%
monocytes:	2%
eosinophiles:	2%
Sedimentation rate:	42 mm/hr
Serum:	
carotene:	110 μg/ml
folate:	10 ng/ml
total protein:	6.0 gm%
albumin:	4.3 gm%
iron:	42 μg%
iron-binding capacity:	412 μg%
SGPT:	18 units
SGOT:	19 units
alkaline phophatase:	165 IU
creatinine:	0.4 mg%
IgG:	1,800 mg%
IgM:	85 mg%
IgA:	110 mg%
IgE:	110 mg%
Urinalysis	negative
Stools:	
reducing substances:	negative
culture:	negative
ova and parasites:	negative
Barium enema:	(Fig. 33.1)
Upper GI - small bowel series:	negative
Proctosigmoidoscopy:	Mild erythema and increased friability to 25 cm
Rectal biopsy:	(Fig. 33.2)

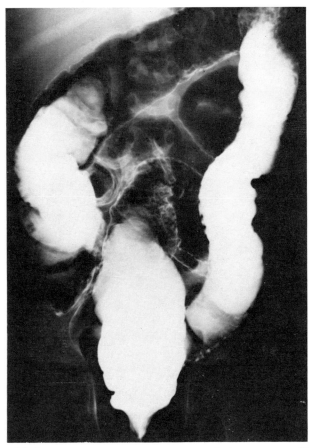

Figure 33.1 Barium enema. Fine spiculations, as well as
probable deeper ulcerations, are shown in the mucosal outline
of the left colon.

QUESTIONS

1. The most likely diagnosis is
    A. duodenal ulcer
    B. cystic fibrosis
    C. celiac disease
    D. Meckel's diverticulum
    E. ulcerative colitis

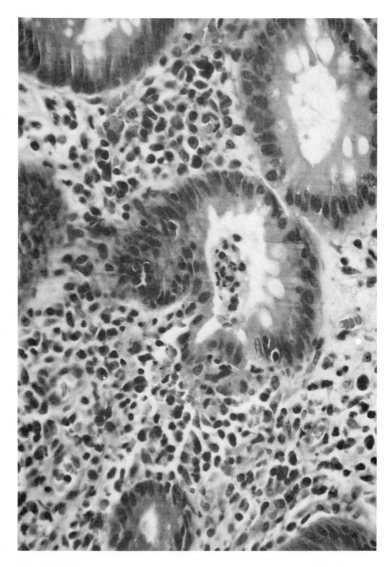

Figure 33.2   Rectum.   A crypt abscess, an accumulation of polymorphonuclear cells in a crypt of Lieberkuhn with wall breakdown, is pictured (H&E, X150).

2. With reference to ulcerative colitis, this condition is
   A. more common in nonwhites than whites
   B. more common between 8 to 15 years of age than in adults
   C. infrequent in more than one family member
   D. present almost exclusively in lower socioeconomic classes
   E. present in Jews with at least a four-to-fivefold increased frequency

3. Current mechanisms of proposed pathogenesis include which of the following?
   A. Infection of colon
   B. Abnormal response to an infective agent
   C. Absence of ganglion cells
   D. Autoimmune response
   E. Primary psychosomatic response

4. Predominant clinical manifestations include which of the following?
   A. Crampy abdominal pain
   B. Jaundice
   C. Diarrhea
   D. Constipation
   E. Rectal bleeding

5. Extraintestinal manifestations include which of the following?
   A. Arthritis
   B. Fatty liver, chronic active liver disease
   C. Conjunctivitis, uveitis
   D. Nephrotic syndrome
   E. None of the above

ANSWERS AND COMMENTS

1. (E) The most likely diagnosis is ulcerative colitis. The presence of diarrhea, hematochezia, abdominal pain associated with bowel movements, and compatible radiological and histological findings strongly suggest the previously mentioned diagnosis and essentially exclude the other answers.

2. (E) Ulcerative colitis is an inflammatory process, located predominantly in the mucosa, involving the colon in 100%, particularly the rectum (95%+), while ileal involvement occurs in only 5 to 10%. (1-4) The annual incidence at all ages varies

between 3 to 6/100,000, the prevalence rate being 44 to 99/
100,000. (1-4) The incidence of Crohn's disease has increased
over the past two decades, while that of ulcerative colitis has
not. (1-5) Whites are affected more commonly than nonwhites.
(1-4) There is no significant sex difference. (1-4) The mean
age at diagnosis is generally between 10 to 11 years. (5) There
is a predominance of patients with ulcerative colitis from a
higher socioeconomic group. (1-4) In addition, there is a four-
to fivefold increased incidence in Jews and other members of
Semitic origin, particularly those living in Europe and North
America, while being less frequent in blacks and Orientals. (1-
5) Familial incidence has been estimated to be 5 to 15%, mainly
in first-degree relatives. (1-4) Finally, 10 to 15% of all cases
of ulcerative colitis occur in the pediatric population. (1-4) The
increased incidence of other conditions, such as eczema and urticaria, in families with one or more members having ulcerative
colitis has not been consistently reported. (1-4)

3.   (A,B,D) A similarity between ulcerative colitis and Shigellosis, i.e., S. dysenteriae, has been recognized for over 50
years. (1,4,6) This observation spurred the continued search
for a bacterial pathogen(s) in this disorder, e.g., E. coli, C.
difficile. (1-6) The results, however, have generally been unrewarding for both aerobic and anaerobic agents. Other transmissible agents, particularly viruses, have been looked for, but
positive results have been few, e.g., cytomegalovirus, Vermont
agent. (4-7) In addition, attention has been directed at the normal bacterial flora, stimulated by the effect of medication, such
as Azulfidine, in decreasing the relapse rate. However, Azulfidine's mode of action has never been confirmed to be by modification of the bacterial flora. (4,6)
     Immunological mechanisms have been most prominently men-
tioned in the pathogenesis of ulcerative colitis. (8) One proposal
has been an abnormal response to an infective agent, either a
pathogen or part of the normal bacterial flora of the gut. (6) Consistent animal models of ulcerative colitis, however, have been
lacking, and it has therefore not been possible to substantiate
this view. In some animals, ingestion of degraded carrageenan
has produced ulcerative disease of the colon. (8) This effect
seems to be species-specific. (8) The "Auer colitis model,"
characterized by antigen-antibody reaction in the colon as a result of nonspecific irritation, has been reasonable experimentally, but whether it is a stereotyped reaction is unresolved. (9)
Use of a 2-4-dinitrochlorobenzene as a sensitizing agent has resulted in similar observations and reservations. (8) Administration of anti-colon serum (antibodies) has resulted in hemorrhagic
colitis in dogs but no chronic disease. (9) Thus, an abnormal

immune response to endogenous bacteria (such as an Arthus'-type reaction in the mucosa), or to infective agents, remains a possibility. (10)

The second immunological proposal involves an allergic reaction to an exogenous protein (antigen). Possible allergy to milk, gluten, or other proteins (antigens) has been scrutinized. However, no consistent relationship to antigen administration or, conversely, to dietary antigen withdrawal, has been observed. (11) In some patients, milk's adverse effect may be a true allergy or could be due to a nonimmunological mechanism, e.g., decreased lactase levels. (4,8) No correlation has been found between antibody titers (milk) and response to a milk-free diet. (8,11) Furthermore, IgE antibodies to milk protein by the red cell-linked antigen-antiglobulin test have not been detected. (8,12) Increased blood and/or rectal eosinophile counts have not been consistently detected either. Increased circulating basophile counts and increased rectal histamine content have been found in a variable number of patients. (13,14) Moreover, the initial reports of favorable response to disodium cromoglycate administration, although not recently confirmed, added to the interest in type I hypersensitivity reactions. (5,8,15)

The third and final immunological proposal has been an autoimmune reaction. (16,19) Associated autoimmune disorders with ulcerative colitis have included systemic lupus erythematosus, pernicious anemia, Hashimoto's thyroiditis, and myasthenia gravis. (8,16) A consistently related augmented incidence of autoantibodies, e.g., gastric parietal cell, smooth muscle, thyroid, or reticulin, has not been found. (17,18) Anticolon antibodies, true autoantibodies reacting with autologous rectal tissue, have been found in children with ulcerative colitis, but only in 25% or less. (19) However, other authors have suggested that this autoimmunization arises from tolerance disruption by cross-reacting bacterial antigens, e.g., anaerobes. (8,16) Serum complement studies have also not produced consistent findings. (20, 21) Therefore, circulating immune complexes (IgG) have been alternatively suggested in the pathogenesis, especially of extraintestinal manifestations. (8,16)

Finally, investigation of cell-mediated immunity, e.g., phytohemagglutinin (PHA) responsiveness, has produced variable results, frequently normal. (22) In ulcerative colitis, most authors feel that there is little evidence for depressed cell-mediated immunity, while there is more evidence for such in Crohn's disease. (22-24) However, altered responsiveness (immunosuppression) can result because of medication and/or recent surgery. (24) Evidence has accumulated to some extent regarding lymphocytes with Fc receptor (null cell) exerting a direct cytotoxic effect on target colon epithelial cells. (12,25)

A primary psychosomatic etiology (E) has not been corroborated. Absence of ganglion cells (C) is characteristic of Hirschsprung's disease or Chagas' disease. (26)

4. (A,C,E) Ulcerative colitis more commonly begins with diarrhea; mild (less than 4 stools daily) or moderate (90 to 96%). (1-5,26-31) The diarrhea may worsen in frequency and associated bright red blood may be noted within weeks or months. (1-4,26,27) These manifestations occur especially during the early morning hours (50 to 65%). If predominantly nocturnal in occurrence, severe disease is usually present. Urgency or actual incontinence may be present in 20 to 30% of cases. (1-4,26,27) Occasionally, constipation occurs, possibly the initial manifestation of the severe form with developing toxic dilatation. (1-4, 26,27) Abdominal pain related to bowel movements is frequently present, usually in the lower abdomen, predominantly leftsided. (1-4,26,27) Food usually aggravates the pain, and defecation produces temporary relief. Tenesmus (urgency of defecation) may be present, too. Anorexia, nausea, and vomiting can also be present, especially during the acute phase and/or severe disease. Growth retardation, delayed sexual maturation, e.g., menstruation, are variable, dependent upon the intensity and duration of disease.

5. (A,B,C) Extraintestinal manifestations are present in the majority of children with ulcerative colitis. (1-4,24-29) They may even precede the onset of common symptomatology by months or even years. (1-4,26,31)

Mucocutaneous lesions occur in 3 to 10% of children. (26) During active phases of disease, erythema nodosum or erythema multiforme can occur. (26) Occasionally, aphthous lesions of the oral cavity are found, but they are more common in Crohn's disease. (26) Pyoderma gangrenosum, a typical lesion of adult ulcerative colitis, is uncommon in children. (28) It is characterized by necrotic, ulcerative, plaque-like lesions of the lower and upper extremities, abdomen, and perineum, particularly legs. (28) These ulcers spread as the colitis worsens.

Musculoskeletal involvement is also quite common. Arthralgia and/or overt arthritis occurs in as many as 25% of children with ulcerative colitis. Four predominant forms are noted: (1) rheumatoid arthritis; (2) rheumatoid spondylitis, changes in the sacroiliac joints with or without spine and peripheral joint involvement; (3) arthralgia only; and (4) "colitic" arthritis, characterized by predominantly large joint involvement, e.g., ankle, knee, elbow. (1-5,26,30) The spondylitic condition has been associated with the histocompatibility antigen HLA-B27. (5,25,32)

Symptomatic hepatic disease occurs in only 10% of patients with ulcerative colitis. (1-4,26,29,30) Inflammatory change of the liver is the most common hepatic abnormality, occurring in almost 70% of patients. (26,29) The histological features include cellular infiltration (lymphocytes especially), variable fibrosis, proliferation of bile ductules, and variable hepatocyte necrosis. (26,29) These lesions are predominantly located in the portal tract areas. (26,29) Two to 3% of patients develop cirrhosis, 1 to 2% a cholestatic syndrome, and 1% develop chronic active liver disease (hepatitis). (26,29) Fatty infiltration is especially common. The presence of liver disease does not correlate with the extent, duration, or activity of disease. Furthermore, hepatic lesions may be present, although liver function tests are normal.

Ocular involvement is also relatively common, including uveitis, 1-2%, conjunctivitis, and keratitis. (1-4,26,27,30) The lesions are usually sterile, responsive to steroids, and may represent hypersensitivity phenomena. (1-4,26,27,30)

Renal lesions, such as glomerulitis, chronic pyelonephritis, and stones, particularly urate, have also been reported in ulcerative colitis. (26,27,30) There is a 100- to 300-fold increased incidence of stones in ulcerative colitis. (26,27,30)

Hematological abnormalities include anemia due to blood loss and/or malabsorption of iron, folic acid, or vitamin B_{12}. (1-4,26,27,30) In addition, Coombs' positive hemolysis has been reported. Thrombophlebitis, thrombocytopenia, and leukopenia have also been reported in 10 to 75% of cases. (1-4,26, 27,30)

Neuropsychiatric manifestations, e.g., neuroses and depression, are relatively common. (26,27,30) Even psychosis has been reported.

Finally, the association with large intestinal carcinoma has been well defined. This predisposition is particularly significant with onset of disease in childhood. (30) This risk increases with duration of disease. After 10 years of disease, the risk is 3 to 7% and increases to 20 to 25% after 20 years of disease. After 20 years of disease, the risk increases 1 to 2% yearly. (33) The risk is particularly prevalent in patients with total colonic involvement. Carcinomas of ulcerative colitis are poorly differentiated, frequently multicentric, can occur anywhere in the colon, and have early metastasis with a 5-year survival rate of 20 to 30%. (5,33)

REFERENCES

1. Davidson, M., Bloom, A.A., Kugler, M.M.: Chronic ulcerative colitis of childhood. J Pediatr 67:471, 1965.

2. Wright, R.: Ulcerative colitis. Gastroenterology 58:875, 1970.

3. Kirsner, J.B.: Clinical observations on inflammatory bowel disease. Med Clin North Am 53:1169, 1969.

4. Ament, M.E.: Inflammatory disease of the colon: Ulcerative colitis and Crohn's colitis. J Pediatr 86:322, 1975.

5. Silverman, A., Roy, C.C.: Pediatric Clinical Gastroenterology, 3rd edition. The CV Mosby Company, St. Louis, 1983, pp. 349, 353.

6. Gorbach, S.L., Nahas, L., Plaut, A.G., et al.: Studies of intestinal microflora. V. Fecal microbial ecology in severity of disease and chemotherapy. Gastroenterology 54:575, 1968.

7. Monteiro, E., Fossey, J., Shiner, M., et al.: Antibacterial antibodies in rectal and colonic mucosa in ulcerative colitis. Lancet 1:249, 1971.

8. Whorwell, P.J., and Wright, R.: Immunological aspects of inflammatory bowel disease. Clin Gastroenterol 5:303, 1976.

9. Ford, H. and Kirsner, J.B.: "Auer colitis" in rabbits induced by intrarectal antigen. Proc Soc Exp Biol Med 116:745, 1964.

10. Goldgraber, M.B. and Kirsner, J.B.: The Arthus' phenomena in the colon of rabbits. Arch Path 67:556, 1959.

11. Jewell, D.P. and Truelove, S.C.: Circulating antibodies to cow's milk proteins in ulcerative colitis. Gut 13:796, 1972.

12. Jewell, D.P. and Truelove, S.C.: Reaginic hypersensitivity in ulcerative colitis. Gut 13:903, 1972.

13. Lloyd, G., Green, F.H.Y., Fox, H., et al.: Mast cells and immunoglobulin E in inflammatory bowel disease. Gut 16:861, 1965.

14. Juhlin, L.: Basophil leukocytes in ulcerative colitis. Acta Med Scand 173:351, 1963.

15. Mani, V., Lloyd, G., Green, F.H.Y., et al.: Treatment of ulcerative colitis with oral disodium cromoglycate. A double-blind controlled trial. Lancet 1:439, 1976.

16. Wright, R. and Truelove, S.C.: Auto-immune reactions in ulcerative colitis. Gut 7:32, 1966.

17. Harrison, W.J.: Thyroid, gastric (parietal cell) and nuclear antibodies in ulcerative colitis. Lancet 1:1350, 1965.

18. Harrison, W.J.: Autoantibodies against intestinal and gastric mucous cells in ulcerative colitis. Lancet 1:1346, 1965.

19. Marcussen, H. and Nerup, J.: Fluorescent anti-colon and organ-specific antibodies in ulcerative colitis. Scand J Gastroenterol 8:9, 1973.

20. Fletcher, J.: Serum complement levels in active ulcerative colitis. Gut 6:172, 1965.

21. Ward, M. and Eastwood, M.A.: Serum complement components C3 and C4 in inflammatory bowel disease. Gut 15:835, 1974.

22. Aas, J., Huizenga, K.A., Newcomer, A.D., et al.: Inflammatory bowel disease: Lymphocytic responses to nonspecific stimulation in vitro. Scand J Gastroenterol 7:299, 1972.

23. Strickland, R.G., Korsmeyer, S., Soltis, R.D., et al.: Peripheral blood T and B cells in chronic inflammatory bowel disease. Gastroenterology 67:569, 1974.

24. Bolton, P.M., James, S.L., Newcombe, R.G., et al.: The immune competence of patients with inflammatory bowel disease. Gut 15:213, 1974.

25. Sachar, D.B., Auslander, M.O., Walfish, J.S.: Aetiological theories of inflammatory bowel disease. Clin Gastroenterol 9:231, 1980.

26. Roy, C.C., Silverman, A., Cozzetto, F.J.: Pediatric Clinical Gastroenterology, 2nd Edition. The CV Mosby Co., St. Louis, 1975, p. 294.

27. Binder, V., Bonnevie, O., Gertz, T.C., et al.: Ulcerative colitis in children: Treatment, course and prognosis. Scand J Gastroenterol 8:161, 1973.

28. Kiel, V.: Pyoderma gangrenosum in ulcerative colitis. Arch Dermatol Syphilol 56:187, 1947.

29. Eade, M.N. and Cooke, W.T.: Hepatobiliary disease associated with ulcerative colitis. Postgrad Med 53:112, 1973.

30. Cavell, B., Hildebrand, H., Meeuwisse, G.W., et al.: Chronic inflammatory bowel disease. Clin Gastroenterol 6:481, 1977.

31. Grand, R.J. and Homer, D.R.: Approaches to inflammatory bowel disease in childhood and adolescence. Pediatr Clin North Am 22:835, 1975.

32. Gitnick, G. L. : Etiology of inflammatory bowel diseases: Are we making progress ? Gastroenterology 78:1089, 1980.

33. Devroede, G.J., Taylor, W.F., Sauer, W.G., et al.: Cancer risk and life expenctancy of children with ulcerative colitis. N Engl J Med 285:17, 1971.

Case 34

INTERMITTENT DIARRHEA AND BLOOD IN
STOOLS IN AN 11-YEAR-OLD BOY

HISTORY

An 11-year-old white male presented with a history of intermittent diarrhea with associated gross blood on top of and mixed in
with the bowel movements for a duration of 4 weeks. The bowel
movements would be as frequent as 7-8 daily, and the amount of
gross blood would be as much as 1 tbsp per bowel movement.
The patient had associated lower abdominal cramping preceding
the bowel movements, which was frequently relieved by bowel
movements. There was no associated history of fever, constipation, melena, jaundice, dysuria, skin lesions, arthralgia, ocular difficulties, or trauma. The patient awoke from sleep in
order to have bowel movements. The past history, developmental history, family history, social history, and review of systems were unremarkable. Appetite and activity were essentially unchanged.

EXAMINATION

He was alert, cooperative, and in no acute distress, with normal vital signs. Height was 132 cm, weight was 37.2 kg. The
remainder of the examination was unremarkable except for mild
tenderness in the left and right lower quadrants of the abdomen,
left greater than right, without rebound tenderness, masses or
distention.

LABORATORY DATA

Hemoglobin:	10.5 gm%
Hematocrit:	32%
White blood cell count:	5,800/mm^3
PMN's:	67%
lymphocytes:	31%
monocytes:	1%
eosinophiles:	1%
Sedimentation rate:	42 mm/hr
Serum:	
sodium:	140 meq/L
potassium:	4.7 meq/L
chloride:	104 meq/L
bicarbonate:	24 meq/L
creatinine:	0.5 mg%
SGOT:	22 units
alkaline phosphatase:	168 IU
total bilirubin:	0.6 mg%
direct bilirubin:	0.4 mg%
total protein:	6.6 gm%
albumin:	4.1 gm%
calcium:	9.4 mg%
glucose:	102 mg%
cholesterol:	158 mg%
prothrombin time:	11.5 seconds
carotene:	116 μg%
Urinalysis:	negative
Stool:	
culture:	negative
ova and parasites:	negative
Barium enema:	(Fig. 34.1)
Upper GI - small bowel series:	mild mucosal irregularity and dilatation of terminal 10 inches of ileum
Proctosigmoidoscopy:	erythema and increased friability up to 25 cm
Rectal biopsy:	(Fig. 34.2)

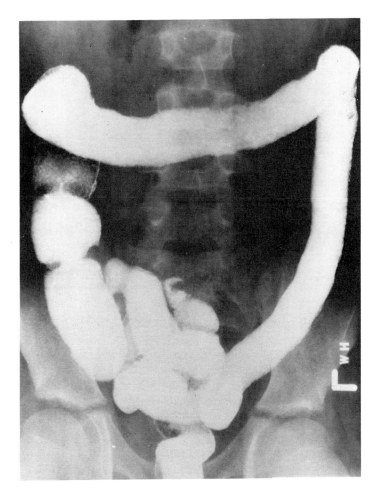

Figure 34.1   Barium enema.   Loss of haustration and the presence of fine spicules are seen throughout the large intestine.

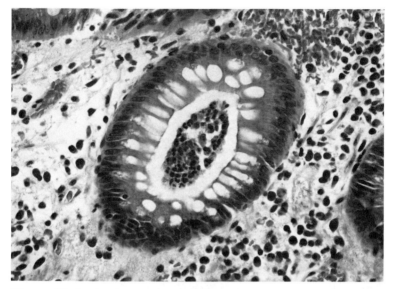

Figure 34.2 Rectum. Acute inflammatory cells have accumulated within a crypt of Lieberkuhn (H&E, X125).

QUESTIONS

1. Which findings would be compatible with the diagnosis of ulcerative colitis?
   A. Pallor of mucosa
   B. Fine venous patterns
   C. Dilatation of rectal lumen
   D. Friability of mucosa to cotton swabs
   E. Erythema of mucosa

2. Which histological features on rectal biopsy are compatible with ulcerative colitis?
   A. Many eosinophiles in lamina propria
   B. Absence of ganglion and myenteric cells of submucosal plexuses
   C. Granuloma(s) in mucosa or submucosa
   D. Absent or diminished goblet cells
   E. Crypt abscesses

3. On the basis of the data provided in answers to questions 1 and 2, which studies would be indicated at this time?
   A. Barium enema
   B. Abdominal ultrasonography
   C. Abdominal computerized tomography
   D. 99mPertechnectate radioisotope scan
   E. None of the above

4. Which measures would probably be indicated in the treatment of this patient?
   A. Milk-free diet
   B. Azulfidine
   C. Corticosteroids
   D. Azathioprine (Imuran)
   E. Surgery

5. Surgery would be indicated under which circumstances?
   A. Age of onset less than 10 years
   B. More than two relapses within first year after onset of symptomatology
   C. Unrelenting rectal bleeding
   D. Presence of pseudopolyps in colon
   E. Duration of disease more than 10 years and epithelial dysplasia of rectal mucosa

6. Which are correct statements regarding prognosis in ulcerative colitis?
   A. The chance of permanent remission after the first episode in children is better than in adults
   B. Regardless of extent of disease, life expectancy is good
   C. The possibility of universal colitis is 10 to 30%
   D. Rate of carcinoma development does not change after 10 years of disease
   E. Mortality rate after 15 years of disease is 15 to 20%

ANSWERS AND COMMENTS

1. (D,E) On sigmoidoscopic examination, the diagnosis of ulcerative colitis is suggested by the following findings: (1) erythema of the mucosa; (2) increased friability of the mucosa, spontaneous and to cotton swabbing; (3) loss or decrease of fine venous structure of the mucosa; (4) ulcerations, usually superficial and symmetrical in location; (5) granularity of the mucosa; (6) pseudopolyps (areas of remaining mucosa between areas of mucosal destruction). (1-6) In the milder forms of the disease, loss of the fine venous pattern, erythema and friability of mucosa

to cotton swabbing, e.g., cotton applicator, are usually the only abnormalities. (1-6) Later in the disease, granular ulcers and pseudopolyps are present. In the chronic state, the colonic configuration will be less flexible and the lumen is decreased. The mucosa may still have a granular appearance, although little else may be present. (3,4)

In Crohn's disease, the rectal mucosa usually appears normal or displays nonspecific findings, such as patchy erythema. However, induration and/or longitudinal, linear ulcerations may be present. An anal fissure, fistula, or abscess may be present. (7-9)

Answers A,B,C are normal findings or variants. They could be present in milder disease but would obviously not be diagnostic or even suggestive.

2. (D,E) Biopsies of the rectal mucosa should always be performed whenever inflammatory bowel disease is suspected. The histological features are essentially the same as in adults.

The histological features in ulcerative colitis are not specific; but in conjunction with the clinical history, X-ray examination, and findings of sigmoidoscopy (or colonoscopy), the diagnosis can be made. (1-7) In the acute phase, inflammatory changes of the mucosa and lamina propria are present. These include disruption of the epithelial (columnar) cell layer, infiltration of the lamina propria with polymorphonuclear leukocytes, as well as lymphocytes and plasma cells, and decreased goblet cell content (see Fig. 35.2). (3,4) The earliest and most typical feature of ulcerative colitis is the crypt abscess, the result of the accumulation of polys in the crypt of Lieberkuhn and the subsequent breakdown of the crypt wall. (3,4) However, this finding can be found in acute bacterial disease, e.g., Shigella, Salmonella, Campylobacter, Yersinia, the latter, more rarely (Y. enterocolitica) amebiasis, and Crohn's disease. (3,7-9) Varying degrees of mucosal destruction, ulceration, and subsequent pseudopolyp formation can be found. Submucosal and mucosal layer involvement can also occur in a smaller number of cases. (3,4,9) In a few cases, vasculitis is found, i.e., vessel wall thickening and thrombi. (3,4,9)

If the biopsy is performed in a more quiescent or healing phase, the inflammatory reaction is reduced and goblet cell content is lessened but present. (3,4,9) Thus, periodic biopsy can be helpful in determining severity of disease, response to therapy, and the presence or absence of epithelial dysplasia, a presumed precancerous change. (1-9)

Eosinophile content (A) can be found in allergic gastrointestinal states, e.g., cow's milk protein intolerance. Absence of ganglion cells (B) is most compatible with aganglionic megacolon

(Hirschsprung's disease). A granuloma (C) is found in certain inflammatory states, particularly Crohn's disease. The latter finding has rarely been reported in ulcerative colitis. (3,4,9)

3. (A) Pediatric patients with ulcerative colitis demonstrate essentially the same radiographic changes as adults. Early changes seem more likely to be present in children. (3,4,8-10) The early changes on barium enema include discrete mucosal abnormality, i.e., small indentations (mottling) and variable loss of haustration. (1-10) Somewhat later, superficial ulcerations (spiculations) of the mucosa may be visualized (see Fig. 35.1). (3,4,8,9) Later changes include thickening of the bowel wall, intestinal shortening, and pseudopolyp formation. (3,4,7-9) The endstage changes, including caliber reduction (lead-pipe colon), are particularly common in long-standing cases. In a few cases, actual stricture formation of segments can occur. In 95%+ of cases, the rectum is involved and the left side of the colon is involved in 60 to 80%. (1-11) The incidence of total colonic involvement has been variably reported, ranging from 10 to 70% of cases, most commonly 5-20%. (3) In 5 to 15% of cases, evidence of distal ileal involvement has been reported, i.e., dilatation and mucosal irregularity of the terminal 5 to 25 inches ("backwash ileitis").

The obvious value of the barium enema is the determination of the extent of disease beyond the reach of the sigmoidoscope, confirmation of the nature of disease, and the demonstration of complications of disease, e.g., stricture. (1-12) Adequate colonic cleansing is a necessity for visualizing the nature and extent of lesions. However, radiographic examination should not be performed in cases where toxic dilatation is suspected or unremitting rectal hemorrhage is present. (1-4,7-9) The increased use of colonoscopy has provided an adjunct, as well as an alternative, to the barium enema examination in determination of extent of disease and potential complications, e.g., stricture, dysplasia. (9,10)

Ultrasonography (B) and CT scan (C) would not be performed unless intra-abdominal extracolonic abnormalities are suspected. ^{99m}Pertechnetate scan (D) would be indicated in suspected cases of Meckel's diverticulum.

4. (B,C) Medication in the management of ulcerative colitis does not differ to any extent from that of Crohn's disease and is the same as in adults with these disease entities. The medication is designed mainly for its anti-inflammatory nature.

Sulfasalazine (Salazopyrin, salicylazosulfapyridine, Azulfidine) has been used in treatment for years. This drug combines a salicylate and a sulfonamide component. (13,14) In the colon, the microflora apparently split this drug. The sulfapyridine is absorbed and excreted in the urine, while 5-aminosalicylic acid is unabsorbed. Recently, the latter component has been suggested to be the main active component. (8) Side effects of this drug include anorexia, nausea, headache, and rash. (8,13,14) Side reactions include serum sickness-like illness, Heinz body hemolytic anemia, colitis, and agranulocytosis. (8,13,14) The side reactions are related not only to dose but also to hepatic acetylation, i.e., slow versus fast acetylator phenotypes. (8,9) Therefore, repeat laboratory examination of the white blood cell count and hemoglobin/hematocrit should be performed every 5 to 7 days for the first 4 to 8 weeks of treatment and every few weeks-to-months thereafter. Frequent checks are also necessary whenever the dose is increased. The initial dose is 1.0 to 1.5 gm daily (with meals) which is increased to 4 gm (infants, children) or 6 gm (adolescents) daily. After a period of 2 to 3 weeks, this loading dose is decreased to a maintenance dose of 1.5 gm (infants) to 2.0 gm (children, adolescents) daily. (8,9, 13,14) This dose is continued indefinitely in order to prevent recurrences. This drug is usually used alone in mild cases (less than 4 stools daily without systemic symptomatology, e.g., fever, weight loss) and in combination with corticosteroids (rectal, oral) in moderate or severe cases. (8,9) Lastly, recent reports have even linked exacerbation(s) of the disease to this drug. (9,15)

As previously mentioned, corticosteroids are used in moderate and severe cases. In severe cases, ACTH or corticosteroids (equal effectiveness) are administered parenterally, i.e., 40 units and 1-2 mg/kg/24 hr, respectively, for 7 to 10 days or until clinical improvement. (1,5,7-9,16) At this time, administration of oral steroids (prednisone, 2 mg/kg/24 hr) are begun and maintained at the same level for 4-6 weeks. The steroids are then reduced in a stepwise fashion; when the dose is 10 to 15 mg daily, Azulfidine treatment is begun. (13,14) Maintenance steroids, 5 to 15 mg/24 hr, are reserved for those cases in which other therapy fails to provide adequate clinical control. (3, 7-9) If future attempts to stop such treatment result in relapses, the choice then becomes long-term steroid administration or surgery, i.e., total colectomy and ileostomy. (7-9) Long-term administration of steroids can be daily, 5 to 15 mg, or on alternate days, 5 to 30 mg. (7-9,18)

However, maintenance steroids, i.e., prednisone, has not been demonstrated to prevent recurrences of adults in remission. (8,9) Corticosteroid retention enemas are particularly valuable in those cases limited to the left side of the colon, e.g., hydrocortisone retention enemas (Cortenema) twice daily for 7 to 10 days, then once daily. The results have been quite rewarding. (7-9,17)

A number of dietary measures have been attempted, including a low-fat diet, milk-free diet, and a low-residue diet. The response usually occurred within days. However, the beneficial value has usually been quite low, 10% or less. (7-9) In severely debilitated patients, oral or parenteral hyperalimentation may be helpful. With reference to oral alimentation, supplementation with either customary or elemental dietary agents, e.g., Vivonex, Travasorb, Precision Isotonic, may be remarkably effective in fecal volume reduction and provision of adequate caloric, protein, and micronutrient intake. In selected patients tube feedings of such elemental liquids can be accomplished, day or night (drip technique). If oral supplementation/intake fails, parenteral nutrition (TPN), peripheral (short-term, less than 2 weeks usually; supplement to oral intake) or central, will be necessary to deliver the needed caloric supply. Once again, especially with TPN, the results have been variable on a long-term basis, but have been encouraging on a short-term basis. (19,21) Home hyperalimentation offers potential long-term benefits. (8-20) Immunosuppressive agents, particularly azathioprine (Imuran), have been used on a temporary basis or chronically. Controlled studies have not demonstrated significant benefit alone or in combination with steroids. However, their use does permit a reduction in steroid dosage, particularly valuable in patients requiring long-term steroid administration for control. (7-9) The usual dose of azathioprine has been 1-2 mg/kg/24 hr.

The indications for surgery, i.e., colectomy/ileostomy or, more recently, colectomy/endorectal anastomosis, are (1) uncontrollable rectal bleeding, (2) perforation or imminent perforation, i.e., toxic dilation, (3) unresponsive fulminant colitis (few days of intensive treatment), (4) retardation of growth and sexual differentiation, (5) continued disease, markedly incapacitating in nature (poor or no response to medical therapy, 1 year or so), (6) disease duration over 10 years with evidence of epithelial dysplasia of the rectal mucosa. (7-9,22,23) The incidence of surgery within 5 years of disease onset has varied from 5 to 30%. (3,8,9)

Finally, other comments regarding treatment are necessary. Activity should be adjusted according to the clinical conditions of the patient. This would include play activity and schoolwork. Anticholinergics can be helpful in reducing dyschezia; opiates and Lomotil (diphenoxylate) are usually not necessary and are variably successful when used. The role of antibiotics, broad-spectrum in type, seems to be restricted to complications. Metronidazole (Flagyl) had promising results in small preliminary trials, but recent, larger trials have not demonstrated a beneficial result. (8) Oral disodium cromoglycate has demonstrated somewhat encouraging results in limited small series. (9,26) Counseling and/or psychotherapy can be quite helpful and are frequently indicated in order to modify environmental factors inducing added stress and to provide better understanding and acceptance of the patient's medical condition.

5.   (C,E) The indications for surgery have been outlined in answer 4.   In ulcerative colitis, surgery is truly curative, obviously a drastic but frequently necessary step.   Total colectomy and ileostomy or total colectomy and endorectal anastomosis remain the preferred surgical procedures.   Colectomy and ileorectal anastomosis in cases with mild to moderate rectal disease continues to be used, mainly in Europe, e. g. , France and England.   (9, 22, 23)   Recurrence of disease and cancer development remain concerns with this type of surgical approach. (9, 22, 23)   More recently, the "continent reservoir ileostomy" and "internal ileal reservoir" techniques have been favorably used in older children and adolescents.   (2, 22, 23, 27-30). Children have adapted quite well to surgical treatment.   A number of ostomy clubs and centers ro continued maintenance care exist successfully throughout the United States.

6.   (C,E)   (Also refer to page 281).   The long-term prognosis is difficult to ascertain on the basis of the severity or extent of the first episode.   In general, onset of disease in children is more severe than in adults.   Furthermore, the possibility of a complete, permanent remission in children is less than in adults, 10% in the latter. (8,9)

In children with milder disease or with distal colon involvement only, life expectancy is good. (8,9,31)   Conversely, total colon involvement (pancolitis) and/or severe disease is characterized by relapses and reduced life expectancy. (8,9,31)   However, more than 50% of pediatric patients respond well to medical treatment and have a normal life style. (8,9,22,23,31)

Those patients with disease limited to the rectosigmoid segment for at least 6 to 12 months have an excellent chance of the disease not extending further caudad, at least 80%. (3,8,9) Conversely, those patients with severe disease have a significant chance of universal colitis (pancolitis), 10 to 30%. (8,9)   The association of cancer of the colon and ulcerative colitis is well established, particularly in patients with disease originating in childhood and adolescence, i.e., 5% at 10 years of disease, 25% at 20 years (refer to case 33, answer 5). (8, 9, 32, 33)

Recent series have disclosed a five-year mortality rate of 15 to 20%. (9)   With more aggressive medical treatment and appropriately performed surgery, this figure should be reduced in the future.

REFERENCES

1. Binder, V., Bonnevie, O., Gertz, T.C., et al.: Ulcerative colitis in children: Treatment, course and prognosis. Scand J Gastroenterol 8:161, 1973.

2. Davidson, M., Bloom, A.A., Kugler, M.M.: Chronic ulcerative colitis of childhood. J Pediatr 67:471, 1965.

3. Ament, M.E.: Inflammatory disease of the colon: Ulcerative colitis and Crohn's colitis. J Pediatr 86:322, 1975.

4. Kirsner, J.B.: Clinical observations on inflammatory bowel disease. Med Clin North Am 53:1169, 1969.

5. Patterson, M., Castiglioni, L., Sampson, L.: Chronic ulcerative colitis beginning in children and teenagers: A review of 43 patients. Am J Dig Dis 16:289, 1971.

6. Wright, R.: Ulcerative colitis. Gastroenterology 58:875, 1970.

7. Grand, R.J. and Homer, D.R.: Approaches to inflammatory bowel disease in childhood and adolescence. Pediatr Clin North Am 22:835, 1975.

8. Cavel, B., Hildebrand, H., Meeuwisse, G.W., et al.: Chronic inflammatory bowel disease. Clin Gastroenterol 6:481, 1977.

9. Silverman, A., Roy, C.C.: Pediatric Clinical Gastroenterology, 3rd edition. The CV Mosby Company, St. Louis, 1983, p. 353.

10. Ein, S.H., Lynch, M.J., Stephens, C.A.: Ulcerative colitis in children under one year: A twenty-year review. J Pediatr Surg 6:264, 1971.

11. Farmer, R.G. and Brown, C.H.: Ulcerative proctitis: Course and prognosis. Gastroenterology 51:219, 1966.

12. Smith, A.H. and MacPhee, I.W.: A clinico-immunological study of ulcerative colitis and ulcerative proctitis. Gut 12:20, 1971.

296 / Case 34

13. Dissanayake, A.S. and Truelove, S.C.: A controlled therapeutic trial of long-term maintenance treatment of ulcerative colitis with sulphasalazine (salazopyrin). Gut 14:923, 1973.

14. West, B., Lendrum, R., Hill, M.J., et al.: Effects on sulphasalazine (salazopyrin) of faecal flora in patients with inflammatory bowel disease. Gut 15:969, 1974.

15. Schwartz, A.G., Targan, S.R., Saxon, A., et al.: Sulfasalazine-induced exacerbation of ulcerative colitis. N Engl J Med 306:409, 1982.

16. Truelove, S.C. and Jewell, D.P.: Intensive intravenous regimen for severe attacks of ulcerative colitis. Lancet 1:1067, 1974.

17. Misiewicz, J.J., Connell, A.M., Lennard-Jones, J.F., et al.: Comparison of oral and rectal steroids in the treatment of proctocolitis. Proc R Soc Med 57:561, 1964.

18. Sadeghi-Nejad, A. and Senior, R.: The treatment of ulcerative colitis in children with alternate-day corticosteroids. Pediatrics 43:840, 1969.

19. Truelove, S.C.: Ulcerative colitis provoked by milk. Br Med J 1:154, 1961.

20. Heird, W.C. and Winters, R.W.: Total parenteral nutrition: The state of the art. J Pediatr 86:2, 1975.

21. Vogel, C.M., Corwin, T.R., Bave, A.E.: Intravenous hyperalimentation in the treatment of inflammatory diseases of the bowel. Arch Surg 108:460, 1974.

22. Hamilton, J.R., Bruce, G.A., Abdourhaman, M., et al.: Inflammatory bowel disease in children and adolescents. Adv Pediatr 26:311, 1979.

23. Kelts, D.G., Grand, R.J.: Inflammatory bowel disease in children and adolescents. Curr Probl Pediatr 10:6, 1980.

24. Jewell, D.P. and Truelove, S.C.: Azathioprine in ulcerative colitis: Final report on controlled therapeutic trial. Br Med J 4:627, 1974.

25. Jones, R.A.: Larger doses of immunosuppressive drugs. Lancet 2:107, 1974.

26. Mani, V., Lloyd, G., Green, F.H.Y., et al.: Treatment of ulcerative colitis with oral disodium cromoglycate. A double-blind controlled trial. Lancet 1:439, 1976.

27. Frey, C.E. and Weaver, D.K.: Colectomy in children with ulcerative and granulomatous colitis. Arch Surg 104: 416, 1972.

28. Kock, N.G.: Continent ileostomy. Progr Surg 12:180, 1973.

29. Fonkalsrud, E.W.: Total colectomy and endorectal ileal pull-through with internal ileal reservoir for ulcerative colitis. Surg Gynecol Obstet 150:1, 1980.

30. Zwiren, G.T., Andrews, H.G., Caplan, D.G.: Total colectomy with ileo-endomuscular pull-through in the treatment of ulcerative colitis in children. J Pediatr Surg 16: 174, 1981.

31. Goel, K.M. and Shanks, R.A.: Long-term prognosis of children with ulcerative colitis. Arch Dis Child 48:337, 1973.

32. Broberg, O. and Lagercrantz, R.: Ulcerative colitis in childhood and adolescence. Adv Pediatr 14:9, 1966.

33. Devroede, G.J., Taylor, W.E., Sauer, W.G., et al.: Cancer risk and life expectancy of children with ulcerative colitis. N Engl J Med 285, 17, 1971.

Case 35

RECURRENT BLOOD IN BOWEL MOVEMENTS IN A 3-YEAR-OLD GIRL

HISTORY

A 3-year-old white female presented with a history of recurrent rectal bleeding, occurring every 1 to 2 days, for 7 weeks' duration. With each bowel movement, 1 tsp or more of blood would be seen, usually mixed with stool. Bowel movements occurred once or twice daily, maximum 3-4 per day, minimum one daily, without associated abdominal pain, fever, nausea, vomiting, skin lesions, apparent ocular difficulty, skin lesions, dysuria, or trauma. Appetite and activity remain unchanged. Hemoglobin and hematocrit determinations revealed apparent decrease from values at 1 and 2 years of age 12.5 and 12.2 gm/100 ml and 37 and 36%, respectively, to 9.0 and 9.2 gm/100 ml and 27 and 28%, respectively. The family history revealed a maternal grandfather with history of peptic ulcer disease and maternal grandmother with history of some type of colitis, now resolved, treatment unknown. The remainder of the past history, developmental history, family history, social history, and review of systems was unremarkable.

EXAMINATION

She was alert, active, and in no apparent distress, with normal vital signs, height 91 cm, weight 14.5 kg, head circumference 48 cm. The remainder of the examination was unremarkable, including abdomen and anorectal area. Anoscopic examination to 4 cm revealed no abnormalities.

LABORATORY DATA

Hemoglobin:	9.0 gm%
Hematocrit:	27.5%
Sedimentation rate:	9 mm/hr
Urinalysis:	negative
Stool:	
reducing substances:	negative
culture:	negative
ova and parasites:	negative
Serum:	
creatinine:	0.4 mg%
Barium enema:	possible lesion at 15 to 20 cm (polyp?)
Fiberoptic colonscopy:	(Fig. 35.1)
Colonic lesion - pathology:	(Fig. 35.2)

QUESTIONS

1. What is the probable diagnosis of this patient?
    A. Meckel's diverticulum
    B. Ulcerative colitis
    C. Colonic polyp
    D. Anal fissure
    E. Nodular lymphoid hyperplasia

2. What is the most common histological type in children?
    A. Adenomatous
    B. Lymphoid
    C. Hamartomatous
    D. Inflammatory (juvenile)
    E. Lipomatous

Questions 3 and 4: Answer true (T) or false (F).

3. This lesion is seen most commonly between 4 and 5 years of age.

4. Most of these defects present with vague abdominal discomfort.

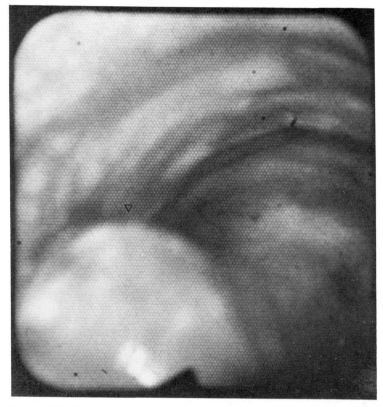

Figure 35.1 Colonoscopy. A round lesion (arrow) is seen in the descending colon.

5. Indicated studies for diagnosis include which of the following?
   A. Barium enema
   B. Proctosigmoidoscopy
   C. ^{99m}Pertechnetate isotope scan
   D. Visceral angiography
   E. Fiberoptic colonoscopy

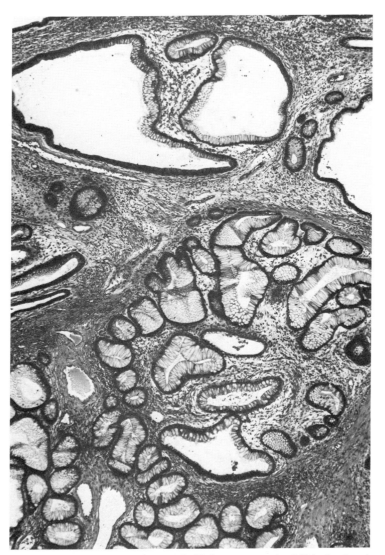

Figure 35.2   Colon. The epithelial component of this lesion is barely perceptible amidst the abundant connective tissue stroma. A single layer of columnar epithelial cells is present, however. Cystic spaces are numerous within the connective tissue stroma, which is infiltrated by a chronic inflammatory reaction (lymphocytes, plasma cells) (H&E, X250).

6. When such a lesion is discovered, it should be
    A. excised if within reach of the proctosigmoidoscope
    B. excised if easily accessible to the fiberoptic colonoscope
    C. excised by laparotomy if not accessible by proctosig-
        moidoscopy or fiberoptic colonoscopy
    D. excised by any means if there is a family history of
        polyposis
    E. never excised under any circumstances because of its
        benign nature

ANSWERS AND COMMENTS

1. (C) The radiographic examination, air-contrast barium enema, demonstrated a polyp in the sigmoid colon. No other lesions are demonstrated. The patient did not have fever, abdominal pain, diarrhea, growth retardation, pain with defecation, or
marked hematochezia. These findings would tend to rule out the
other possibilities.

2. (D) Inflammatory polyps are also termed retention or juvenile polyps. On gross appearance, they have a round or oval
configuration with a smooth surface and are attached to a thin
stalk. (1-6) Microscopically, the stalk is covered by normal
colonic mucosa. (1-6) The polyps are composed of a fibrous
stroma which is infiltrated by inflammatory cells, both acute
and chronic (round cells, polys). Throughout this stroma, there
are cystic spaces which are lined with mucus-secreting epithelial cells. (1-6) This composition has a branching cystic appearance. (1-6) The surface of the polyp does not have an epithelial
covering. (1-6) The epithelial changes do not have any sem-
blance of neoplastic activity. (1,3-6)

3. (T) Juvenile polyps are uncommon before 1 to 2 years of
age. The usual age range is 2 to 30 years, with 75 to 80% occurring in the first decade of life. (1-10) The maximum frequency occurs between 4 and 5 years of age. (1-10) There is a
slight male preponderance (3:2). (1-10)

4. (F) The predominant presentation is as bright red blood in
the stools (95-100%). (1-11) Usually the bleeding is mild and intermittent, on top of or mixed in with the stools. Usually the
bleeding has been present for at least one month before diagnosis, 55 to 60%. (1,3-6,8-11) Profuse bleeding is seen in 5 to
15% of cases, although exsanguination is rare. (1,3-6,8,11) Occult bleeding with anemia is equally uncommon. (1,3-6,8-11)
The hemoglobin level is usually above 11 gm% (85 to 95%).

Some juvenile polyps may have a long stalk, and prolapse through the rectum or even intussusception is possible. (1-11) Crampy abdominal pain may be associated in some cases. (1-11) A change in the bowel habit pattern (constipation or diarrhea) can occur and does so in a small percentage of cases. (1, 3-6, 8-11) Fever, vomiting, and growth disturbance do not occur.

Juvenile polyps have been found in siblings. (1-11) Yet, there is no significant increased familial incidence or apparent genetic predisposition. (1-11)

5. (A, B, E) The vast majority of juvenile polyps, 75 to 85%, are within the reach of the proctosigmoidoscope, one-half to two-thirds being within the first 10 cm. (1-11) These polyps can be excised through the proctosigmoidoscope in order to confirm their histological nature.

A barium enema should be performed in essentially all cases. Air-contrast or double contrast studies are more definitive than routine barium enemas. Unfortunately, most radiological units do routine barium enemas. The positive results of radiological examination in proven cases of juvenile polyposis range between 30 and 85%, usually 65 to 80%. (1-11) Usually juvenile polyps are solitary (65 to 70%). (1-11)

In those cases where the radiological examination is equivocal, negative, or demonstrates a lesion beyond the reach of the proctosigmoidoscope, fiberoptic colonoscopy is indicated. The latter procedure has been used with increasing frequency in children during the last 5 years. General anesthesia is usually required in younger children, while sedation with diazepam, meperidine, and promethazine or chlorpromazine may be satisfactory in older children and adolescents. The patient must be prepared adequately so that the colon is essentially free of contents. The fiberoptic colonoscope, such as the Olympus CF-MB (110 cm) or CF-LB (187 cm), is inserted and advanced under direct vision. Small amounts of air can be inserted in order to aid visualization. As the colonoscope is withdrawn, the mucosa is examined by moving the flexible tip of the instrument and twisting the instrument itself. Superficial biopsies can be taken, brush cytology performed, lavage cytology performed with sterile saline, and polyps of less than 3-4 cm in diameter, having a stalk or sessile in some cases, can be removed. Limiting factors include the size of the colonoscope (only adult instruments are available), adequacy of colonic cleansing for proper visualization, and experience of the endoscopist. (12-16) With increasing experience, this method of examination, as well as of treatment, may become as routine, efficient, and safe as in adults.

Furthermore, a recent report by Euler, et al. (17) emphasized that patients with a negative sigmoidoscopic examination,
as well as those with previous rectal polyps (polypectomy) and
recurrent hematochezia, should have fiberoptic colonoscopy performed, since the barium enema examination failed to demonstrate polyps in 5 of 14 patients. This author, however, must
sound a note of caution because of the cost-effectiveness and
morbidity of such procedures and considering the natural history
of juvenile polyps.

6. (A,B,D) Any polyp within the reach of the proctosigmoidoscope should be excised for examination. If histological examination confirms that it is of an inflammatory nature (juvenile),
and not adenomatous (tubular glandular), nothing else should be
done. If no lesions are seen at proctosigmoidoscopy, a barium
enema examination should be done. If this examination is negative or positive for a polyp, fiberoptic colonoscopy should be
performed if possible. If a lesion is found, removal should be
attempted if adequate control and experience of the endoscopist
permits. A snare loop is passed through the biopsy channel,
then opened, looped over the polyp, the loop closed, and the
stalk cauterized. The polyp is retrieved by suction and sent for
examination. All areas of the colon are within the possible
reach of the colonoscope. The morbidity is relatively low, although lacerations and perforations have been reported. (12-18)
The mortality is essentially zero. The procedure allows the diagnosis and treatment of an age group previously left alone or
subjected to laparotomy, the latter unwarranted for polyps of
benign nature. More conservative treatment is warranted unless intussusception is present, bleeding is excessive, or there
is a family history of polyposis (adenomatous) with malignant potential.

REFERENCES

1. Holgersen, L.O., Miller, R.E., Zintel, H.A.: Juvenile
polyps of the colon. Surgery 69:288, 1971.

2. Louw, J.H.: Polypoid lesions of the large bowel in children with particular reference to benign lymphoid polyposis. J Pediatr Surg 3:195, 1968.

3. Franklin, R. and McSwain, B.: Juvenile polyps of the colon and rectum. Ann Surg 175:887, 1972.

4. Mazier, W. P. , Bowman, H. E. , Ming Sun, K. , et al. : Juvenile polyps of the colon and rectum. Dis Colon Rectum

17:523, 1974.

5.   Harris, J. W. : Polyps of the colon and rectum in children. Dis Colon Rectum 10:267, 1967.

6.   Shermeta, A. W. , Morgan, W. W. , Eggleston, J. , et al. : Juvenile retention polyps. J Pediatr Surg 4:211, 1969.

7.   Bussy, H. J. R. : Gastrointestinal polyposis. Gut 11:970, 1970.

8.   Veale, A. M. O. , McColl, I. , Bussey, H. J. R. , et al. : Juvenile polyposis coli. J Med Genet 3:5, 1966.

9.   Smith, W. G. : Familial multiple polyposis. Dis Colon Rectum 11:17, 1968.

10. Duhamel, J. and Bauchel, P. : Polyps of the colon beyond the reach of the sigmoidoscope. Arch Dis Child 10:173, 1965.

11. Toccalino, H. , Gustavind, E. , DePini, F. , et al. : Juvenile polyps of the rectum and colon. Acta Paediatr Scand 62:337, 1973.

12. Deyhle, P. : Colonoscopy in the management of bowel disease. Hosp Pract 9:121, 1974.

13. Gans, S. , Ament, M. E. , Christie, D. , et al. : Pediatric endoscopy with flexible fiberscopes. J Pediatr Surg 10:375, 1975.

14. Liebman, W. M. : Fiberoptic endoscopy of the gastrointestinal tract in infants and children. II. Fiberoptic colonoscopy and polypectomy in 15 children. Am J Gastroenterol 68:452, 1977.

15. Cadranel, S. , Rodesch, P. , Peters, J. P. , et al. : Fiberendoscopy of the gastrointestinal tract in children. Am J Dis Child 131:41, 1977.

16. Gleason, W. A. , Jr. , Goldstein, P. D. , Shatz, B. A. , et al. : Colonoscopic removal of juvenile colonic polyps. J Pediatr Surg 10:519, 1975.

17. Douglas, J. R. , Campbell, C. A. , Salisbury, D. M. , et al. : Colonoscopic polypectomy in children. Br Med J 281:1386, 1980.

18. Daum, F. , Zucker, P. , Boley, S. J. , et al. : Colonoscopic polypectomy in children. Am J Dis Child 131:566, 1977.

Case 36

ALTERED BOWEL HABIT PATTERN IN A 4-YEAR-OLD BOY

HISTORY

A 4-year-old white male presented with a history of altered bowel habit pattern for approximately three years. Frequency of bowel movements had decreased to once every 2 to 3 days; stools were frequently hard, and there was associated anorectal discomfort at the time of defecation. There was occasional abdominal protuberance, firm and large in nature.

Diet had been variable but without change in its composition. Activity had been essentially unchanged. There was no associated history of abdominal pain, vomiting, anorexia, fever, diarrhea, melena, hematochezia, jaundice, dysuria, or trauma. Pertinent family history included maternal grandfather with peptic ulcer disease and sister with hay fever and bronchial asthma. The remainder of the past history, developmental history, family history, social history, and review of systems was unremarkable.

EXAMINATION

He was alert, cooperative, and in no distress, with normal vital signs, height 108 cm, weight 19 kg, and head circumference 52 cm. Examination was unremarkable except for definite abdominal protuberance, with no palpable masses or tenderness of liver, kidney, and spleen. Active bowel sounds were present with no bruits.

The anorectal evaluation revealed an intact perianal reflex, good external sphincter tone, and no masses or fissures. There was soft, brown stool, small in amount, in the distal rectal vault which did not feel narrowed. Stool hemoccult examination was negative.

LABORATORY DATA

Hemoglobin:	12.1 gm%
Hematocrit:	36%
White blood cell count:	7,400/mm^3
PMN's:	42%
lymphocytes:	56%
monocytes:	1%
eosinophiles:	1%
Urinalysis:	negative
Serum:	
total protein:	6.6 gm%
albumin:	4.6 gm%
SGPT:	19 units
alkaline phosphatase:	110 IU
creatinine:	0.6 mg%
carotene:	120 μg%
Plain films - abdomen:	feces in large intestine
Barium enema:	(Fig. 36.1)
Rectal biopsy:	(Fig. 36.2)

QUESTIONS

Questions 1-12: From the historical and radiological details answer true (T) or false (F).

1. The probable diagnosis is Hirschsprung's disease (aganglionic megacolon).

2. This disorder frequently occurs in the first decade of life.

3. This disorder is more frequent in females.

4. Diarrhea may be the initial presentation in some patients with this disorder.

5. Soiling never occurs in this disorder.

6. Radiological examination is usually specific for this disorder.

7. If this disorder is suspected, a prepared colon study must be performed.

8. Definitive diagnosis requires rectal biopsy.

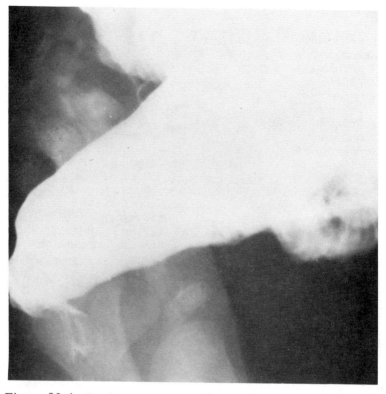

Figure 36.1   Barium enema. Irregular narrowed rectosigmoid segment with abrupt dilatation proximal to this narrowed region is shown.

9.   Short-segmental involvement is usually diagnosed by biopsy.

10.   80 to 90% of cases involve the rectum and rectosigmoid segment.

11.   Once the diagnosis is established, a trial of medical treatment is indicated.

12.   In infants less than 6 to 12 months of age, definitive surgical reconstruction is mandatory.

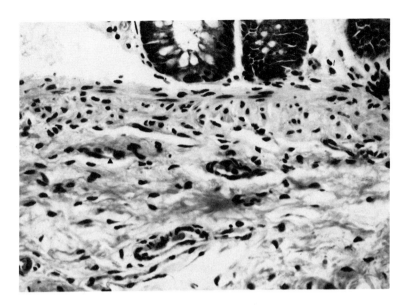

Figure 36.2   Rectum (7 cm from anal verge). Absence of ganglion cells in the submucosa (Meissner's plexus) and the presence
of hyperplastic nonmyelinated nerve fibers (arrow) are pictured
(H&E, X250).

ANSWERS AND COMMENTS

1.   (T) Hirschsprung's disease must be considered whenever
difficulties in defecation begin in the neonatal or early infantile
periods.

2.   (T) In fact, early onset of manifestations is the rule. Despite this continued emphasis, the diagnosis is often delayed, and
serious consequences, including death, can result. Estimated
mortality in the first year of life has been as high as 50%, principally due to secondary enterocolitis. (1-9) A recent review by
Tobon and Schuster (4) confirmed the onset of symptomatology
in 33 of 40 patients (83%) in the first month of life and in 38 of
40 (96%) in the first year. Furthermore, they emphasize that
the majority have discernible difficulty in defecation during the
first week of life.

3.   (F) A male preponderance (4:1) has been recognized since
the initial descriptions of this disorder. (1-9) However, long

segmental involvement is almost as common in females as in males. (1-9) Familial occurrence is low (4-5%). (6,9) Associated conditions include Down's syndrome, malrotation, and diaphragmatic hernia. (9)

4. (T) Occasionally a severe form of enterocolitis may develop, especially in infants, characterized by frequent watery stools, fever, abdominal distention, dehydration, and even shock. (1,5,7,9) This entity can develop at any age, however, and can occur before or after surgery. (1,5,7,9) The mortality can be quite high, 30 to 50%. The bowel itself displays both inflammatory and ischemic changes, leading to necrosis, even perforation. Sepsis is frequent. Careful and frequent clinical observation and radiological studies are paramount in appropriate management. Saline irrigations through a carefully positioned rectal tube remain the predominant form of treatment. (1,5,7,9)

5. (F) Many studies have stated that soiling (encopresis) does not occur in Hirschsprung's disease. (1-9) However, if the aganglionic involvement is limited to the internal sphincter or to a very short segment distally, soiling may result. (1-9)

6. (T) Plain radiographic films, anteroposterior and lateral abdominal views in particular, should be performed and will demonstrate the presence or absence of stool or gas in the rectal ampulla, as well as distention throughout the bowel. Thereafter, barium examination should be performed, even during the first few days of life. The radiographic findings will depend upon the extent of involvement, the tone of the areas above and below the junction of dilatation and stenosis, and the level at which the junction exists. In the usual case, the rectum and distal aspect of the sigmoid are narrowed, and there is abrupt dilatation of segments directly above this level, usually coinciding with the upper sacrum. (9-14) In cases of long segmental involvement, the rectum may appear normal with the remaining segments of involvement appearing narrowed. (9-14) The clinician must remember that in the neonatal period the radiological, as well as the clinical picture, may not be obvious. Five types of correlative radiographic and histological types have been defined: type I, the entire rectosigmoid segment being aganglionic but the proximal segment only being narrowed; type II, the entire aganglionic segment being narrowed; type III, stenosis only at the junction of the aganglionic and ganglionic segments; type IV, a lesser degree of stenosis at the aganglionic and ganglionic segments; and type V, two narrowed segments with an intervening dilated segment. (9-14) After the barium examination has

been completed, the diagnostic evaluation is not concluded, because an early and reliable sign of aganglionic megacolon is the
failure of evacuation of the barium enema, even on delayed examination at 24 to 48 hours. (1,9-14) This sign is particularly
valuable in neonates and young infants.

7. (F) If aganglionosis is suspected, an unprepared colon
study is indicated. The radiological examination depends upon
the demonstration of the transition from normal or narrowed
(aganglionic) to dilated colon (innervated). (1,9-14) With removal of fecal matter prior to the barium enema, the demonstration
of this transitional zone becomes more difficult. (1,9-14) As
previously described in answer 6, failure of evacuation 24 to 48
hours later is a valuable sign, as is the mixing of fecal matter
with barium. (1,9-14)

8. (T) The diagnosis of Hirschsprung's disease depends on
histological evidence and, in particular, on the absence of ganglion cells in the myenteric and submucosal plexuses. (1,3,8,9,
15-17) Thus, rectal biopsy is necessary. Many have employed
the rectal suction biopsy, using the multipurpose biopsy tube
(Quinton Instruments Company, Seattle, Washington), while others have continued to perform a full-thickness surgical biopsy
of the rectum. The former has advantages of ease, need for no
or only local anesthesia, reduced cost, and high accuracy. At
least two biopsies must be performed, a minimum of 3 cm from
the anal margin. These specimens should be processed like a
small intestinal biopsy. Multiple sections of each specimen
must be examined for the presence of ganglion cells in the submucosal plexus. (1,3,8,9,15-17) Examination for ganglion cells
in the myenteric plexus requires more experience and patience.
(1,3,8,9,15-19) Additionally, submucosal hyperplastic neural
elements will be present, except in newborns. The pathologist
must remember that the junctional area (1-2 cm in length) between the anus and rectum may have few or essentially no ganglion cells and must rely on an accurate assessment by the clinician as to a satisfactory site for biopsy.
    Other techniques of histological examination have incorpor-
ated cholinesterase histochemical staining, as well as the actual
measurement of acetylcholinesterase activity in the rectal biopsies. (15-17) Higher enzyme activity is found in biopsies of patients with aganglionosis. (15-17,19)

9. (F) The biopsy results depend upon the site of biopsy versus
the site of aganglionic involvement. In short segmental involvement, the usual site of biopsy, 3 to 5 cm from the anal margin,
contains ganglion cells. (1,3,5,8,9,15-19) The radiological

study is frequently equivocal or normal. (1,3,5,8,9-14) Fortunately, in 1968, Tobon, et al. (20) described a manometric technique for diagnostic use in Hirschsprung's disease. A double balloon instrument obtained simultaneous pressure readings from the internal and external anal sphincteric regions in response to rectal distention produced by a third balloon. (9,18) In normals, rectal distention produces contraction of the external anal sphincter and relaxation of the internal anal sphincter. In aganglionosis, there is contraction, rather than relaxation, of the internal sphincter. A note of caution must be that the experience of the investigator is paramount in achieving accurate recordings and interpretation, such as the 100% accuracy of Tobon and Schuster. (9,18-20) My own experience has been less satisfactory, specifically, 67% accuracy.

10. (T) Many series have documented the overwhelming preponderant involvement of the rectum and sigmoid areas, 80-90% to be exact. (1-9,21) More proximal involvement has been reported in 5 to 20% of cases, total colonic involvement being present in 1 to 5%. Short segmental involvement, usually the proximal rectum or distal sigmoid colon, comprises 1 to 5% of cases. (1-9,19) Involvement of only the internal anal sphincter is rare, 1%. (1,3,5,8,9)

11. (F) Once the diagnosis is established, surgical treatment is indicated. Medical treatment (including enemas, high-roughage diets, mineral oil or other types of laxatives) provides only temporary relief, and may be associated with an increased incidence of enterocolitis and with possible fluid and electrolyte disturbances as a complication of enemas, which are frequently necessary in the management. (1-9,22,23) Examples of the latter problem include water intoxication with tap-water enemas and hypernatremic dehydration, with and without hyperphosphatemia, after using hypertonic phosphate enemas, such as Fleet's. (23)

12. (F) In neonates and young infants (less than 6 to 12 months of age), a preliminary colostomy is performed (decompression). In those with a preliminary colostomy, a definitive reconstructive repair is performed at one year of age. (1,3,5,8,9,22,24-27) In older infants and children, a definitive repair is performed. (1,3,5,8,9,22,24-27) Three main, definitive operations are commonly used. These are (1) the Swenson operation, in which the aganglionic segment is resected and the ganglionic bowel is pulled down or through the pelvis and anastomosed to the anus; (2) the Soave operation, in which the bowel is transsected at the rectosigmoid junction, all aganglionic bowel rectum

is discarded, ganglionic bowel is brought down through the remaining rectal muscle layer, and anastomosis is performed just proximal to the dentate margin (mucosa to mucosa); and (3) the Duhamel operation, in which the rectum is transected as low as possible, the proximal aganglionic segment is resected, the retrorectal space is enlarged, ganglionic bowel is brought down through the retrorectal space, and an anastomosis is made (mucosa to mucosa); the posterior anastomosis is between ganglionic bowel and the anal canal, while the anterior anastomosis consists of the anal canal and the ganglionic bowel as well as the rectum and the ganglionic bowel superiorly. (22-24,26) Other procedures have and do include Martin's procedure (side-to-side anastomosis), Rehbein's procedure (deep anterior resection), posterior sphincterotomy, and rectal myotomy. (27-29) Good results have generally been obtained, ranging between 70 and 90%, i.e., correction of constipation and the lack of induced soiling (incontinence) or other problems. (1,3,5,8,9,22,27) The latter would include delayed bowel obstruction (2.2 to 4.4%), diarrhea (2 to 15%). (28-30)

REFERENCES

1. Ehrenpreis, T.: Hirschsprung's disease. Am J Dig Dis 16:1032, 1971.

2. Fraser, G.L. and Wilkinson, A.W.: Neonatal Hirschsprung's disease. Br Med J 3:7, 1967.

3. Nixon, H.H.: Hirschsprung's disease. Br J Hosp Med 5: 199, 1971.

4. Tobon, F. and Schuster, M.M.: Megacolon: Special diagnostic and therapeutic features. Johns Hopkins Med J 135: 91, 1974.

5. Corkery, J.J.: Hirschsprung's disease. Clin Gastroenterol 4:531, 1975.

6. Bodian, M. and Carter, C.O.: A family study of Hirschsprung's disease. Ann Hum Genet 26:261, 1963.

7. Bill, A.H., Jr. and Chapman, N.D.: The enterocolitis of Hirschsprung's disease. Am J Surg 103:70, 1972.

8. Howard, E.R.: Hirschsprung's disease: A review of the morphology and physiology. Postgrad Med J 48:471, 1972.

9. Roy, C.C., Silverman, A., Cozzetto, F.J.: Pediatric
   Clinical Gastroenterology, 2nd Edition. The CV Mosby
   Co., St. Louis, 1975, p. 799.

10. Franken, E.A., Jr.: Gastrointestinal Radiology in Pedi-
    atrics. Harper and Row, Hagerstown, 1975, p. 323.

11. Berman, C.Z.: Roentgenographic manifestations of con-
    genital megacolon (Hirschsprung's disease) in early in-
    fancy. Pediatrics 18:227, 1956.

12. Kilcoyne, R.F. and Taybi, H.: Conditions associated with
    congenital megacolon. Am J Roentgen Rad Ther Nucl Med
    108:615, 1970.

13. McDonald, R.G. and Evans, W.A., Jr.: Hirschsprung's
    disease: Roentgen diagnosis in infants. Am J Dis Child
    87:575, 1954.

14. Keefer, G.P. and Mokrohisky, J.F.: Congenital mega-
    colon (Hirschsprung's disease). Radiology 63:157, 1954.

15. Garrett, J.R. and Howard, E.R.: Histochemistry and the
    pathology of Hirschsprung's disease. Proc R Microscop
    Soc 4:76, 1969.

16. Gannon, B.J., Burnstock, G., Noblett, H.R., Campbell,
    P.E.: Histochemical diagnosis in Hirschsprung's disease.
    Lancet 1:894, 1969.

17. Boston, V.E., Dale, G., Riley, K.W.A.: Diagnosis of
    Hirschsprung's disease by quantitative biochemical assay
    of acetylcholinesterase in rectal tissue. Lancet 2:951,
    1975.

18. Kekomaki, M., Rapola, J., Louhimo, I.: Diagnosis of
    Hirschsprung's disease. Acta Paediatr Scand 68:893,
    1979.

19. Liebman, W.M.: Constipation and fecal incontinence in
    children: Clinical and therapeutic considerations. Post-
    grad Med 66:105, 1979.

20. Tobon, F., Reid, N.C.R.W., Talbert, J.L., Schuster,
    M.M.: Non-surgical test for the diagnosis of Hirsch-
    sprung's disease. N Engl J Med 278:188, 1968.

21. Meier-Ruge, W. : Das Megacolon. Seine Diagnose und Pathophysiologie. Virchows Archiv Abteilung A: Patholog Anat 344:67, 1968.

22. Swenson, O.: Congenital megacolon. Pediatr Clin North Am 14:189, 1967.

23. Moseley, P.K. and Segar, W.E.: Fluid and serum electrolyte disturbances as a complication of enemas in Hirschsprung's disease. Am J Dis Child 115:714, 1968.

24. Swenson, O. and Bill, A.H., Jr.: Resection of rectum and rectosigmoid with preservation of the sphincter for benign spastic lesions producing megacolon. Surgery 24: 212, 1948.

25. Soave, F.: Hirschsprung's disease: A new surgical technique. Arch Dis Child 35:38, 1960.

26. Duhamel, B.: A new operation for the treatment of Hirschsprung's disease. Arch Dis Child 35:38, 1960.

27. Thomas, C.G., Jr., Bream, C.A., DeConnick, P.: Posterior sphincterotomy and rectal myotomy in the management of Hirschsprung's disease. Ann Surg 171:796, 1970.

28. Ott, W.R., Joppich, I.: Late postoperative complications in Hirschsprung's disease. Z Kinderchir 32:115, 1981.

29. Holschneider, A.M. (Ed): Hirschsprung's Disease. Hippokrates Verlag, Stuttgart; Thieme-Stratton, Inc. , New York, 1983, p. 189.

30. Khan, D., Nixon, H.H.: Results following surgery for Hirschsprung's disease: A review of three operations with a reference to neorectal capacity. Br J Surg 67:436, 1980.

Case 37

ANAL PAIN AND CONSTIPATION IN A 4-YEAR-OLD BOY

HISTORY

A 4-year-old white male presented with a history of anorectal
pain, crying with bowel movements, and decreased frequency of
bowel movements, now every 3-7 days, since the age of 20
months. The pertinent prior history revealed harder bowel
movements every 1-3 days since 4 to 6 weeks of age, requiring
the initial usage of Maltsupex, as much as 1 tbsp daily, until almost one year of age. Softer bowel movements, occurring every
one to two days, were produced by this regimen. In addition, increased irritability, decreased appetite and activity, with variable abdominal protuberance, accompanied the present clinical
pattern. Prior medication included Senokot and mineral oil without effect. However, consistent usage of this medication with
appropriate adjustments had not occurred. There was no history
of blood in the stools, abdominal pain, nausea, vomiting, or fever.

The family history included a mother with history of constipation in early childhood, surgery for possible anal fissure, and
maternal grandfather with history of peptic ulcer disease.

EXAMINATION

He was alert, height 103.5 cm and weight 18.9 kg, with normal
vital signs. The remainder of the examination, including the
abdomen, was unremarkable. At the time of examination, anoscopy was negative.

LABORATORY DATA

Hemoglobin:	12.8 gm%
Hematocrit:	38%
White blood cell count:	8,100/mm^3
PMN's:	42%
lymphocytes:	52%
monocytes:	4%
eosinophiles:	2%
Urinalysis:	negative
Stool:	
occult blood:	negative
reducing substances:	negative
Barium enema:	dilated colon with feces

QUESTIONS

1. What is the most likely diagnosis of this patient?
    A. Celiac disease
    B. Regional enteritis
    C. Ulcerative colitis
    D. Aganglionic megacolon (Hirschsprung's disease)
    E. Fecal retention syndrome

Question 2: Answer true (T) or false (F).

2. The most common cause of constipation/fecal retention in children is Hirschsprung's disease.

3. Factors implicated in functional fecal retention include
    A. anal canal disease
    B. patient's developmental stage
    C. medication
    D. toilet training experience
    E. all of the above

4. Symptoms commonly associated with fecal retention include
    A. inactivity
    B. anorexia
    C. abdominal pain
    D. irritability
    E. none of the above

5. Studies indicated in evaluation of this patient include
   A. history, physical examination
   B. family interview
   C. barium enema
   D. anorectal manometry
   E. rectal biopsy

6. Treatment of this patient (and condition) should include
   A. parental counseling
   B. initial colonic cleansing
   C. stool softener
   D. stimulant cathartic
   E. surgery

ANSWERS AND COMMENTS

1. (E) Fecal retention syndrome (functional) is the most likely diagnosis. It is characterized mainly by the passage of enormous stools every few days to 1-2 weeks. This stool passage
will usually obstruct the toilet. With fecal accumulation, various postures, e.g., crossing legs, squatting in the corners, are
assumed.

The presence of constipation, the age of onset (1-1/2 years),
and normal growth and development would make Hirschsprung's
disease and celiac disease less likely. The lack of diarrhea, hematochezia, fever, and growth retardation make regional enteritis and ulcerative colitis less likely.

2. (F) The most common cause of constipation/fecal retention
is functional or idiopathic, accounting for 80 to 90% of cases.
(Tables 37.1 and 37.2). (1-8) The remainder of cases include
Hirschsprung's disease (1 to 5%), intestinal pseudo-obstruction
syndrome, endocrine, metabolic, and pharmacologic disorders,
e.g., hypothyroidism, codeine-containing analgesics, intestinal
smooth muscle disorders, e.g., scleroderma and anal/rectal
stenosis. (2-5)

3. (E) The functional fecal retention syndrome is infrequently
due to a single cause, but usually to a constellation of factors.
These factors include (1) lack of parental comprehension of a
normal or regular bowel habit pattern, i.e., once every 3 to 4
days to 3 to 4 stools daily; (2) infant's temperament, variable
fussiness and parental response thereto; (3) anal canal disease,
producing pain; (4) developmental stage, which will influence patient's understanding of defecation and the parental response to
his or her efforts; (5) quality of the parent-child relationship,

TABLE 37.1   Classification of Constipation

I.   Fecal Retention:

   A.   Organic:

      1. Hirschsprung's disease
      2. Hyperparathyroidism
      3. Hypothyroidism
      4. Intestinal pseudo-obstruction
      5. Anal/rectal stenosis
      6. Medication, e.g., phenothiazines
      7. Lead poisoning (chronic)
      8. Abdominal muscle defect
      9. Scleroderma (rare in children)

   B.   Functional

II.   No Fecal Retention:

   A.   Organic:

      1. Cryptitis, proctitis
      2. Anal fissure
      3. Inadequate dietary bulk

Modified from Liebman. (4)

i.e., understanding of parents and ability to respond in a comforting, helpful manner; (6) the cultural background of the parents, as well as experience; and (7) socioeconomic environment, e.g., marital discord, separation, or divorce, parental illness, financial matters. (2-4,8-12) Comfort, security, lack of preoccupation with bowel habits, or use of excessive force, punishment, and/or anxiety are necessary to ensure a normal bowel movement pattern. (1-11)

4. (E) With continued, increasing fecal accumulation, certain symptomatology occurs with relative frequency. Symptomatology includes (1) posturing, e.g., crossing of lower extremities, squatting; (2) irritability; (3) decreased play activity; (4) recurrent abdominal pain, variable in intensity, frequency, duration and location; (5) decreased appetite; (6) less so, nausea; and (7) infrequently, emesis. (2-6,8,11) In addition, pallor is described

TABLE 37.2 Differences Between Hirschsprung's Disease and
Fecal Retention Syndrome

	Hirschsprung's Disease	Fecal Retention Syndrome
Age of onset	Usually less than 3-6 months	Usually over 1-1/2 years
Symptoms	Constipation, anorexia, poor nutrition and growth, and variable nausea, vomiting. Essentially no soiling. Abdominal distention	Constipation, anorexia variable nausea, vomiting. Frequent soiling. Variable abdominal distention
Anorectal examination	Usually empty rectal ampulla	Usually full rectal ampulla
Barium enema examination	Dilated proximal colon; narrowed distal segment of colon; poor evacuation	Colon dilatation with feces throughout; good evacuation
Rectal biopsy	Absence of ganglion cells (submucosa, myenteric)	Ganglion cells present (submucosa, myenteric)
Anorectal manometry	Failure of internal sphincter relaxation	Normal
Treatment	Surgery	Medical

in 10 to 25%, while gross blood (stripes, spots) is found in only 5 to 10%. (8,11) In essentially every series, 1 to 5% of patients have had associated enuresis, too. (4,8,11) Diagnostic evaluation of this latter symptom has usually been unrevealing as to a specific organic basis. (8,11) A positive family history of constipation has been found in 15 to 35% of cases. (1-8,11)

5. (A,B) The most important aspect of evaluation of constipation is the clinical history. As alluded to in other answers, an appropriate history must include data regarding (1) parental concern and attitudes about bowel habits and irregularities,

(2) parental idea of an appropriate toilet training program, (3) parental interrelationships, (4) family illness or death, (5) school performance and peer interrelationships, (6) ethnic derivation and idiosyncrasies. The physical examination is usually of limited value, although abdominal protuberance, palpable fecal matter in the abdomen, especially the left lower quadrant, presence or absence of fecal matter in the rectal ampulla, assessment of external anal sphincter tone, presence or absence of the perianal reflex, caliber of the rectal ampulla, and appearance of the perianal area may possibly be helpful. As previously mentioned, one or more family interviews are necessary to ascertain the psychosocial milieu of the patient, correct improper attitudes, provide counseling and support, and form a strong link for continued dialogue and trust.

Further diagnostic studies are frequently indicated in those patients with onset before 6 to 12 months of age, failure to thrive, associated systemic disease, or musculoskeletal anomaly (Table 37.3). The barium enema is a cornerstone of diagnosis under such circumstances. The presence of an area or areas of narrowing, malrotation, or inflammation, as well as size (diameter) of the colon, is assessed. If Hirschsprung's disease cannot be excluded, a rectal biopsy should be considered. The author has used the suction biopsy technique, employing the Quinton tube and rectal capsule, and found this technique to be satisfactory for determining the presence or absence of ganglion cells in the submucosa. Special stains or even assay of acetylcholinesterase activity can be used to augment histological examination. (2-5,8,11-14)

If ganglion cells are absent, a full-thickness surgical biopsy is indicated. (4,8,11) If short-segmental or internal sphincter involvement is suspected, the barium enema examination and rectal suction biopsy may be nondiagnostic. In these cases (1-10%), anorectal motility study may be of value. (15,16) A modified technique of Tobon, et al. (15) can be used. In those patients with Hirschsprung's disease, failure of internal anal sphincter relaxation with rectal balloon distention is diagnostic. (15,16) However, adequate experience with this technique is mandatory for its satisfactory performance and interpretation.

This patient's age of onset, presence of adequate growth and development, and physical examination findings would mediate against the performance of those procedures listed as C, D, E.

6. (A, B, C) The management of apparently nonorganic constipation/fecal retention requires most importantly an empathetic, available, and patient physician. The physician must identify, understand, and then explain to the parents the psychological and physical factors that are responsible for their child's

TABLE 37.3   Diagnostic Evaluation

A. Common

   1. Complete blood count
   2. Stools for occult blood, culture, ova and parasites
   3. Glucose
   4. Sedimentation rate
   5. Calcium, phosphorus
   6. Barium enema
   7. Rectal suction biopsy
   8. Anorectal manometry

B. Less Common

   1. Proctosigmoidoscopy
   2. Upper gastrointestinal/small bowel series
   3. Colonoscopy

C. Uncommon

   1. Skull series
   2. Electroencephalogram
   3. Myelogram
   4. Surgery

problem. Specific steps in treatment must be carefully prepared and then explained to the parents and child, as possible. The problem is stressed as being unacceptable, not the child, since the self-worth of the child must be preserved. The solution to the problem must be consistent yet reasonable.

The medical treatment of constipation should consist of an initial cleansing of the fecal mass and/or impaction. Usually enemas will be required, e.g., pediatric Fleet's. These enemas can be administered every hour, 2 or 3 times, in the evening. The dose is 1/2 to 1 ounce per 10 lbs of body weight. (2, 4, 8, 11, 17-21) Two to 4 days constitute the usual duration of administration. After this phase of treatment, an orally administered laxative, i.e., stool softener/lubicant, should be initiated. Taste and age of the patient are important considerations in laxative choice. Acceptable agents include mineral oil, mineral oil/flavored (Neo-cultol, chocolate), mineral oil plus dioctyl sodium sulfosuccinate (Milkinol), dioctyl sodium sulfosuccinate (Colace). Stimulant cathartics (D), e.g., cascara sagrada, castor oil, should be avoided. (2,4,11) The effective dose is frequently 2 or 3 times the recommended amount, e.g., mineral oil, 1 or more tablespoonfuls daily. (4) The goal is 2 to 4 looser bowel movements daily. Thereafter, the amount is reduced until 1 to 2, soft to firm, bowel movements are achieved. Continued adjustments are necessary to maintain this pattern. Ultimately, a gradual reduction in dose over weeks to months is accomplished. These adjustments will require frequent telephone contact and occasional, brief outpatient visits. In addition, the child is encouraged to have regular potty or toilet periods. There must be firm support for the feet on the floor or on a stool.

In a few cases, where significant emotional factors are identified, referral to a clinical psychologist or psychiatrist may be indicated. The purpose of this referral must be clearly defined for the family.

Biofeedback involves the use of an instrument which provides information regarding physiological mechanisms of a patient so that the patient may learn to control these mechanisms. Therefore, voluntary control of some or all of these mechanisms can occur through biofeedback techniques. (22-24) These techniques have been applied with reasonable success to constipation, as well as incontinence (soiling). The biofeedback techniques involve initial anorectal manometry, confirmation of sensation of rectal distention with the balloons, adequate patient cooperation, and then conditioning sessions, e.g., external anal sphincter contraction and increased pressure. Positive results, specifically, significant improvement or cure, have been noted in 50 to 75% of cases. (22,23,25)

Regardless of the total treatment plan, a patient, understanding, and available physician must be involved in management in a consistent manner.

Surgery (E) is rarely, if ever, necessary in treatment of constipation/fecal retention syndrome.

REFERENCES

1. Clayden, G.S.: Constipation and soiling in childhood. Br Med J 1:515, 1976.

2. Mercer, R.D.: Constipation. Pediatr Clin North Am 14: 175, 1967.

3. Fleisher, D.R.: Diagnosis and treatment of disorders of defecation in children. Pediatr Ann 5:700, 1976.

4. Liebman, W.M.: Constipation and fecal incontinence in 123 children: Clinical and therapeutic considerations. Postgrad Med 66:105, 1979.

5. Schnaufer, I., Kumer, A.P.M., White, J.J.: Differentiation and management of incontinence and constipation problems in children. Surg Clin North Am 50:895, 1970.

6. Davidson, M., Kugler, M.M., Bauer, O.H.: Diagnosis and management in children with severe and protracted constipation and obstipation. J Pediatr 62:261, 1963.

7. Bently, J.F.R.: Progress report. Constipation in infants and children. Gut 12:85, 1971.

8. Fitzgerald, J.F.: Difficulties with defecation and elimination in children. Clin Gastroenterol 6:283, 1977.

9. Bell, A.I. and Levine, M.I.: The psychologic aspects of pediatric practice. I. Causes and treatment of chronic constipation. Pediatrics 14:259, 1954.

10. Spock, B. and Bergen, M.: Parents' fear of conflict in toilet training. Pediatrics 34:112, 1964.

11. Silverman, A., Roy, C.C.: Pediatric Clinical Gastroenterology, 3rd edition. The CV Mosby Co., St. Louis, 1983, p. 392.

12. Keokami, M., Rapola, J., Louhimo, I.: Diagnosis of Hirschsprung's disease. Acta Paediatr Scand 68:893, 1979.

13. Campbell, P.E. and Noblett, H.R.: Experience with rectal suction biopsy in the diagnosis of Hirschsprung's disease. J Pediatr Surg 4:410, 1969.

14. Alridge, R.T. and Campbell, R.E.: Ganglion cell distribution in the normal rectum and anal canal. J Pediatr Surg 3:475, 1968.

15. Tobon, F., Reid, N., Talbert, J., et al.: Nonsurgical test for the diagnosis of Hirschsprung's disease. N Engl J Med 278:188, 1968.

16. El Shaffie, M., Suzuki, H., Schnaufer, I., et al.: A simplified method of anorectal manometry for wider clinical application. J Pediatr Surg 7:230, 1972.

17. Duthie, H.L.: Progress report. Anal continence. Gut
     12:844, 1971.

18. Hata, Y., Duhamel, M., Pages, R., et al.: Megarectum
     de l'enfnat. Ann Chir Infant 15:65, 1974.

19. Fitzgerald, J.F.: Encopresis, soiling, constipation: What's
     to be done? Pediatrics 56:348, 1975.

20. Benson, J.A., Jr.: Simple chronic constipation. Post-
     grad Med 57:55, 1975.

21. Lawson, J.O.N. and Clayden, G.S.: Physiological as-
     pects and treatment of severe chronic constipation. Arch
     Dis Child 49:245, 1974.

22. Wald, A.: Biofeedback therapy for fecal incontinence. Ann
     Int Med 95:146, 1981.

23. Olness, K., McFarland, F.A., Piper, J.: Biofeedback:
     A new modality in the management of children with fecal
     soiling. J Pediatr 96:505, 1980.

24. Orne, M.T.: The efficacy of biofeedback therapy. Ann
     Rev Med 30:489, 1979.

25. Sondheimer, J.M., Gervaise, E.P.: Lubricant versus
     laxative in the treatment of chronic functional constipation
     of children: A comparative study. J Pediatr Gastroenterol
     Nutr 1:273, 1982.

Case 38

ACUTE DIARRHEA, ABDOMINAL PAIN, AND BLOOD
IN STOOLS IN A 27-MONTH-OLD BOY

HISTORY

A 27-month-old white male presented with an 8-day history of
diarrhea, associated abdominal pain, and infrequent bright red
blood streaks within the bowel movements. In addition, there
was associated intermittent low-grade fever, up to 101°F orally,
generalized malaise, and decreased appetite. The diarrhea consisted of 5-8 loose to watery bowel movements daily, infrequently containing mucus with streaks of bright red blood. The abdominal pain was midabdomen in location, and was associated
or not associated with bowel movements. Defecation frequently
relieved the pain.

   Prior to the presenting complaint, the patient had had altered bowel habit pattern of 5-6 months' duration. The bowel
movements had become harder, occurring every 4-5 days, in
comparison to previous ones of every 2-3 days. In addition,
there was associated lower abdominal discomfort preceding the
bowel movements and generally relieved by having a bowel
movement. There was a 2-month history of apparent, sudden,
lancinating, anorectal discomfort, both associated and not associated with these bowel movements. There was no history of
hematemesis, melena, diarrhea, nausea, vomiting, or anorexia. Appetite had been unchanged. Social history was unremarkable. The pertinent family history included father with history
of apparent spastic colon and maternal grandmother with history
of diverticulitis. Treatment included mineral oil, 3 tsp maximum daily, without relief.

EXAMINATION

He was small, alert, cooperative, and in no distress, with normal vital signs. Weight was 12.2 kg and height 91 cm. The remainder of the examination was unremarkable, including the abdomen, anus, and rectum.

LABORATORY DATA

Hemoglobin:	12.2 gm%
Hematocrit:	37%
White blood cell count:	7,400/mm^3
PMN's:	38%
lymphocytes:	58%
monocytes:	3%
eosinophiles:	1%
Urinalysis:	negative
Serum:	
total protein:	6.0 gm%
albumin:	4.2 gm%
SGOT:	20 units
SGPT:	18 units
alkaline phosphatase:	170 IU
carotene:	135 μg%
folate:	11 ng/ml
IgG:	570 mg%
IgA:	32 mg%
IgM:	80 mg%
Barium enema:	negative
Proctoscopy:	negative except for a small rent at 1 cm from anal verge, 6 o'clock position
Rectal biopsy:	negative

QUESTIONS

Question 1: Answer true (T) or false (F).

1. Anal fissure is the most common cause of blood in the stools
    in childhood.

2. Which age group is most commonly affected by this disorder?
   A. Newborns
   B. 2 months to 2 years
   C. 2 to 5 years
   D. 5 to 10 years
   E. 10 to 15 years

3. Which are the predominant manifestations of this disorder?
   A. Melena
   B. Occult blood in stools
   C. Discomfort with stools
   D. Diarrhea
   E. Bright red blood on top of stools

4. The diagnosis is confirmed by which studies?
   A. Anal examination
   B. Sedimentation rate
   C. Barium enema
   D. Anoproctoscopy
   E. Colonoscopy

5. The treatment of this disorder includes
   A. stool softener, such as dioctyl sodium sulfosuccinate
   B. digital anal sphincter dilatation
   C. Azulfidine
   D. topical anesthetic agent
   E. sitz baths

ANSWERS AND COMMENTS

1. (T) The most common cause of hematochezia in infants and children is anal fissure. (1-5) The blood is usually small in amount, bright red in color, and usually appears on the outside of the stool, most commonly as a stripe or spots. In addition, a drop or two of blood may be seen on the diaper or in the toilet bowl.

2. (B) The predominant age of involvement is postneonatal, 2 months of age to 2 years of age. There is still a significant percentage of cases up to 5 years of age, but it is uncommon thereafter. (1-5) It is infrequent in older children or teenagers. In the latter group, consideration of special types of proctitis, e.g., herpes simplex (HSV; homosexual males) should not be forgotten. (6)

3. (C,E) The infant or younger child will cry with defecation and will attempt to withhold feces. He may be irritable with possible abdominal discomfort ("colic"). Tenesmus may also be present. Small amounts of bright red blood will begin to appear with defecation, on top of the stools, on the diaper or toilet paper and possibly 1 or 2 drops in the toilet bowl immediately after defecation. (1-5)

4. (A,D) The most important diagnostic study is direct examination of the anal canal. To aid the examination, the patient can be placed in a knee-chest or left lateral position (Sims position) to allow visualization of the mucocutaneous region. Anterior, lateral, and usually more than one tear are most commonly deomonstrated. An increased incidence of posterior tears are seen in older children. (1,3,4,7) If no lesion is demonstrated, a digital examination is performed. Lastly, an anoproctoscopy should be performed if further localized examination is negative, and the clinical history is suggestive. For the performance of anoproctoscopy in infants and younger children, sedation may be necessary. This sedation can be chloral hydrate orally, 30 to 60 minutes before examination, or parenteral medication, such as diazepam, meperidine, phenergan, or chlorpromazine (0.4-1.0 mg/kg). A pediatric proctoscope should be used. If one is not available, an otoscope with a large speculum can be used with confidence. The use of a test tube and light source cannot be recommended.

5. (A,B,D,E) Anal fissures should be treated promptly and vigorously. Because constipation is frequently present, further augmenting formation of and persistence of fissures, the treatment should consist of (1) stool softening with agents, such as dioctyl sodium sulfosuccinate, 5-10 mg/kg/day, administered with feedings, (2) gentle anal dilatation by the mother with a finger cot 2 or 3 times daily, (3) topical anesthetic ointment with anesthetic and/or anti-inflammatory agent(s), e.g., xylocaine, Anusol® , and Proctofoam® with or without hydrocortisone, after each bowel movement or 2 to 4 times daily, (4) sitz bath after each bowel movement in older infants and toddlers. (1-12) If there is accompanying external irritation (erythema), caution must be exercised with reference to topical anesthetic agents due to the potential of local sensitization. Usually a minimum of 2 to 3 weeks of treatment must be expected before satisfactory healing. If there is essentially no response to the previously mentioned regimen within 4 to 6 weeks, cauterization with silver nitrate (0.5%) or other agent must be contemplated. Uncommonly, surgery will be necessary, especially when the fissure lies within scar tissue, presumably due to an accompanying cryptitis. (1,3,4,8,10)

Surgery is reserved for infrequent, resistant cases and for complications, e.g., extension.

REFERENCES

1. Silverman, A., Roy, C.C.: Pediatric Clinical Gastroenterology, 3rd edition. The CV Mosby Co., St. Louis, 1983, p. 413.

2. Mercer, R.D.: Constipation. Pediatr Clin North Am 14: 175, 1967.

3. Duhamel, J. and Ngo, Q.B.: Anal fissures in children: Report of 100 cases. Arch Fr Pediatr 24:1131, 1970.

4. Arminski, T.C. and McLean, D.W.: Proctologic problems in children. J Am Med Assoc 194, 1195, 1965.

5. The Roche Handbook of Differential Diagnosis: Constipation. Hoffman-LaRoche, Inc., Nutley, New Jersey, 1970, p. 5.

6. Goodell, S.E., Quinn, T.C., Mkrtichian, E., et al.: Herpes simplex virus proctitis in homosexual men. Clinical, sigmoidoscopic, and histopathological features. N Engl J Med 308:868, 1983.

7. Brash, I.M.: Examination of the proctologic patient. Pract Gastroenterol 4:36, 1980.

8. Bentley, J.F.R.: Constipation in infants and children. Gut 12:85, 1971.

9. Fleisher, D.R.: Diagnosis and treatment of disorders of defecation in children. Pediatr Ann 5:699, 1976.

10. Ellison, F.S.: Anal fissure occurring in infants and children. Dis Colon Rectum 3:161, 1960.

11. Benson, J.A., Jr.: Constipation: A stage of arrested motion. Warren-Teed GI Tract 4:4, 1974.

12. Schapiro, S.: Proctologic conditions in children: A pictorial review. Hosp Med 5:53, 1969.

Case 39

RECURRENT ABDOMINAL PAIN IN A 10-YEAR-OLD GIRL

HISTORY

A 10-year-old white female presented with a history of recurrent abdominal pain of 3 months' duration. It was sharp to gnawing in nature, occurring every 1-2 days, without association
with meals, food types, time of day, position, and/or bowel movements. There was infrequent nausea but no vomiting, fever, anorexia, diarrhea, constipation, dysuria, skin lesions or trauma. Her appetite and activity remained unchanged. The family
history included a brother and sister with bronchial asthma. The
remainder of the past history, developmental history, family
history, social history, and review of systems was noncontributory. Ethnic derivation was English. There had been no related
trips outside of her area of residence, a big city, during the preceding 2 years.

EXAMINATION

She was in no apparent distress, with normal vital signs, weight
31.8 kg, height 137 cm. The remainder of the examination, including the abdomen, was negative.

LABORATORY DATA

Hemoglobin:	12.5 gm%
Hematocrit:	36%
White blood cell count:	6,600/mm^3
PMN's:	55%
lymphocytes:	40%
monocytes:	3%

eosinophiles:	2%
Serum:	
sodium:	138 meq/L
potassium:	4.2 meq/L
chloride:	104 meq/L
bicarbonate:	23 meq/L
total protein:	6.8 gm%
albumin:	4.7 gm%
SGOT:	23 units
alkaline phosphatase:	105 IU
creatinine:	0.4 mg%
carotene:	132 μg%
calcium:	9.6 mg%
Urinalysis:	negative
Stool:	
occult blood:	negative
reducing substances:	negative
culture:	negative
ova and parasites:	negative
Barium enema:	negative
Upper GI - small bowel series:	negative
IVR:	negative
Oral cholecystogram:	negative
Fiberoptic upper endoscopy:	negative
Duodenal biopsy:	
histology:	negative except for the presence of a protozoan agent (Fig. 39.1)

QUESTIONS

1. The most likely diagnosis of this patient is
   A. duodenal ulcer
   B. Meckel's diverticulum
   C. ulcerative colitis
   D. giardiasis
   E. celiac disease

Questions 2 and 3: Answer true (T) or false (F).

2. Man is the only host and reservoir for this agent.

3. Widespread variability in symptomatology and geographic distribution characterizes this agent.

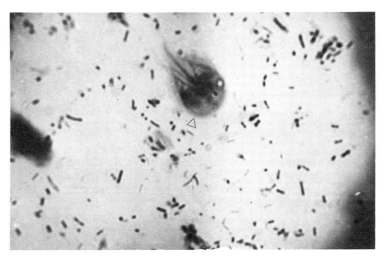

Figure 39.1   Duodenal fluid.   Motile, flagellate organism is shown (arrow).

4.   Which of the following characterize this agent?
  A.   Trophozoites are present in the upper small intestine
  B.   It can attack the fuzzy coat of the microvilli
  C.   It is a nonflagellated protozoa
  D.   Transmission is by ingestion of trophozoites
  E.   Achlorhydria alters host susceptibility

5.   The clinical picture of infestation includes
  A.   no symptomatology
  B.   anorexia, nausea, epigastric discomfort, diarrhea
  C.   chronic diarrhea
  D.   steatorrhea with marked weight loss
  E.   all of the above

Question 6:   Answer true (T) or false (F).

6.   Diagnosis rests upon stool examination but can be augmented by duodenal fluid examination.

7. Which of the following drugs have been demonstrated to be effective in treatment?
   A. Quinacrine (Atabrine)
   B. Metronidazole (Flagyl)
   C. Tetracyclines
   D. Tinidazole (Fasigyn)
   E. Furazolidone (Furoxone)

ANSWERS AND COMMENTS

1. (D) Giardiasis is the most likely diagnosis. The type of pain, the lack of fever, hematochezia, melena, occult blood in stools, and of dietary relationships would mediate against the other diagnostic considerations.

2. (T) Man is the only host and reservoir for this intestinal protozoa. (1,2) Refer to answer 4.

3. (T) An estimate of worldwide distribution has been 5 to 10%. (1,2) In the United States, the prevalence rate has been estimated as 7.4%, based on at least 23 epidemiologic surveys. (3) Infestations are particularly common in children, but outbreaks have been reported in the elderly as well as in nurseries. (1-√) The clinical pattern can range from no symptomatology (most common), to acute infection, mimicking an acute gastroenteritis, to a chronic malabsorption-like syndrome or even protein-losing enteropathy. (1-9)

4. (A,B,E) Giardia lamblia is a flagellated protozoa. (1,2,8) Trophozoites are found in the upper part of the small intestine, adjacent to the mucosa. (1,2,8) These trophozoites can be present in the secretory tubules of the mucosa and can rarely enter the biliary tree. (1,2,8) The parasite has a sucking disk which can produce mechanical irritation and can provide the capability for attacking the fuzzy coat of the microvilli. (2,6) Additionally, mucosal invasion has been demonstrated. The cyst form is the "means" by which G. lamblia is transmitted, occurring by intimate contact with an infected person or ingestion of food or water contaminated with infected feces. (1-8) Yet, the reason for the range of symptomatology in infected persons remains unexplained.

In experimentally induced infection in volunteers with as many as 10,000 times the necessary cysts for infection, minimal or no symptomatology was produced. (1,2,8)

Thus, attention has been directed at host susceptibility in order to explain the variability of individual response. One of

the identified predisposing factors is achlorhydria. (1,2,8) In
addition, an altered immune mechanism has been demonstrated
to be a major factor. (2,10,12) Various humoral immunological
disorders, such as low or absent immunoglobulin G, have been
frequently associated with giardiasis. (2,10-12) Cell-mediated
immunological disorders per se have not frequently been associated with G. lamblia. (2,10-12) The altered immunological
status may diminish host resistance in the intestinal mucosa and
lead to larger and more severe infestations. Recently, diminished secretory IgA levels in intestinal fluid have been implicated in giardiasis. (12)

5. (E) The majority of individuals with G. lamblia are asymptomatic. Of the symptomatic "patterns," the most consistent
has been anorexia, nausea, epigastric discomfort, diarrhea,
and minimal or no weight loss. The diarrhea can be watery or
loose, explosive, malodorous, with an abrupt onset. Less frequently present are vomiting, fever, chills, and significant generalized malaise. Blood and pus are absent in stools, and aid
in diagnostically separating giardiasis from bacterial forms of
dysentery. (1-7,13,14) This acute form may last days to weeks.
(1-7,13) It will uncommonly evolve into the chronic form with a
malabsorptive clinical pattern. The "symptomatic" latent period of such infections has averaged 15 days in travelers, e.g.,
in the Soviet Union. (13)

Some patients may even have a subacute pattern, lasting
months, or, rarely, years. (1-7) In addition to the altered bowel habit pattern (diarrhea), steatorrhea, distention, and significant weight loss, some may have features of the acute phase infection. Urticaria can rarely be present, too. The laboratory
evaluation may disclose evidence of malabsorption and/or immunoglobulin deficiency, such as IgG or IgA. In addition, oral
disaccharide tolerance tests may be abnormal, lactose in particular. The small intestinal (jejunal) biopsy may reveal findings ranging from normal to severe flattening of the villous pattern with marked inflammatory reaction within the lamina propria, predominantly polymorphonuclear leukocytes. (2,5,6) Mucosal invasion by the trophozoites may be identified. (1-8) There
are minimal or no changes in the surface epithelial cells. However, these morphological changes frequently do not correlate
with the severity or even presence of symptomatology. (1-7) Intestinal mucosal enzyme (disaccharidase) assays have revealed
deficiencies of lactase and sucrase, particularly the former,
which returns to normal with treatment but more slowly than sucrase. (2,5,6) Caution must be used in ascribing lactose intolerance to giardiasis, and future reevaluation for an acquired lactose intolerance (primary) must be undertaken.

6. (T) G. lamblia infection is frequently diagnosed by stool examinations, using a direct smear zinc sulfate concentration, or formol-ether. (2,4,7,15) The problem with stool examination is the periodicity of parasite (cyst) passage. (2,5,7,15) Even with three or more examinations on alternate days, the false negative rate is still 30 to 50%. (2,5,7,15) Trophozoites are usually not discovered in the stools unless rapid transit time is present. (2,5,7,15)

If the stools are negative after a minimum of three examinations as previously suggested, duodenal fluid examination should be enacted. Duodenal fluid intubation and aspiration is completed using a rubber or plastic nasogastric tube in younger children or longer intestinal tube in older children. An alternative has recently been provided by the development of a string in a gelatin capsule (Enterotest®). An adult-sized capsule and string (140 cm) and pediatric-sized capsule and string (90 cm) have been developed and evaluated. The Enterotest results have been comparable to intubation and aspiration. Both methods provide 85 to 95% accuracy. (8, 9, 16) However, the most accurate method is examination of the small intestinal biopsy's mucus (superficial) layer, providing essentially 100% accuracy. (15)

Other laboratory studies are nonspecific, as are the radiological findings of edema and segmentation of the upper small intestine. (17)

7. (A,B,D,E) Treatment with metronidazole (Flagyl) is and has been quite successful (symptomatic, morphological, and parasite elimination) in practically all cases. In children, the dosage varied from 250 to 750 mg daily (10 days). With one course of treatment, the failure rate has varied from 15 to 30%, and additional courses of treatment have lowered this rate to 5 to 20%. (1-8,17-21) However, since this drug has been suggested experimentally to be mutagenic and carcinogenic, other forms of treatment must be contemplated. A newer therapeutic agent, Furazolidone (Furaxone), a nitrofuran derivative, 5 mg/kg/24 hours, for 7 days (4 divided doses daily) has been demonstrated to be equally effective in most studies, is available in liquid suspension form, has a reasonable taste, but is more expensive than the other preparations. (17-22) Therefore, the present treatment of choice seems to be quinacrine hydrochloride (Atabrine), 5-10 mg/kg/24 hours, for 10 days (3 divided doses daily). The failure rate of one course of treatment has ranged from 25 to 35%. (1-7,18,19) Additional courses of treatment have lowered this rate to 5 to 23%. (1-6,18-23) Other successful therapeutic agents, although utilized less often, include chloroquine and paromomycin. (18,19) Lastly, a new agent tinidazole (Fasigyn) has been used in Europe and the Far East, achieving almost 90% cure

rates, but is presently not available for use in the United States. (21,24) Single dose and 1-day treatment schedules have been recently investigated, less successful cure rates, 30 to 60% being achieved. (21) None of the previously mentioned primary drugs should be used during pregnancy, unless mandatory due to severity of disease. (2,24)

REFERENCES

1. Marsden, P.D. and Schultz, M.G.: Intestinal parasites. Gastroenterology 57:724, 1969.

2. Brandborg, L. L. : Parasitic diseases. In: Gastrointestinal Disease. Sleisenger, M.H. and Fordtran, J.S. (Eds). WB Saunders Co. , Philadelphia, 1973, p. 989.

3. Stevens, D.P.: Giardiasis. Clinical presentation, diagnosis, and treatment. Pract Gastroenterol 4:52, 1980.

4. Hoskins, L.C., Winawer, S.J., Broitman, S.A., et al.: Clinical giardiasis and intestinal malabsorption. Gastroenterology 53:265, 1967.

5. Ament, M.E.: Diagnosis and treatment of giardiasis. J Pediatr 89:633, 1972.

6. Barbieri, D., DeBrito, T., Hoshino, S., et al.: Giardiasis in childhood. Absorption tests and biochemistry, histochemistry, light and electron microscopy of jejunal mucosa. Arch Dis Child 45:466, 1970.

7. Wolfe, M.S.: Giardiasis. J Am Med Assoc 233:1362, 1975.

8. Belding, D.L.: Textbook of Parasitology, 3rd Edition. Appleton-Century-Crofts, New York, 1965, p. 124.

9. Sherman, P., Liebman, W.M.: Protein-losing enteropathy associated with giardiasis. Am J Dis Child 134:893, 1980.

10. Brown, W.R., Butterfield, D., Savage, D., et al.: Clinical, microbiological and immunological studies in patients with immunoglobulin deficiencies and gastrointestinal disorders. Gut 13:441, 1972.

11. Ament, M.E. and Rubin, C.E.: Relation of giardiasis to abnormal intestinal structure and function in gastrointestinal immunodeficiency syndromes. Gastroenterology 62: 216, 1972.

12. Zinneman, H.H. and Kaplan, A.P.: The association of giardiasis with reduced intestinal secretory immunoglobulins. Am J Dig Dis 17:793, 1972.

13. Walzer, P.D., Wolfe, M.S., Schultz, H.G.: Giardiasis in Russia. J Infect Dis 124:235, 1971.

14. Babb, R.R., Peck, O.C., Vescia, F.G.: Giardiasis: A cause of traveler's diarrhea. J Am Med Assoc 217, 1359, 1971.

15. Kamath, K.R. and Murugasu, R.: A comparative study of 4 methods for detecting Giardia lamblia in children with diarrheal disease and malabsorption. Gastroenterology 66:16, 1974.

16. Rosenthal, P., Liebman, W.M.: Comparative study of stool examinations, duodenal aspiration and Entero-Test-Pediatric for giardiasis in children. J Pediatr 96:279, 1980.

17. Marshak, R.H., Ruoff, M., Lindner, A.E.: Roentgen manifestations of giardiasis. Am J Roentgenol Radium Ther Nucl Med 104:557, 1968.

18. Most, H.: Treatment of common parasitic infections of man encountered in the United States. N Engl J Med 287: 495, 1972.

19. Kay, R., Barnes, G.L., Townley, R.R.W.: Giardia lamblia infestation in 154 children. Aust Paediat J 13:98, 1977.

20. Lerman, S.J., Walker, R.A.: Treatment of giardiasis. Literature review and recommendations. Clin Pediatr 21: 409, 1982.

21. Wolfe, M.S.: The treatment of intestinal protozoan infections. Med Clin North Am 66:707, 1982.

22. Craft, J.C., Murphy, T., Nelson, J.D.: Furazolidone and quinacrine. Comparative study of therapy for giardiasis in children. Am J Dis Child 135:164, 1981.

23. Report of the Committee on Infectious Diseases, American Academy of Pediatrics, 19th edition, Evanston, Illinois, 1982, p. 163.

24. Anderson, T., Forssell, J., Sterner, G.: Outbreak of giardiasis: Effect of a new antiflagellate drug, tinidazole. Br Med J 2:449, 1972.

Case 40

ACUTE DIARRHEA IN A 23-MONTH-OLD BOY

HISTORY

A 23-month-old white male presented with a history of diarrhea
of almost 4 weeks' duration, consisting of 4 to 6 loose bowel
movements daily. There was associated vague abdominal cramping frequently related to bowel movements but unassociated with
time of day, meals, or food types. There was no associated
vomiting, fever, melena, hematochezia, skin lesions, jaundice,
dysuria, upper respiratory tract infection, or any drug, unusual
food, or unusual plant exposure. The patient's appetite was initially decreased but more recently returned almost to normal.
After the onset of the diarrhea, the patient was switched by his
private physician to Pedialyte without significant improvement
in the diarrhea. Subsequently, a soybean formula was added,
but this change also did not result in alleviation of the previous
symptomatic pattern. No other family member or friend had
similar clinical pattern at or prior to the onset of this patient's
problem. The family history included a maternal uncle with
bronchial asthma and paternal aunt with apparent cow's milk intolerance. The remainder of the past history, developmental
history, family and social history, and review of systems was
noncontributory.

EXAMINATION

He was relatively alert, active and in no distress with normal
vital signs. Head circumference was 46 cm, length 78 cm,
weight 10 kg, birth weight, 2.5 kg. The remainder of the physical examination was unremarkable, including the abdomen and
anorectal area. Stool hemoccult examination was negative.

340

LABORATORY DATA

Hemoglobin:	12.8 gm%
Hematocrit:	39%
White blood cell count:	10,500/mm^3
PMN's:	58%
lymphocytes:	40%
monocytes:	1%
eosinophiles:	1%
sedimentation rate:	18/mm/hr
Platelets:	215,000/mm^3
Urinalysis:	negative
Serum:	
sodium:	137 meq/L
potassium:	4 meq/L
chloride:	100 meq/L
bicarbonate:	20 meq/L
creatinine:	0.6 mg%
total protein:	6.0 gm%
albumin:	4.0 gm%
Stool:	
occult blood:	negative
reducing substances:	negative
ova and parasites:	negative
cultures:	negative

QUESTIONS

1. Which of the following is the probable diagnosis of this patient?
    A. Infectious diarrhea
    B. Duodenal ulcer
    C. Ulcerative colitis
    D. Cystic fibrosis
    E. Celiac disease

2. Which of the following studies would be indicated in this patient at this time?
    A. Stool smear (white and red blood cells)
    B. Stool culture
    C. Proctosigmoidoscopy
    D. Barium enema examination
    E. Barium swallow examination

3. If a diagnosis of Campylobacter is suggested, which of the following studies would be needed to establish the diagnosis?
   A. Stool isolate serotyping
   B. Adrenal tumor cell assay
   C. Stool filtration/columbia agar study
   D. Guinea pig conjunctivae (Sereny test)
   E. RAST test

4. Treatment of this agent includes which of the following measures?
   A. Antiperistaltic agents, e.g., Lomotil
   B. Cholestyramine
   C. Antacids
   D. Antibiotics in all patients
   E. Antibiotics in selected patients

ANSWERS AND COMMENTS

1. (A) An infectious diarrhea is suggested by the abrupt, acute onset, presence of diarrhea, no blood in the stools, variable abdominal discomfort (pain), and age of onset. The other choices would be less likely.

2. (A,B) A stool specimen or rectal swab should be obtained and examined by Wright or methylene blue stain for the presence of white blood cells (WBC) and red blood cells (RBC). If polys are present, especially if many, a culture must be performed. Standard procedures (media) are used. Although SS agar may be satisfactory for salmonellae, it may be too inhibitory for Shigellae; MacConkey agar or XLD agar should be more favorable for Shigellae. (1) If Shigellae grow from stools, the diagnosis is established. Serum agglutinins can be determined, with a fourfold or greater rise in agglutinins in paired sera also establishing the diagnosis. In salmonellosis, the stool culture will be positive initially but then may become negative, coinciding with bloodstream invasion. (1) Serotyping, as with Shigellae, is of interest but is of little value in the treatment of patients. However, epidemiologically and for establishing the presence of Group D Salmonellae, including S. typhi, serotyping can be important. On blood agar, thio-blood agar and other agars, Campylobacters will grow under appropriate atmospheric conditions, i.e., reduced oxygen tension (5 to 6% usually), 25°C to 43°C. (1,2)

3. (C) The designation of Campylobacter as a Vibrio species
was made on the basis of morphologic similarity. (1, 2) Campylobacter is also a motile, "curved," gram-negative rod, but
does not ferment or oxidize carbohydrates. They are micro-
aerophilic (anaerobic), possess a guanine/cystosine content of
30 to 36%. In comparison, e.g., true Vibrios ferment selected
carbohydrates, and their guanine/cystosine content is 40 to 50%.
(1-3)
    There are three species within the genus Campylobacter.
(1-3) There are three subspecies of C. fetus that are considered of importance in animal and human disease, specifically,
ss. fetus, ss. intestinalis and ss. jejuni. (1-3)
    Campylobacters can grow on blood agar, Brucella agar,
Mueller-Hinton agar, columbia agar, thio-blood agar, less so.
MacConkey's agar, trypticase soy broth. They require reduced
oxygen tension for growth, 5 to 60%. Modified agars have al-
lowed for growth at oxygen content up to 21% in investigative
studies. (1, 2) Growth occurs at 25°C to 43°C. (1-3)
    Clinical syndromes with Campylobacter include enteritis
and colitis. (1-11) Estimated incubation period is 2 to 11 days.
(4-11) Clinical features consist of fever and abdominal pain for
1 to 3 days, followed by diarrhea with or without blood (10 to
92%). (4-10) Acute diarrhea is the usual complaint, but chronic
diarrhea for months has been noted. (4-10)
    The diagnosis consists of the suggestive clinical features
(suspicion) but requires fecal isolation. Stool filtration is not
necessary, but, as previously mentioned, the use of blood agar
or columbia agar with added antimicrobials (fecal flora suppression) and at reduced oxygen tension will allow accurate, "speedy"
fecal isolation of Campylobacter. Clinically, an atmosphere of
5% oxygen and 42°C to 43°C enhance the isolation of ss. jejuni.
(1-3) Karmali and Fleming (5) reported the potential use of direct phase fecal microscopy for identification.

4. (E) Erythromycin has been the suggested treatment, based
on in vitro sensitivities. (1, 10-13) Controlled studies of the
treatment of Campylobacter enteritis, colitis have not been accomplished. The natural history of these clinical syndromes
with reference to the effect of antimicrobial therapy has not been
established, either.
    Therefore, treatment should consist of (1) maintenance of
adequate fluid, acid-base, and electrolyte status (oral sucrose
or glucose solutions versus intravenous fluid therapy); (2) avoidance of antiperistaltic agents, such as Lomotil (Kaolin preparations, e.g., Kaopectate may be used); and (3) antimicrobial
treatment, i.e., erythromycin, 25 to 50 mg/kg/day (3 to 4 divided doses) for 7 to 14 days. In mild cases clinically, antimicrobial therapy need not be used. (1, 10-12)

REFERENCES

1. Rettig, P.J.: Campylobacter infections in human beings. J Pediatr 94:855, 1979.

2. Smibert, R.M.: The genus campylobacter. Ann Rev Microbiol 32:673, 1978.

3. White, F.H., Walsh, A.F.: Biochemical and serological relationships of isolants of Vibrio fetus from man. J Infect Dis 121:471, 1970.

4. Dale, B.: Campylobacter enteritis. Br Med J 2:318, 1977.

5. Karmali, M.A., Fleming, P.C.: Campylobacter enteritis in children. J Pediatr 94:527, 1979.

6. Taylor, D.N., Porter, B.W., Williams, C.A., et al.: Campylobacter enteritis: A large outbreak traced to commercial raw milk. West J Med 137:365, 1982.

7. Tanner, E.I., Bullin, C.H.: Campylobacter enteritis. Br Med J 2:579, 1977.

8. Butzler, J.L., DeKeyser, P., Detrain, M., et al.: Related Vibrio in stool. J Pediatr 82:493, 1975.

9. Heyman, M.B., Paterno, V.I., Ament, M.E.: Campylobacter colitis. A cause of chronic diarrhea in children. West J Med 137:243, 1982.

10. Guandalini, S., Cucchiara, S., deRitis, G., et al.: Campylobacter colitis in infants. J Pediatr 102:72, 1983.

11. Report of the Committee on Infectious Disease, American Academy of Pediatrics, 1982, pp. 56, 57.

12. Chow, A.W., Patten, V., Bednor, A.D.: Susceptibility of campylobacter fetus to twenty-two antimicrobial agents. Antimicrob Agents Chemother 13:415, 1978.

13. Vanhoof, R., Vanderlinden, M.P., Dierck, X.R., et al.: Susceptibility of campylobacter fetus subsp jejuni to twenty-nine antimicrobial agents. Antimicrob Agents Chemother 14:553, 1978.

Case 41

ACUTE DIARRHEA IN A 2-YEAR-OLD BOY

HISTORY

A 2-year-old boy presented with a history of loose to watery
bowel movements of 5 days' duration. The bowel habit pattern
had changed from 1 bowel movement daily to 5 to 8 bowel movements daily. There was associated anorectal discomfort and
occasional lower abdominal cramping but without fever, nausea,
vomiting, melena, hematochezia, skin lesions. Appetite and
activity were decreased. There was no relationship to food
types or meals. There was no significant weight loss. The patient has been treated with ampicillin for a right otitis media,
completing the 7th day of antibiotic administration at the onset
of diarrhea. The remainder of the past history, developmental
history, family history, social history, and review of systems
was noncontributory.

EXAMINATION

He was alert, active, and in no apparent distress, with normal
vital signs, weight 9.9 kg, height 78 cm, head circumference
46.5 cm. The remainder of the examination, including the abdomen and anorectal area, was unremarkable. Stool hemoccult
testing was negative.

LABORATORY DATA

Hemoglobin:	12.1 gm%
Hematocrit:	36%
White blood cell count:	11,300/mm^3
PMN's:	73%

lymphocytes:	22%
monocytes:	3%
eosinophiles:	2%
Sedimentation rate:	28 mm/hr
Serum:	
sodium:	137 meq/L
potassium:	4.1 meq/L
chloride:	100 meq/L
bicarbonate:	21 meq/L
creatinine:	0.5 mg%
Urinalysis:	negative
Stool:	
occult blood:	negative
white blood cells	5-10/HPF
culture:	pending
ova and parasites:	negative

QUESTIONS

1. This disorder's cause could be determined by which of the
   following studies?
   A. Urine culture
   B. Stool culture and cytotoxin
   C. Serology (complement-fixing antibody)
   D. String test
   E. Barium enema examination

Questions 2-6: Answer true (T) or false (F).

2. Transmission of these agents seems mainly to be from contaminated water and/or food.

3. Erythromycin and tetracycline have been the most commonly implicated antibiotics in this disorder.

4. In milder cases, the antimicrobial therapy need not be discontinued.

5. Vancomycin is the treatment of choice for this disorder.

6. Relapse does not occur after appropriate treatment has been
   accomplished.

ANSWERS AND COMMENTS

1. (B) Precise diagnosis depends upon the isolation of Clostridium difficile (C. difficile) from the stool and the presence of fecal cytotoxin. The latter is required for making the association of toxin-positive colitis, enteritis, or enterocolitis. (1-3) The finding of a toxin can be accomplished by a cytotoxicity assay, since tissue culture assay is time-consuming and not cost-effective. (1-5)

No radiological studies are pathognomonic for this disorder, instead demonstrating mucosal edema, ulcerations, e.g., on barium enema examination. (1-3,5-8) The latter may demonstrate pseudomembrane-like formation on occasions. (5-8) However, proctosigmoidoscopic examinations more strongly may suggest the diagnosis, i.e., edema, erythema, increased friability of the mucosa and the characteristic yellow-white, raised plaques. (1-3,5-9) Rectal biopsy may demonstrate the pseudomembrane, which actually consists of fibrin, epithelial debris, white blood cells (polys), and mucin. (1-3,5-9) However, the proctosigmoidoscopic examination and rectal biopsy may actually be normal or demonstrate nonspecific findings in a small percentage of cases, 5 to 20%. (1,7,8) Colonoscopic examination may only demonstrate abnormality(ies). (1,7,8)

2. (F) Clostridia are thought to proliferate during the antibiotic treatment and apparently reduce the remainder of normal small intestinal microflora. As the clostridia increase in number, an increasing amount of toxin is produced. This toxin then has a direct action on the intestinal mucosa, resulting in the pathophysiological changes, manifested by symptoms, such as diarrhea. Pseudomembranes are formed, pathologically consisting of white blood cells (polys), fibrin, and cellular debris. (1,2,8)

The toxin isolated in stools of patients with antibiotic-associated pseudomembranous colitis has been characterized as heat labile, lethal for hamsters, cell cytotoxic in tissue culture, and neutralized by sordelli antitoxin. (1,4,7,8) The latter indicates antigenic cross-reactivity.

3. (F) Clindamycin and ampicillin, the latter in particular, have been the most implicated antibiotics and also the most extensively studied to allow any reasonable conclusions regarding causality and frequency. Tedesco, et al. (2) reported a 10% incidence of pseudomembranous colitis, almost 21% incidence of diarrhea, in a prospective study of 200 patients receiving clindamycin, while reporting no cases of pseudomembranous colitis,

4.5% incidence of diarrhea, in another study of 200 patients receiving ampicillin. (3) Conversely, Christie and Ament (9) reported a pediatric case of ampicillin-associated colitis. Despite the above-mentioned studies and others, clindamycin has rarely been associated with pseudomembranous colitis in children. (6, 7) Ampicillin has been implicated as cause more often in children. (8)

Other antimicrobial agents have been implicated as cause, too. (Table 41.1) Agents have included penicillin, cephalothin, and carbenicillin. Total dose of drug, duration of treatment, and age of patient have not been related to the development of colitis.

4. (T) If the diarrhea is mild, the antimicrobial agent need not be discontinued. (1,7,8) However, the patient should be closely monitored. Should the diarrhea worsen, the antibiotic should be stopped.

Severe cases can be characterized by severe diarrhea, fever, nausea, vomiting, and abdominal distention. Abdominal pain, crampy in nature, usually will occur. Dehydration and acid-base imbalance will then result, and blood in the stools, toxic dilatation of the colon, even peritonitis and/or sepsis can result should the antibiotic be continued. (1-3, 5-9)

TABLE 41.1 Antibiotics Associated with Pseudomembranous Colitis

Ampicillin
Clindamycin
Lincomycin
Penicillin
Tetracycline
Oxacillin
Carbenicillin
Dicloxacillin
Cephalothin
Cephaloridine
Cefazolin
Cephalexin
Cephradine
Chloramphenicol
Novobiocin
Streptomycin

5. (T) A number of therapeutic regimens have been utilized in the treatment of antibiotic-associated colitis during the last 10 to 15 years. However, only vancomycin and cholestyramine have been objectively confirmed as effective (curative). (1-3,5-8,11,12) Steroids, e.g., prednisone, antispasmodics, anticholinergics, e.g., Lomitol, have not been confirmed as effective. (1-3, 5-8, 10-13)

Oral as well as parenteral vancomycin has been effective. A specific pediatric dose has not been formulated, but an adult dose of 2 grams daily, i.e., 2,000 mg/1.73 m^2/24 hours, has been established. (1-3,5-8,11) The pediatric equivalent would be obtained by using the patient's body surface area in relationship to the adult equivalents of surface area and dosage. Treatment is required for 10 to 14 days.

Cholestyramine, an anion-binding resin, has been found to effectively bind clostridial toxin in the stool, too. In one study, cholestyramine was administered for only a few days before the diarrhea ceased, and was continued for one week after the diarrhea disappeared. (12) Thus, cholestyramine shortened the duration of illness, regardless of the timing of initiation of treatment. (12) Further controlled studies are needed, especially in view of lack of protection by colestipol administration in the hamster model. (12) The role of metronidazole (Flagyl) is being studied. (11)

As with other causes of diarrhea, intravenous fluid therapy, selective use of colloid administration, and oral carbohydrate (glucose, sucrose)-electrolyte solutions are an important part of the therapeutic program. Close monitoring of intake (intravenous and/or oral) and of output (insensible, urine, stool, vomitus) is mandatory. (13)

6. (F) Relapse occurs in 15 to 20% of children treated with vancomycin, a rate similar to that in adults. (7) The factors in the presence or absence of a relapse have not been delineated, although reexposure to C. difficile, on or off of antibiotic treatment at the onset of diarrhea, have been mentioned. (1, 7, 8)

Mortality has varied from 0 to 25%. As mentioned in the answer to question 4, significant dehydration, toxic dilatation of the colon, peritonitis, and sepsis have been reported. (1,5,7,8)

REFERENCES

1. Bartlett, J.G.: Antibiotic associated pseudomembranous colitis. Rev Infect Dis 1:530, 1979.

2. Tedesco, F.J., Barton, R.W., Alpers, D.H.: Clinda-
    mycin-associated colitis: A prospective study. Ann In-
    tern Med 81:429, 1974.

3. Tedesco, F.J.: Ampicillin-associated diarrhea - A pros-
    pective study. Am J Dig Dis 20:295, 1975.

4. Chang, T.W., Lavermann, M., Bartlett, J.G.: Cytotox-
    icity assay in antibiotic-associated colitis. J Infect Dis
    140:765, 1979.

5. Barlett, J.G. : Antibiotic-associated colitis. Clin Gastro-
    enterol 8:783, 1979.

6. Randolph, M.F., Morris, K.E.: Clindamycin-associated
    colitis in children. Clin Pediatr 16:722, 1977.

7. Viscidi, R.P., Bartlett, J.G.: Antibiotic-associated pseu-
    domembranous colitis in children. Pediatrics 67:381, 1981.

8. Prince, A.S., Neu, H.C.: Antibiotic-associated pseudo-
    membranous colitis in children. Pediatr Clin North Am
    26:261, 1979.

9. Christie, D.L., Ament, M.E.: Ampicillin-associated
    colitis. J Pediatr 87:657, 1975.

10. Mirdh, P.A., Helin, I., Collene, I., et al. : Antibiotic-
    associated colitis. Acta Paediatr Scand 71:275, 1982.

11. Report of the Committee on Infectious Diseases, American
    Academy of Pediatrics, Nineteenth Edition, American
    Academy of Pediatrics, Evanston, 1982, pp. 292, 297.

12. Kreutzer, E.W., Milligan, F.D.: Treatment of antibiotic-
    associated colitis with cholestyramine resin. Johns Hop-
    kins Med J 143:67, 1978.

13. Hirschhorn, N.: The treatment of acute diarrhea in chil-
    dren: A historical and physiological perspective. Am J
    Clin Nutr 33:637, 1980.

Case 42

ACUTE ABDOMINAL PAIN AND VOMITING
IN A 5-YEAR-OLD GIRL

HISTORY

A 5-year-old white female presented with a 5-day history of mid-abdominal pain, with associated nausea and vomiting. The pain was crampy, without radiation and not related to meals, food type, position, urination, or bowel movements. The pain would last minutes to hours and could recur during the same day. With one of the episodes of vomiting, dark material was noted on the third day, and there was one questionable episode of a pinkish tinge of the urine. There was no history of associated arthralgia, fever, diarrhea, constipation, melena, hematochezia, pyrosis, skin lesions, oral or ocular lesions, or dysuria. The appetite and activity were decreased. The past medical history included DT immunization 8 days beforehand because of a superficial laceration. The remainder of the past history, developmental history, family history, social history, and review of systems was unremarkable.

EXAMINATION

She was alert but in mild abdominal distress, with normal vital signs, height 105 cm, weight 21 kg. The remainder of the examination was unremarkable except for (1) several punctate 5-6 mm maculopapular, purple lesions of the left shoulder area and gluteal areas bilaterally and (2) midabdominal tenderness without rebound tenderness, masses, or organomegaly.

LABORATORY DATA

Hemoglobin:	12.1 gm%
Hematocrit:	35%
White blood cell count:	9,000/mm^3
PMN's:	72%
lymphocytes:	14%
monocytes:	11%
eosinophiles:	3%
Sedimentation rate:	31 mm/hr
Urinalysis:	negative except 1+ protein, 0-4 RBC, 2-5 WBC/HPF
Serum:	
sodium:	136 meq/L
potassium:	3.6 meq/L
chloride:	97 meq/L
bicarbonate:	19 meq/L
creatinine:	0.8 mg%
SGOT:	46 KU
alkaline phosphatase:	230 IU
total protein:	5.4 gm%
albumin:	3.1 gm%
amylase:	43 units
IgG:	1,590 mg%
IgM:	96 mg%
IgA:	190 mg%
Stool:	
hemoccult:	trace
culture:	negative
ova and parasites:	negative
rotazyme assay:	negative
Plain films of chest:	negative
Plain films of abdomen:	dilated bowel loops; no free air, obstruction

QUESTIONS

1. The most likely diagnosis in this child is
   A. gastroesophageal reflux
   B. duodenal ulcer
   C. giardiasis
   D. acute viral gastroenteritis
   E. anaphylactoid purpura

2. Which one of the following studies would be indicated in this patient?
   A. pH Probe test
   B. String test
   C. Upper gastrointestinal-small bowel series
   D. Proctosigmoidoscopy
   E. Colonoscopy

3. Treatment of this patient might include which of the following?
   A. Antacids
   B. Cimetidine
   C. Anticholinergics
   D. Antibiotics
   E. Steroids

4. Which of the following are indications for surgical treatment of this condition?
   A. Respiratory insufficiency
   B. Dysphagia
   C. Abdominal pain
   D. Massive intestinal hemorrhage
   E. Intussusception

ANSWERS AND COMMENTS

1. (E) Anaphylactoid purpura (Henoch-Schönlein purpura; H-SP) is an "allergic vasculitis," characterized by colicky abdominal pain (50 to 75% of patients), skin lesions, predominantly lower extremity in location and petecchial to nodular purpuric in type, and the presence of arthralgia with or without frank arthritis (30 to 70%). (1-8) The onset can be acute with the simultaneous appearance of several manifestations or insidious with manifestations occurring over several weeks to months. (1-8) The gastrointestinal symptomatology may precede the skin, joint, and/or renal components. (1-8) Any part of the gastrointestinal tract can be involved, although esophageal involvement has not been well substantiated. (1-8) This patient most likely has this condition (H-SP) since there has not been pyrosis, dysphagia, epigastric or substernal pain (A), recurrent pain with different features, e.g., meal, food type, or time of day associations (B), diarrhea with different pain features, e.g., severity (C), nor diarrhea, different pain features, associations, e.g., severity, bowel movements, or fever (D).

2. (C) The differential diagnosis does include other conditions producing an acute abdomen, e.g., infectious gastroenteritis and enterocolitis, inflammatory bowel disease, but the lack of certain features, e.g., fever, diarrhea, hematochezia, make certain possibilities less likely, including those previously mentioned, e.g., inflammatory bowel disease, particularly ulcerative colitis. Careful monitoring of the patient's clinical course, with appropriate, selective studies would be the best approach. However, a helpful diagnostic procedure could be the small intestinal X-ray study. (1-3,5) The small bowel series frequently demonstrates suggestive changes in the proximal small intestine, specifically thickening, prominence, and dilation of the valvulae conniventes. (1-3,5,7) "Thumbprinting" can be present, too, representing blood accumulation between the mucosal and deeper layers of the wall, e.g., submucosal hemorrhage (Table 42.1). Similar changes can occur in any area of the gastrointestinal tract, e.g., colon, particularly the splenic flexure region. (1-3,5,7-9)

The pH probe test (A) would be of value in gastroesophageal reflux, while the string test (B) could be used for small intestinal fluid analysis, e.g., parasites (giardia lamblia), culture. The performance of a proctosigmoidoscopy (D) might have been useful, even in this patient, particularly if inflammatory bowel disease was suspected; at the same time, examination of stool for WBC, RBC, culture, ova and parasites could be accomplished. In patients with Henoch-Schönlein purpura, the proctosigmoidoscopy is usually normal or may reveal nonspecific

TABLE 42.1   Henoch-Schönlein Purpura

Purpura (Nonthrombocytopenic)
Abdominal pain, colicky
Arthralgia, knee and ankle (Schunlein)
Renal (glomerulonephritis)
    nephrotic syndrome

Renal
  subendothelial granular and nodular deposition
    IgA, IgG, complement, glomerular basement membrane

Gastrointestinal
  Hemorrhage, intestinal wall edema, submucosa and mucosa
    scalloping, thumbprinting on X-ray mucosal ulceration
    (arteriolitis, fibrinoid necrosis)
  Intussusception

---

edema of the mucosa. (1-3,5,7,8) A rectal biopsy would reveal normal findings, a nonspecific, mild inflammatory reaction of the lamina propria, or, less so, submucosal hemorrhage. (1-3, 5,7) Colonoscopy, more so, could be utilized to assess the integrity of the entire colon and/or terminal ileum, e.g., splenic flexure area. However, the preparation needed for an adequate examination, the sedation or general anesthesia required, the cost in relation to positive results, and the morbidity of the procedure would surely not justify its routine utilization. This author is not aware of any colonoscopic studies in children in Henoch-Schönlein purpura at this time.

With reference to laboratory studies not mentioned previously, serum complement components have been assessed, and low CH_{50} and properdin values have been noted. (10) Conversely, high C4 and C3 values have also been found. (10) Thus, complement activation is thought to be a feature of acute Henoch-Schönlein purpura, while the low properdin values in 30% or more of patients reflect involvement of the alternative pathway (complement). (10,12) Increased IgA levels and also IgA complexes, as well as IgG complexes, have been found in Henoch-Schönlein purpura, but whether the actual disease is produced by deposition of complexes per se, modulation of polymorphonuclear leukocyte function, or other mechanisms remains unknown. (10-12) Therefore, an immune complex mechanism is likely present in this condition.

Recently, Saulsbury and Kesler (13) reported the association of thrombocytosis (67%) and the presence of abdominal pain and bleeding in Henoch-Schönlein purpura. Unfortunately, no diagnostic laboratory test or tests have been found in this disease entity.

3. (D,E) There is no satisfactory modality of treatment for the common manifestations of this disease entity. Any suspected antigen (allergen) should be avoided and/or removed from the patient's environment, e.g., drugs (sulfas, etc.). If a streptococcal infection, or other agent infection, e.g., mycoplasma, are confirmed, specific treatment, e.g., antibiotics, should be instituted. Streptococcal infection is a relatively common forerunner of Henoch-Schönlein purpura and should be looked for in each patient. (1-8)

The severity of abdominal pain will dictate whether an intravenous route of fluid and nutrient administration is necessary or not (NPO or not). Hypertension associated with other signs of renal involvement, e.g., hematuria, proteinuria, must be closely looked for, since nephritis occurs in approximately 50% or more of patients. Gastrointestinally, microscopic blood is present in approximately 50% of patients, while gross blood is

noted in 15 to 30% of patients. (1-3,5,7,8) Massive intestinal
hemorrhage occurs in 1 to 10%. (1,5,8) Intussusception occurs
in as many as 3 to 5% of patients. (1,5,8) However, steroids,
e.g., hydrocortisone, prednisone, have been found to be beneficial for abdominal pain, producing partial or total relief within
the first 12 to 24 hours of administration. (3,8) A gradual but
progressive weaning from the steroid therapy is accomplished
after an initial 10 to 21-day course. (3,8) The severity and/or
persistence of the abdominal pain determines whether steroids
are used or not. Steroid therapy has not been confirmed as beneficial for gastrointestinal hemorrhage, or the cutaneous, renal,
or arthritic components, either. (3,8)

Antacids (A), cimetidine (B), and anticholinergics (C) would
not be indicated in such patients.

4. (D,E) As previously mentioned in question 3, massive gastrointestinal hemorrhage occurs in 1 to 10% of patients, and surgery would be indicated and necessary in the vast majority. (1,
3,8) Medication, i.e., steroids, have not produced consistent
beneficial results with regard to hemorrhage.

Intussusception, as mentioned also in question 3, occurs in
1 to 5% of patients, and surgery would be indicated and necessary in the majority. (1,3,8) The underlying vasculitis and intestinal wall changes apparently predispose to invagination, possibly by altered resistance relationships in adjacent bowel segments. Although the abdominal pain (C) may be quite severe in
Henoch-Schönlein purpura, even requiring exploratory laparotomy, this symptom by itself is not an indication for surgery.
Respiratory insufficiency (A) and dysphagia (B) are not applicable to this entity.

REFERENCES

1. Rodriguez-Erdmann, F., Levitan, R.: Gastrointestinal
   and roentgenological manifestations of Henoch-Schönlein
   purpura. Gastroenterology 54:260, 1968.

2. Sahn, D.J. and Schwartz, A.D.: Schönlein-Henoch Syndrome: Observations of some atypical clinical presenta-
   tions. Pediatrics 49:114, 1972.

3. Silber, D.L.: Henoch-Schönlein syndrome. Pediatr Clin
   North Am 19:1061, 1972.

Case 42 / 357

4. Allen, D.M., Diamond, L.K., Howell, D.A.: Anaphylactoid purpura in children (Schönlein-Henoch syndrome), Am J Dis Child 99:833, 1960.

5. Feldt, R.H. and Stickler, G.B.: The gastrointestinal manifestations of anaphylactoid purpura in children. Proc Mayo Clin 37:465, 1961.

6. Grossman, H., Berdon, W.E., Baker, D.H.: Abdominal pain in Schönlein-Henoch syndrome. Am J Dis Child 108: 67, 1964.

7. Byrn, J.R., Fitzgerald, J.F., Northway, J.D., et al.: Unusual manifestations of Henoch-Schönlein Syndrome. Am J Dis Child 130:1335, 1976.

8. Roy, C.C., Silverman, A., Cozzetto, F.J.: Pediatric Clinical Gastroenterology, 2nd Edition. The CV Mosby Company, St. Louis, 1975, p. 291.

9. Ockner, R.K.: Vascular diseases of the bowel. In Gastrointestinal Disease. Sleisenger, M.H., Fordtran, J.S. (Eds). WB Saunders Company, Boston, 1978, p. 1907.

10. Garcia-Fuentes, M., Martin, A., Chantler, C., et al.: Serum complement components in Henoch-Schönlein purpura. Arch Dis Child 53:417, 1978.

11. Levinsky, R.J., Barratt, T.M.: IgA immune complexes in Henoch-Schönlein purpura. Lancet 2:1100, 1979.

12. Sams, W.M., Jr.: Allergic vasculitis. Postgrad Med 70: 193, 1981.

13. Saulsbury, F.T., Kesler, R.W.: Thrombocytosis in Henoch-Schönlein purpura. Clin Pediatr 22:185, 1983.

Case 43

ACUTE DIARRHEA AND WEIGHT LOSS
IN A 7-YEAR-OLD BOY

HISTORY

A 7-year-old Mexican-American male presented with diarrhea
of 2-1/2 weeks' duration. He had also experienced a weight loss
of 3-1/2 pounds. There was no associated history of vomiting,
preceding constipation, melena, jaundice, skin lesions, or trauma. The patient had been born and resided in the United States,
but he had visited Mexico with his parents approximately 3 weeks
before the onset of the present symptomatic pattern. However,
no other member of the family was ill at the time of presentation. The remainder of the past history, developmental history,
family history, social history, and review of systems was unremarkable.

EXAMINATION

He was alert and in no significant distress, with normal vital
signs except for temperature of 37.9°C orally. The height was
133 cm and the weight was 22.8 kg. The remainder of the examination was unremarkable, except for mild generalized abdominal tenderness with no rebound tenderness, distention, or
masses. The liver, spleen, and kidneys were not palpable. Active bowel sounds were present with no bruits.

LABORATORY DATA

Hemoglobin:	12.0 gm%
Hematocrit:	37%
White blood cell count:	11,700/mm^3

PMN's:	72%
lymphocytes:	24%
monocytes:	1%
eosinophiles:	3%
Sedimentation rate:	19 mm/hr
Urinalysis:	negative
Stool:	
reducing substances:	negative
occult blood:	negative
culture:	negative
ova and parasites:	cyst-like structures
Serum:	
sodium:	138 meq/L
potassium:	4.5 meq/L
chloride:	103 meq/L
bicarbonate:	21 meq/L
creatinine:	0.4 mg%
Plain films, abdomen:	air within loops of small and large intestine

QUESTIONS

1. The probable diagnosis of this patient is which one of the following?
   A. Enterobiasis
   B. Amebiasis
   C. Eosinophilic gastroenteritis
   D. Tuberculous enteritis
   E. Ulcerative colitis

Question 2: Answer true (T) or false (F).

2. Incidence of this agent being harbored by the world's population has been estimated at 20%.

3. How many cycles does this agent have?
   A. One
   B. Two
   C. Four
   D. Three
   E. Six

Question 4: Answer true (T) or false (F).

4. The site of predilection for this agent is the small intestine.

5. In its invasive form, it will principally involve which organs?
    A. Heart
    B. Large intestine
    C. Small intestine
    D. Pancreas
    E. Liver

6. The clinical findings usually include which of the following?
    A. Diarrhea
    B. Abdominal pain
    C. Blood and mucus in stools
    D. Headache
    E. Jaundice

7. Which of the following are extra-intestinal forms of this disease?
    A. Cerebral abscess or meningoencephalitis
    B. Pericarditis
    C. Chronic hepatitis
    D. Anterior uveitis
    E. Glomerulonephritis

8. How many stool examinations must be performed before 75% accuracy is assured?
    A. Two
    B. Three
    C. One
    D. Five
    E. Six

Question 9: Answer true (T) or false (F).

9. Serologic examination is positive in at least 75% of asymptomatic cyst carriers and over 90% of patients with colitis or liver abscess.

10. The treatment of the intestinal form includes which of the following?
    A. Erythromycin
    B. Tetracycline
    C. Paromomycin (Humatin)
    D. Metronidazole (Flagyl)
    E. Chloroquine

11. The treatment of the extra-intestinal form includes which of the following?
    A. Chloroquine
    B. Metronidazole (Flagyl)
    C. Tetracycline
    D. Emetine
    E. Nystatin

ANSWERS AND COMMENTS

1. (B) Amebiasis is the probable diagnosis, considering the clinical presentation and studies.

2. (T) An estimated 20% of the world's population is believed to harbor E. histolytica. (1-4) In the United States, this figure is closer to 5%, and 20% in its neighbor, Mexico. (1-4)

3. (B) E. histolytica has two cycles: (1) noninvasive, in which the parasite is present in the intestine, forms cysts which can be excreted and transmit disease; and (2) invasive, in which there is penetration of the colonic wall by the trophozoite form. (1-5) Trophozoites have destructive ability but are not capable of transmitting disease. Cysts are the form capable of transmitting infection. (1-5)

4. (F) The large intestine is the site of predilection. (1-5) Refer to answer 5.

5. (B,E) Invasive amebiasis principally involves the large intestine and the liver. E. histolytica may pass through the intestinal wall and travel to the lungs, pericardium, and brain, as well as to the liver (most common). (1-9)

6. (A,B,C) Amebic disease consists of a broad spectrum of disease from mild chronic gastrointestinal symptomatology to an acute fulminant, hemorrhagic diarrheal state. (1-5,10,11) "Acute" amebic dysentery, the usual symptomatic form, consists of a more gradual onset of diarrhea with blood and mucus in the stools. The number of stools can exceed 5 to 10 daily. (1-5,10,11) Abdominal cramping, tenesmus, nausea, and low-grade fever, 101°F or less, can be present. (1-5,10,11) Variable, abdominal tenderness is present, and secondary hepatic involvement is a possibility. If this state is untreated, the symptomatology may improve, fluctuate for weeks or months, or may progress to one of many potential complications, intestinal or extra-intestinal. Refer to answer 7. The intestinal complications

include perforation with peritonitis or localized abscess, hemorrhage, stricture, ameboma (right colon usually), or so-called
postdysenteric colitis, resembling ulcerative colitis. (1-5,10)
    A significant percentage of patients with E. histolytica re-
main asymptomatic throughout, estimated at 10 to 50%. (1-5)
However, these individuals are at risk of overt colitis, hepatic
involvement, or certainly can transmit the organism to others.

7. (A,B,C) Those factors which favor invasion of the intestinal wall and subsequent intestinal and extra-intestinal features
are not known, e.g., immunological. However, the invasion is
initiated at the base of the crypts, extends to the mucosa, resulting in the characteristic flask-shaped ulceration as well as inflammatory reaction. (1-5,10) Once mucosal invasion occurs,
transmission via venous channels is possible, especially to the
portal vein and liver. (1-6) In the liver, the amebae are destroyed or can initiate subsequent abscess formation. The latter
only occurs in a very small percentage of patients with amebic
colitis, 1 to 5%. (1-6) Less than half of patients with liver abscess have E. histolytica in stools or a history of diarrhea. (1-
6) Other extra-intestinal areas of involvement, although infrequent, include the lungs, brain, skin, and perineum. (1-10)
    The most frequent extra-intestinal site of involvement is the
liver. Amebic liver abscesses are usually single and usually
located in the right lobe. The clinical features of amebic liver
abscess vary with the size, location, and number of lesions.
Thus, the onset can be gradual or more acute with fever and
chills. (1-6) Pain is almost always present with possible radiation to the shoulder with diaphragm involvement. (1-6) Fever
occurs in most patients, usually low-grade in type, and may be
accompanied by sweating and chills. Other symptomatology includes nausea, vomiting, anorexia, weight loss, weakness, and
nonproductive cough. (1-6) Physical examination may reveal
tenderness and/or enlargement of the liver. Laboratory studies
are frequently not helpful. Liver function testing, including
SGOT, SGPT, and alkaline phosphatase, may be normal or may
demonstrate mild alteration, while the total bilirubin level is
usually within normal limits. (1-6) The complete blood count
will usually reveal a leukocytosis, generally below 25,000 per
mm^3. (1-6,13,14) Most helpful tests have been (1) serologic
examination, such as indirect hemagglutination, complement fixation and agar diffusion identification, positive in over 90% with
invasive amebiasis; and (2) liver scan, technetium [99m]sulfide
colloid and gold[198] colloid, in particular. (1-6,13,19) The former has been most widely used, has little associated radiation
dose, 1 rad or less, and provides high diagnostic accuracy, both
individually and serially. (5,6,17-19) The size of the lesion

must usually be at least 1.0 cm in diameter to be detected. (17-19) Ultrasonography or computerized tomography have not been utilized in a large series. Complications of amebic liver disease include penetration into adjacent organs, spaces, or to the exterior of the trunk, such as the pleural space, pericardium, biliary tract, or renal pelvis. (5,6,17-19) Infrequently, there is hematogenous spread and the grave complication of a cerebral abscess. (9)

There has been one relatively large series from Durban reporting amebic pericarditis, as well as amebic peritonitis. (17, 19) Cerebral amebiasis (not abscess) has also been reported, apparently due to free-living soil amebae. (19) Infrequent observations have included cutaneous and perineal amebiasis. (19) Controversy continues to surround the disputed existence of amebic hepatitis. (6,17-19)

8. (B) The cornerstone of diagnosis is still the demonstration of the organism. The means of identification have included wet mounts, concentration techniques (for cysts), and permanently stained slides, such as with Gomori's trichrome stain. (13,14) Fresh stool specimens may be examined, obtained at the time of sigmoidoscopic examination and examined fresh, as well as after fixation in Schaudin's solution or alternative fixatives. (13, 14) If a biopsy is performed, the organism may be demonstrated; Best's carmine stain or PAS are particularly helpful in this regard. Despite the best of preparations, an experienced examiner must review these studies in order to maximize the results. Thirty percent positive identifications are made on the first stool specimen, while an additional 45 to 65% are made by two further specimens. (13,14)

9. (F) As previously mentioned in answer 7, invasive amebiasis is characterized by over 90% positive serologic examination. However, in asymptomatic patients, serologic examination is only approximately 50% positive. (15,16) Other serologic tests, including complement fixation, countercurrent electrophoresis, are available but do not provide additional accuracy, are not commercially available, and/or are expensive. (12) Since amebiasis has mainly a cosmopolitan distribution, not tropical, a high index of suspicion is essential.

10. (B,C,D,E) There are many drugs available for the treatment of amebiasis, as well as a myriad of drug combinations. Unfortunately, difficulty continues in defining the best combination since long-term studies, uniform criteria for successful treatment (cure), and controlled studies are few or nonexistent. The drugs generally employed include: (1) Diiodohydroxyquinoline

(Diodoquin), 7-10 mg/kg/day; particularly useful in eliminating amebae from the intestinal lumen, little is absorbed, and should be avoided in patients sensitive to iodides; (2) chloroquine diphosphate (Aralen), 15-20 mg/kg/day, particularly valuable in extra-intestinal forms, though prolonged usage should be avoided, considering possibility of rentinal and lens damage; (3) tetracycline, 25-50 mg/kg/day, particularly useful in symptomatic reduction in intestinal forms; (4) paromomycin (Humatin), 15-20 mg/kg/day, very effective in acute or chronic intestinal amebiasis; (5) metronidazole (Flagyl), 25-50 mg/kg/day, useful in intestinal (mild to severe) and extra-intestinal amebiasis, e.g., hepatic abscess, although recent concern has been raised, due to reports of mutagenic and carcinogenic effects. (1-5,10, 12,17-22) The usual combinations utilized for intestinal amebiasis are paromomycin for 5 to 7 days, then metronidazole for 5 to 7 days, and finally chloroquine for 10 to 14 days, the above with tetracycline substituted for paramomycin, or rarely (in very severe cases) addition of emetine hydrochloride, parenterally, 1 mg/kg/day, for 10 days. (19,21) In asymptomatic patients, metronidazole alone or a combination of diiodohydroxyquinoline for 21 days and chloroquine for 14 days are suggested. (19,21) The purpose of these combinations is to eliminate amebae from the intestine, eliminate symptomatology, and prevent formation of liver abscess. Surgery is reserved for the complications that are described in answer 6.

11. (A,B,D) Refer to answer 10 for dosage schedule. Once the diagnosis of amebic abscess is suspected, treatment must be initiated as soon as possible. Response within 48 to 72 hours is to be expected if amebic in origin; the promptness of starting treatment may negate the need for a surgical approach. (1,4,17, 21) The medical treatment consists of chloroquine for 2 weeks, maximum 4 weeks, metronidazole for 10 to 14 days, emetine hydrochloride, 1 mg/kg/day for 10 days, or metronidazole for 10 to 14 days followed by chloroquine for 2 weeks. (1,4,12,17-22) Surgical drainage is rarely indicated. Controversy continues regarding needle aspiration of an amebic abscess, even under fluoroscopic or ultrasound control. (1,4,17-24) Obviously, preparations for possible emergency surgery must be arranged before attempts at aspiration. In addition, approximately 10 to 20% of amebic liver abscesses become secondarily infected and will require surgical drainage. (1,4,17-24) Since this complication is difficult to recognize, the usual approach is to wait for 48 to 72 hours in order to obtain a response or nonresponse with antiamebic therapy. (1,4,19,21) If colitis is present too, then chloroquine and metronidazole or chloroquine and emetine are administered for 10 to 14 days. Resolution of these abscesses

may require many months. Serial scans as well as the clinical course and laboratory studies, can be utilized effectively in the followup of such patients. A persistent defect in the liver scan for even one year does not warrant retreatment. (1,4,17-21)

In patients with pulmonary, pericardial, or cerebral involvement, a combination of emetine (same dose as previously described) and chloroquine (also same dose as previously described) for 10 to 14 days is recommended. (4,19,21) Radiological examinations or scans can be used to confirm the clinical response and then to follow the patient serially.

REFERENCES

1. Marsden, P.D. and Schultz, M.G.: Intestinal parasites: Gastroenterology 57:724, 1969.

2. Pittman, F.E., Hashimi, W.K., Pittman, J.C.: Studies of human amebiasis. I. Clinical and laboratory findings in eight cases of acute amebic colitis. Gastroenterology 65:581, 1967.

3. Brandt, H. and Perez, T.R.: Pathology of human amebiasis. Human Pathol 1:351, 1970.

4. Mahmoud, A.A.F. and Warren, K.S.: Algorithms in the diagnosis and management of exotic diseases. XVII. Amebiasis. J Infect Dis 134:639, 1976.

5. Turrill, F.F. and Burnhamn, J.R.: Hepatic amebiasis. Am J Surg 111:424, 1966.

6. Doxiades, T., Candreviotis, N., Yiotas, Z.D., et al.: Chronic amebic hepatitis. Clinical and experimental observations. Arch Int Med 11:137, 1963.

7. Macleod, I.N., Wilmot, A.J., Powell, S.J.: Amoebic pericarditis. Q J Med 35:293, 1966.

8. Butt, C.G.: Primary amebic meningoencephalitis. N Engl J Med 274:1473, 1966.

9. Orbison, J.A., Reeves, N., Leedham, C.L., et al.: Amebic brain abscess. Medicine 30:247, 1951.

10. Pardo, G.A., Perez, A.N., Zavala, B.: Differential diagnosis of nonspecific and amebic ulcerative colitis. Dis Colon Rectum 15:147, 1972.

11. Cardoso, J.M., Kimura, D., Stoopen, M., et al.: Radiology of invasive amebiasis of the colon. Am J Roentgenol 128:935, 1977.

12. Report of the Committee of Infectious Diseases, American Academy of Pediatrics, 19th edition, Evanston, Illinois, 1982, p. 150.

13. Stamm, W.P.: The laboratory diagnosis of clinical amebiasis. Trans R Soc Trop Med Hyg 51:306, 1957.

14. Healy, G.R.: Laboratory diagnosis of amebiasis. Bull NY Acad Med 47:478, 1971.

15. Junipei, K., Jr., Worrell, C.L., Minshew, J.C., et al.: Serologic diagnosis of amebiasis. Am J Trop Med Hyg 21: 157, 1972.

16. Healy, G.R. and Karft, S.C.: The indirect hemagglutination test of amebiasis in patients with inflammatory bowel disease. Am J Dig Dis 17:97, 1972.

17. Cowie, R.L., Hichman, R., Saunders, S.J., et al.: Amoebic liver disease in Cape Town. SA Med J 46:1917, 1972.

18. Reynolds, R.B.: Amoebic abscess of the liver. Gastroenterology 60:952, 1971.

19. Silverman, A., Roy, C.C.: Pediatric Clinical Gastroenterology, 3rd edition. The CV Mosby Co., St. Louis, 1983, p. 431.

20. Cohen, H.G. and Reynolds, T.B.: Comparison of metronidazole and chloroquine for the treatment of amoebic liver abscess; a controlled trial. Gastroenterology 69:35, 1975.

21. Powell, S.J.: New developments in the therapy of amebiasis. Gut 11:967, 1970.

22. Wolfe, M.S.: The treatment of intestinal protozoan infections. Med Clin North Am 66:707, 1982.

23. Crane, P.S., Lee, Y.T., Seel, D.J.: Experience in the treatment of two patients with amebic abscess of the liver in Korea. Am J Surg 123:332, 1972.

24. Ribaudo, J.M. and Oshsner, A.: Intrahepatic abscesses: Amebic and pyogenic. Am J Surg 125:570, 1973.

Case 44

CHRONIC DIARRHEA IN A 2-YEAR-OLD GIRL

HISTORY

A 2-year-old white female presented with a 3-month history of
looser bowel movements, generally 2 to 5 per day. There was
no associated fever, vomiting, constipation, melena, hematochezia, dysuria, anorexia, skin lesions. The appetite and activity remained unchanged. There was no relationship to food
types. There was no apparent weight loss. The remainder of
the past history, developmental history, family history, social
history, and review of systems was noncontributory.

EXAMINATION

She was alert, active, and in no apparent distress, with normal
vital signs, weight 12.1 kg, height 8.5 cm. The remainder of
the examination, including the abdomen and anorectal area, was
unremarkable. Stool hemoccult testing was negative.

LABORATORY DATA

Hemoglobin:	12.2 gm%
Hematocrit:	37%
White blood cell count:	7,800/mm^3
PMN's:	44%
lymphocytes:	54%
monocytes:	2%
Sedimentation rate:	9 mm/hr
Serum:	
sodium:	138 mg/L
potassium:	4.4 meq/L

chloride:	102 meq/L
bicarbonate:	23 meq/L
creatinine:	0.4 mg%
total protein:	6.5 gm%
albumin:	3.9 gm%
calcium:	9.6 mg%
Urinalysis:	negative (pH 5.5)
Stool:	
occult blood:	negative
reducing substances:	negative
fat:	0-1 globule/HPF
culture:	negative
ova and parasites:	negative

QUESTIONS

1. Which of the following is the most likely diagnosis of this patient?
   A. Chronic nonspecific diarrhea of infancy
   B. Regional enteritis
   C. Ulcerative colitis
   D. Celiac disease
   E. Cystic fibrosis

2. Which of the following studies would be indicated in this patient at this time?
   A. Proctosigmoidoscopy
   B. Upper gastrointestinal series
   C. Barium enema examination
   D. Small intestinal biopsy and aspiration
   E. None

Question 3: Answer true (T) or false (F).

3. Failure to thrive is present in the majority of patients with chronic diarrhea.

4. Treatment of this condition includes which of the following?
   A. Diet revision
   B. Anticholinergics
   C. Antacids
   D. Antibiotics
   E. Cholestyramine

ANSWERS AND COMMENTS

1. (A) The presence of chronic diarrhea, but less than 6 bowel movements daily, with normal growth and development and without other symptomatology strongly suggests the diagnosis of chronic nonspecific diarrhea of infancy (CNSD). (1-1) The lack of systemic complaints, e. g. , fever, blood in the bowel movements, and the normal growth and development, make the other possibilities unlikely.

2. (E) Evaluation of the patient with chronic diarrhea begins with a careful, concise history and physical examination. The keynotes of the history are a thorough diet diary (record), growth parameters (height, weight, and head circumference in chronology), history of exposure regarding water and food supply, large groups, travel areas, and medication/environmental agents, as well as family history, and, last but not least, stool pattern (number, consistency, content, odor). The keynotes of the physical examination are the measurements of height, weight, and head circumference, signs, positive or negative, of nutrient deficiency, e. g. , dermatological (dryness, petecchiae, ecchymoses), and examination of stool, including smear for WBC, RBC, and fat droplets, and testing for reducing substances (WBC, RBC -methylene blue stain; sudan stain-fat droplets; Clinitest tablets-reducing substances). (1-6) Of significant importance at this point is the presence or absence of failure to thrive. Without significant weight loss, extensive evaluation for malabsorption is unnecessary and unwarranted. Reassurance of parents and comprehensive follow-up are the requisites, particularly future dietary records, and weight/height measurements.

3. (F) The overwhelming majority of patients with chronic diarrhea do not have associated failure to thrive, i. e. , 70 to 75%. (1-3) As previously mentioned in question 2, parental reassurance is paramount.

In the 25 to 30% with failure to thrive, further evaluation is indicated (Table 44. 1). As stated by Walker, (1) 75% with weight loss have iatrogenic failure to thrive, the "sequence of events" including fluid and electrolyte treatment of the diarrhea on a recurrent basis, resulting in caloric deprivation. The remainder will not respond to simple dietary management by weight increase, and more extensive malabsorptive studies will be indicated (refer to Case 25).

4. (A, B) The treatment of CNSD has included two main components: (1) diet, (2) medication, particularly anticholinergic agents. (1-5, 7-11)

With reference to diet, higher fat intake, particularly polyunsaturated fat (LCT) substitution, has been found to be effective in CNSD, unfortunately only in a minority. (1, 2, 7, 8) Walker

TABLE 44.1   Management of Chronic Diarrhea

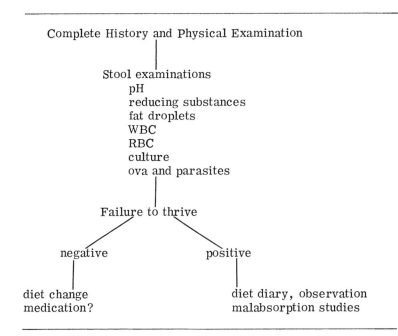

Complete History and Physical Examination

Stool examinations
   pH
   reducing substances
   fat droplets
   WBC
   RBC
   culture
   ova and parasites

Failure to thrive

negative — diet change / medication?

positive — diet diary, observation / malabsorption studies

(1) suggested that fat in the small or large intestine may decrease motility. Other dietary changes have included the use of nonlactose, nonsucrose formulas/liquids which are iso- or hypotonic, e.g., ProSobee®, RCF®. At times, a nonlactose formula/liquid with simpler protein and fat content which are iso- or hypotonic have been helpful, e.g., Precision Isotonic®, Travasorb®, Osmolite®. For supplementation, if necessary, the "special" or variably "elemental" (predigested) formulas/liquids can be used as previously mentioned, but also Polycose (glucose polymer; 2 cal/ml), medium-chain triglyceride oil (MCT), 9 cal/ml, and similar agents can be used. (1-2, 4, 7-10)

With reference to medication, anticholinergic agents, e.g., Donnatal®, Probanthine®, have been utilized in order to decrease motility in the small and large intestine. (1, 2, 4, 10) Antidiarrheal agents, e.g., opiates, provide temporary aid generally and commonly have side effects. Binding agents, e.g., anion resin (cholestyramine), antacids (aluminum type), have been used with variable success. (1, 10) Presumably bile acids are bound and, therefore, are not able to irritate the colonic mucosa. (1, 2, 10) These agents, unfortunately, are not tasty, cost excessively, i.e., cholestyramine, and are not uniformly beneficial.

Antibiotics are not of value with any consistency and presumably alter bowel microflora, both positively and negatively. Lactinex granules have not had confirmed value, either. (1) Therefore, standard medication is not routinely recommended because of common side effects, limited palatability, cost, and lack of practical value in clinical experience. Therefore, parental reassurance, patience, and adequacy of follow-up (availability, counseling, dietary suggestions) are the critical factors in a successful outcome of the treatment program.

REFERENCES

1. Walker, W.A.: Benign chronic diarrhea of infancy. Pediatr Rev 3:153, 1981.

2. Ament, M.E. and Barclay, G.N.: Chronic diarrhea. Pediatr Ann 11:124, 1982.

3. Davidson, M. and Wasserman, R.: The irritable colon of childhood. J Pediatr 69:1027, 1966.

4. Gall, D.G. and Hamilton, J.R.: Chronic diarrhea in childhood: A new look at an old problem. Pediatr Clin Am 21:1001, 1974.

5. Phillips, S.F.: Diarrhea: A current view of the pathophysiology. Gastroenterology 63:495, 1972.

6. Moore, J.G., Englert, E., Byler, A.H., et al.: Simple fecal tests of absorption: A prospective study and critique. Am J Dig Dis 16:97, 1971.

7. Lloyd-Still, J.D.: Chronic diarrhea of childhood and the misuse of elimination diets. J Pediatr 95:10, 1979.

8. Cohen, S., Lake, A.M., Mathis, R.K., et al.: Perspectives on chronic non-specific diarrhea: Dietary management. Pediatrics 61:808, 1979.

9. Walker-Smith, J.A.: Toddler's diarrhea. Arch Dis Child 55:329, 1980.

10. Liebman, W.M. and Thaler, M.M.: Life-threatening diarrhea states in early infancy. In: Gastrointestinal Disease. Sleisenger, M. H. and Fordtran, J. S. (Eds). WB Saunders Co., Philadelphia, 1978, p. 1730.

11. Anderson, C.M.: Malabsorption in children. Clin Gastroenterol 6:355, 1977.

Case 45

CHRONIC DIARRHEA IN AN 18-MONTH-OLD BOY

HISTORY

An 18-month-old white male presented with a 6-week history of looser, more frequent bowel movements. The bowel habit pattern had changed from 1 to 2 bowel movements daily to 5 to 10 bowel movements daily, loose to watery in nature. There was an associated weight loss of 3 pounds. There was no associated vomiting, melena, hematochezia, skin lesions, dysuria, respiratory difficulty, or jaundice. The appetite and activity were decreased. There was also a history of vague abdominal distress unrelated to meals, food types, bowel movements, time of day, or position. Milk and soy elimination had produced no apparent effect. The remainder of the past history, developmental history, family history, social history, and review of systems was noncontributory.

EXAMINATION

He was reasonably alert and active, with minimal fussiness, vital signs, weight 9.0 kg, height 76 cm, and head circumference 46.5 cm. The remainder of the examination, including the abdomen and anorectal area, was unremarkable and stool hemoccult testing was negative.

LABORATORY DATA

Hemoglobin:	11.1 gm%
Hematocrit:	33%
White blood cell count:	8,700/mm^3
PMN's:	38%

lymphocytes:	50%
monocytes:	9%
eosinophiles:	3%
Sedimentation rate:	11 mm/hr
Serum:	
sodium:	136 meq/L
potassium:	3.6 meq/L
chloride:	98 meq/L
bicarbonate:	20 meq/L
creatinine:	0.6 mg%
calcium:	8.7 mg%
total protein:	5.7 gm%
albumin:	3.2 gm%
T4:	8.6 μg%
Urinalysis:	negative
Stool:	
occult blood:	negative
reducing substances:	trace
culture:	negative
ova and parasites:	negative
Chest X-ray:	negative
Right wrist X-ray:	appropriate for chronological age

QUESTIONS

Questions 1-8: Answer true (T) or false (F).

From the historical, laboratory, and radiological details you may assume that

1. the probable diagnosis is celiac disease.

2. this disease entity occasionally occurs in the first decade of life.

3. the diarrhea is usually of less than 2 weeks' duration.

4. mucosal injury with associated absorptive deficiency is the underlying common pathophysiology.

5. small intestinal biopsy and analysis will demonstrate pathognomonic findings.

6. treatment is directed at correction of fluid, electrolyte, and nutrient deficiency.

7. elemental diets are not helpful in this entity.

8. if intractable to dietary management, total parenteral nutrition is indicated and is effective in the vast majority of patients.

ANSWERS AND COMMENTS

1. (F) The diarrhea is chronic, since formless stools had been passed for more than 14 days. The age of onset, lack of significant growth deficiency, i.e., weight less than third to fifth percentile (25.0) with associated stunted height, and lack of prior difficulty with gluten-containing foods make the diagnosis of celiac disease less likely but not eliminated. At this point, the probable diagnosis is persistent or chronic diarrhea of infancy, becoming intractable. (1-6)

Intractable diarrhea of infancy was originally defined by Avery et al. (2) and included infants less than 3 months of age with diarrhea over 2 weeks and without evidence of an identifiable infectious agent (stool studies).

2. (F) As mentioned in question 1, the original definition of Avery et al. (2) included only infants less than 3 months of age. Infants older than 3 months of age, as well as older children, may also develop significant diarrhea less than or more than 2 weeks in duration and manifest a clinical course, "life-threatening" in nature. Therefore, the disease entity is actually a syndrome, and mucosal injury (insult) is a common feature and "cause" of certain features, i.e., diarrhea, nutrient-electrolyte-fluid loss. Any age may be involved, generally less than 8 to 10 years of age, particularly the young infant. However, the syndrome can include older children and adolescents, e.g., inflammatory bowel disease, immunodeficiency states. (1-8)

3. (F) As previously mentioned in questions 1 and 2, the diarrhea was longer than 2 weeks in the initial definition by Avery et al. (2), and this time period has continued to be a part of the syndrome, too. (1-6) Life-threatening diarrhea is possible in less than 2 weeks' duration, but the overwhelming majority have the diarrhea longer than 2 weeks with the resultant malnutrition in so many. (1-5,7-12)

4. (T) Small intestinal mucosal injury is the common denominator, the result of the offending agent, e.g., infectious agent, result of celiac disease, inflammatory bowel disease. Due to the mucosal injury, enzyme deficiency occurs, e.g.,

disaccharidases, and subsequently, secretory and reabsorptive function can be disturbed, e.g., electrolytes and proteins/peptides, respectively. (1,4,6,8) As a result of the nutrient disturbances, calorie sources and protein are lost, with adverse effects on mucosal regeneration/turnover, exocrine function, e.g., pancreatic. Bacterial overgrowth also frequently occurs at this point. (1-6,8-11) Bile salt malabsorption and deconjugation with resultant fat malabsorption, principally long-chain triglyceride, can then occur. (Table 45.1) As Rossi and Lebenthal (8) note, a vicious repetitive cycle is certainly in effect.

5.   (F) Small intestinal biopsy (mucosal) and duodenal (jejunal) fluid analysis for culture, ova and parasites, and enzyme analysis (pancreatic) can be helpful in delineating the degree of mucosal injury or conversely, recovery, enzyme deficiency, and bacterial overgrowth, respectively. However, the specificity of the type of changes is lacking since malnutrition per se or a number of clinical entities, e.g., celiac disease, cystic fibrosis, immunodeficiency syndromes, can cause mild (grade I) to severe (grade IV) mucosal changes, e.g., altered villous/crypt ratio, lamina propria cellularity. (1-8)

6.   (T) The initial treatment phase is directed toward restoration of fluid (plasma volume), electrolyte and acid-base deficiencies. (1-6,8-11) (Table 45.2) Usually intravenous fluid therapy is required to accomplish these goals. At this time, oral nutrient intake can be attempted. When oral intake is not possible and/or not tolerated, parenteral nutrition becomes necessary.

7.   (F) As indicated in question 6, oral nutrient intake is attempted after intravenous fluid therapy for correction of plasma volume, electrolyte, and acid-base deficiencies. The initial oral intake should be simple or "elemental," consisting of monosaccharides or oligosaccharides (carbohydrate), medium-chain triglycerides (fat), and protein hydrolysates or amino acids (protein), as well as minerals, vitamins, trace metals. These formula require minimal digestion, less mucosal absorptive surface, are reasonably low solute load gastrointestinally. (1-4,6, 8,13) Examples of commercial elemental diets include Vivonex®, Pregestimil®, Precision Isotonic®, Vital®, Travasorb®, Osmolite®. Most provide 1 cal/ml, while a few, e.g., Pregestimil®, provide 2/3 cal/ml. Some, however, do have a high osmolality at full concentration and must initially or always be diluted, e.g., Vivonex®, regular nitrogen content (N), 550 milliosmols, Vital®, 450 milliosmols. (1-4,6,8,13) The amounts

TABLE 45.1   Diagnostic Evaluation of Patients with
Intractable Diarrhea

(Persistent) Chronic Diarrhea
|

complete blood count
sedimentation rate
urinalysis
serum electrolytes, calcium, glucose, cholesterol,
total protein/albumin
quantitative immunoglobulins
blood, urine, stool cultures (bacterial, viral)

positive   negative
| |
appropriate treatment   sweat test
for condition   24-hr urine for amino acids,
                                       catecholamines 5 HI AA
                                       urine and stool for chloride analysis
                                       breath tests (hydrogen) for
                                       disaccharides or disaccharide tol-
                                       erance tests orally |

                                                    negative

                                       upper gastrointestinal-small bowel
                                       series
                                       barium enema
                                       proctosigmoidoscopy and rectal bi-
                                       opsy
                                                    |

                                                    negative

                                       duodenal aspirate for culture (par-
                                       asites, aerobic/anaerobic) and for
                                       file acids, pancreatic enzymes
                                       small intestinal biopsy for histology
                                       and disaccharidase assay
                                                    |

                                                    negative

                                       serum gastrin
                                       serum vasoactive intestinal
                                       polypeptide (VIP)

TABLE 45.2   Treatment of Intractable Diarrhea of Infancy

Intractable Diarrhea
|
Intravenous fluid therapy (fluids, electrolytes, colloid)

positive response

Begin oral diet (initially elemental,
hypo- or iso-osmolar)

negative response
(continued diarrhea)

positive response   negative response
(diarrhea subsides)

advance oral diet   consider continuous
   slowly   nasogastric drip (elemental diet)
(initially elemental at   or
increased concentration,
then sucrose-containing)   parenteral hyperalimentation

peripheral   continuous nasogastric
hyperalimentation   drip (elemental diet)

negative response	positive response	negative response	positive response
central hyperalimentation	Begin oral diet, (initially elemental diet, hypo- or-iso-osmolar)	Parenteral* hyperalimentation	Begin oral diet, (initially elemental diet, hypo- or iso-osmolar)

cessation of diarrhea
weight increase

Begin oral diet (initially
elemental, hypo- or iso-osmolar)
(decrease hyperalimentation)

*Parenteral = peripheral or central

administered are adjusted according to fluid and calorie requirements. Stools are weighed and tested for reducing substances
(Clinitest), pH, and occult blood. The patient's weight and the
caloric intake are monitored daily, too. These simple parameters serve as the basis for changes in dietary fluid and nutrient content.

8. (T) When oral intake of simple nutrients (elemental diet) is
not possible or tolerated, total parenteral nutrition (TPN) is indicated. As always, adequate caloric intake is a must (carbohydrate, fat), and amino acids, or protein hydrolysates are administered in order to achieve positive nitrogen balance (protein
sparing). (1-4, 6, 8-12) For short-term administration, 2 weeks
or less, a peripheral vein can be used, while usually a central
vein is used for longer therapy or, practically, for ease and consistency of intravenous access. Meticulous attention to catheter care
is mandatory to prevent infection or other complications. (9-13)
Nutritional requirements, e.g., 65 to 150 cal/kg/24 hr, 1.5 to
4.0 gm of protein/kg/24 hr (positive nitrogen balance), provide
the guidelines for the composition and volume of TPN administered daily. Intravenous fat, e.g., 10 to 20% Intralipid (soybean), Liposyn (safflower), is used for caloric needs and also
to provide fat as long-chain triglyceride (CT; include essential
fatty acids, e.g., linoleic acid). As with oral nutrient intake,
daily weight of the patient, stool weight, fluid intake and output
are assessed. As the stool pattern returns to normal, the patient's weight increases, and other parameters, e.g., laboratory studies, including protein/albumin levels, return to or
toward normal, oral intake can be considered. Oral tolerance
tests, glucose or sucrose, can be accomplished to provide additional information for gradual oral nutrient intake. (1-4, 6, 8-12)
    Gavage, enterostomy, and tube (nasogastric, nasoduodenal,
nasojejunal) feedings are periodically used in intractable (persistent) diarrheal states, but are more utilized in anatomic defects and postsurgical conditions of the gastrointestinal tract,
e.g., short bowel syndromes. (1, 4, 8, 14) Elemental diets are
generally delivered through these routes, bolus or intermittent/
continuous drip method.
    Medication has generally been ineffective in intractable diar-
rhea of infancy, e.g., opiates, anticholinergics. (1, 4, 8) Antibiotics, corticosteroids, and even prostaglandin inhibitors have
not demonstrated a consistent beneficial effect, either. (1, 4, 6)
However, cholestyramine, an anion-binding resin of bile acids,
enterotoxin, bacteria, has been reported to have a significant
beneficial effect in some cases. (1, 4, 6, 15) The positive effect is
generally noted in the first 48 to 72 hours. (1, 4, 6, 15) Lastly, a
recent report by Sandhu et al. (16) noted a positive effect in each

of 6 infants with protracted diarrhea by Loperamide (Imodium®),
an opiate analogue, presumably by its action on smooth muscle/
intestinal motility.

With the introduction of total parenteral nutrition (TPN) and
special oral (elemental) diets, the prognosis has been favorably
affected. Prior mortality rates of 40 to 90% have been reduced
to 5 to 20%. (1, 4, 6) Longer-term growth and development seems
also to be favorably influenced, e.g., approaching or reaching
normal, but additional studies and follow-up will be necessary
to fully delineate expected outcome. (4, 6)

REFERENCES

1. Sunshine, P., Sinata, F.R., Mitchell, C.H.: Intractable
   diarrhea of infancy. Clin Gastroenterol 6:445, 1977.

2. Avery, G.B., Villavicencio, D., Lilly, J.R., et al.: Intractable diarrhea in early infancy. Pediatr 41:712, 1968.

3. Hyman, C.J., Reiter, J., Rodman, J., et al.: Parenteral
   and oral alimentation in the treatment of the nonspecific protracted diarrhea syndrome in infancy. J Pediatr 78:17,
   1971.

4. Liebman, W.M. and Thaler, M.M.: Life-threatening diar-
   rhea states in early infancy. In: Gastrointestinal Disease,
   Sleisenger, M.H. and Fordtran, J.S. (Eds). WB Saunders
   Co., Philadelphia, 1978, p. 1730.

5. Liebman, W.M., Thaler, M.M., DeLorimier, A., et al.:
   Intractable diarrhea of infancy due to intestinal coccidiosis.
   Gastroenterology 78:579, 1980.

6. Greene, H.L., McCabe, D.R., Merenskin, G.B.: Protracted diarrhea and malnutrition in infancy: Changes in intestinal morphology and disaccharidase activities during
   treatment with total intravenous nutrition or oral elemental
   diets. J Pediatr 87:695, 1975.

7. Ament, M.E.: Immunodeficiency syndrome and gastrointestinal disease. Pediatr Clin Aames 22:807, 1975.

8. Rossi, T.M. and Lebenthal, E.: Intractable diarrhea of
   infancy. In: Textbook of Gastroenterology and Nutrition in
   Infancy, Lebenthal, E. (Ed). Raven Press, New York,
   1981, p. 987.

9. Heird, W.C. and Winters, R.W.: Total parenteral nutrition: The state of the art. J Pediatr 86:21, 1975.

10. Hamilton, R.F., Davis, W.C., Stephenson, D.V., et al.: Effects of parenteral hyperalimentation on upper gastrointestinal tract secretions. Arch Surg 102:348, 1971.

11. Lloyd-Still, J.D., Shwachman, H., Filler, R.: Protracted diarrhea of infancy treated by intravenous alimentation. I. Clinical studies of 16 infants. Am J Dis Child 125:358, 1973.

12. Corand, A.G.: Parenteral nutrition in infants and children. Surg Clin North Am 61:1089, 1981.

13. Poley, J.R. : Liver and nutrition: Hepatic complications of total parenteral nutrition. In: Textbook of Gastroenterology and Nutrition in Infancy, Lebenthal, E. (Ed). Raven Press, New York, 1981, p. 743

14. Christie, D. L. and Ament, M. E. : Dilute elemental diet and continuous infusion technique for management of short bowel syndrome. J Pediatr 87:705, 1975.

15. Tamer, M.A., Santora, T.R., Sandberg, D.H.: Cholestyramine therapy for intractable diarrhea. Pediatrics 53:217, 1974.

16. Sanhu, B.K., Tripp, J.H., Milla, P.J., et al.: Loperamide in severe protracted diarrhea. Arch Dis Child 58:39, 1983.

Case 46

ALTERED BOWEL HABIT PATTERN AND
ANAL PRURITUS IN A 9-MONTH-OLD GIRL

HISTORY

A 9-month-old white female presented with a 6-month history of an altered bowel habit pattern, which consisted of discomfort, including itching, with the passage of bowel movements. However, the number of bowel movements supposedly remained 1 to 2 daily, firm, occasionally soft in nature, with no gross blood being noted. There was no associated history of fever, vomiting, diarrhea, anorexia, melena, apparent dysuria, or trauma. Dietary history consisted of Enfamil, with subsequent addition of cereals, lamb, and applesauce at 3 months of age, and other baby foods for the next 2 months. Subsequent to 5 months of age, the patient was placed on table food, prepared in a blender; bowel movement changes did not appear to be related to this dietary history. The remainder of the past history, developmental history, family history, social history, and review of systems was unremarkable.

EXAMINATION

She was alert and in no apparent distress, weight 8.3 kg, length 71 cm, head circumference 43 cm. The remainder of the examination was unremarkable except for mild erythema in the perianal area. Anoscopic examination to 4 cm was unremarkable.

LABORATORY DATA

Hemoglobin:	11.9 gm%
Hematocrit:	35%
White blood cell count:	6,800/mm^3
PMN's:	40%
lymphocytes:	56%
monocytes:	2%
eosinophiles:	2%
Urinalysis:	negative
Stool:	
reducing substances:	negative
culture:	negative
ova and parasites:	(Fig. 46.1)

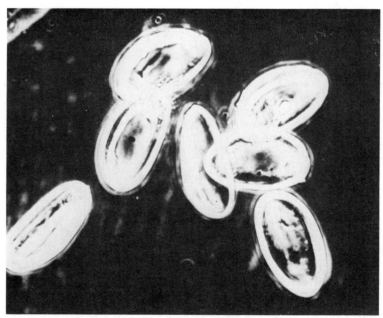

Figure 46.1 Stool. Several ova, oval in shape, are seen. A double membrane-like structure is apparent.

QUESTIONS

1. The most likely diagnosis in this patient is which one of the following?
   A. Regional enteritis
   B. Giardia lamblia
   C. Strongyloides stercoralis
   D. Enterobius vermicularis
   E. Ulcerative colitis

Questions 2-5: Answer true (T) or false (F).

2. Children are more susceptible to this agent than adults.

3. This agent is the most common helminthic infection in the temperate areas of the world.

4. Mating of these worms occurs in the jejunum or ileum of the human intestine.

5. Eggs are deposited in the rectum and then pass out of the anus at night.

6. The usual symptomatology produced by this agent includes
   A. anal pruritus
   B. diarrhea
   C. hematochezia
   D. vaginitis
   E. fissure-in-ano

7. Diagnosis can be made by
   A. stool examination
   B. microscopic examination of perianal cellulose tape
   C. anoscopy
   D. fiberoptic colonoscopy
   E. barium enema

8. Treatment should consist of which of the following?
   A. Treat family household members
   B. Pyrvinium pamoate
   C. Piperazine citrate
   D. Silver nitrate cauterization
   E. Hydrocortisone acetate enemas

ANSWERS AND COMMENTS

1.   (D) The most likely diagnosis of this patient is Enterobius
vermicularis.
     The presence of anal pruritus only, without diarrhea, fever,
abdominal pain, melena, hematochezia, anorexia, or weight
loss, would make the other answers less likely.

2.   (T) Enterobiasis (oxyuriasis) has worldwide distribution
and is estimated to be present in as many as 30 to 40% of school-
age children. (1,3-7) In addition, children seem to be more susceptible than adults. (1,3-7) The reason for this increased susceptibility is unknown. There is no sex predilection and no apparent seasonal variation, either. (8) In the United States, the
incidence has been estimated at 5 to 15%. (8)

3.   (T) The pinworm is easily the most common helminthic infection in the temperate areas of the world. (1,3-7) Refer to
answer 2.

4.   (F) E. vermicularis, a nematode, attaches to the mucosa
of the appendix and cecum. The male and female worms under-
go mating in the immediate cecal area. The gravid female worm,
about 2 inches in length, then migrates to the anorectal region,
subsequently making its way outside the anal margin.

5.   (F) The eggs are deposited outside the anal margin, i.e.,
in the perineal and perianal regions. (1-9) Ingestion of these
eggs (fecal-oral route) completes the life cycle. (1-9) These
eggs are football shaped, have a transparent, flattened shell,
and motile larvae may be within. (1-9) The ingested eggs will
hatch in the duodenum, and the liberated larvae will migrate to
the cecum, even possibly invading the appendix. (1-9)

6.   (A,D) The only well-confirmed symptom of this worm's infestation is anorectal pruritus. (1-9) Localized, secondary infection of the perianal area may result from the intense pruritis.
(1-9) In females, vaginitis and salpingitis, have been reported.
Other symptomatology attributed to E. vermicularis infestation
has included restlessness, irritability, nightmares, and night
terrors, as well as recurrent abdominal pain. (1-9) These clinical parameters have not been adequately confirmed.

7.   (A,B) Examination of stool is a less efficient means of diagnosis and is usually not positive. (1-9) Instead, the diagnosis is
best made by examination of a piece of transparent cellulose or
adhesive tape applied to the perianal surface upon awakening in

the morning. After 15 to 60 seconds, the tape is removed and placed upon a slide covered with toluene. (4-7) Microscopic examination will reveal the eggs described in answer 5.

The other listed methodology will be unproductive, unless fecal material is obtained for examination or the adult worms are visualized. These studies are cumbersome, expensive, and generally an unproductive means of making a diagnosis of this benign condition.

8. (A,B,D) The treatment program must consist of cleaning all contaminated objects, such as clothing and sheets. Usually all family members are treated, as well as the patient. Effective treatment consists of mebendazole (Vermox, 100 mg as a single dose, repeated in 2 weeks), pyrvinium pamoate (Povan, 5-10 mg/kg, as a single dose), or piperazine citrate (65 mg/kg/ 24 hr for 7 days). (1,4,6,9,10) The previously mentioned cleaning must be performed and the family should be given a second course of treatment after 2 weeks. The latter is usually necessary since reinfection is common during the cleaning phase. In addition, a repeated course of treatment may be necessary for some patients (5 to 10%). (1,4,6,9,10)

REFERENCES

1. Brandborg, L.L.: Parasitic diseases. In: Gastrointestinal Disease. Sleisenger, M.H. and Fordtran, J.S. (Eds). W.B. Saunders Co., Philadelphia, 1973, p. 989.

2. Marsden, P.D. and Schultz, M.G.: Intestinal parasites. Gastroenterology 57:724, 1969.

3. Hunter, G.W., Swartzwelder, J.C., Clyde, D.F.: Tropical Medicine. WB Saunders Co., Philadelphia, 1976.

4. Beeson, P.D. and McDermott, W. (Eds): Protozoal and helminthic diseases. In: Textbook of Medicine. 14th Edition, WB Saunders Co., Philadelphia, 1975, p. 471

5. Marcial-Rojas, R.A. (Ed): Pathology of Protozoal and Helminthic Diseases with Clinical Correlations. Williams and Wilkins Co., Baltimore, 1971.

6. Silverman, A., Roy, C.C.: Pediatric Clinical Gastroenterology, 3rd edition. The CV Mosby Co., St. Louis, 1983, p. 436.

7. Jelliffe, D.B. : Diseases of Children in the Subtropics and Tropics, 2nd Edition. The CV Mosby Co., St. Louis, 1975, p. 355.

8. Report of the Committee on Infectious Diseases, American Academy of Pediatrics, 19th edition, Evanston, Illinois, 1982, p. 160.

9. Jones, T.C.: Parasitic diseases you're likely to encounter. Resident Staff Physician, November 1977, p. 173.

10. Most, H.: Treatment of common parasitic infections of man encountered in the United States. N Engl J Med 287: 495, 698, 1972.

Case 47

ALTERNATING CONSTIPATION AND DIARRHEA IN
A 13-MONTH-OLD BOY

HISTORY

A 13-month-old white male presented with a history of altered
bowel habit pattern of 3 months' duration. The frequency of
bowel movements varied from 0 to 4-5 bowel movements daily,
loose to soft in nature. In addition, there was probable associated increased flatus passage on occasions. There was no history of fever, vomiting, abdominal pain, melena, hematochezia,
skin lesions, anorexia, jaundice, or dysuria. Appetite and activity remained good. Growth pattern, height, and weight, remained within normal limits. There was no relationship of the
bowel movements with meals, time of day, or food types. The
parents had eliminated milk products on their own, but this produced no effect. The remainder of the past history, developmental history, family history, social history, and review of systems was noncontributory. Medications have included Lactinex
granules without apparent effect.

EXAMINATION

He was alert, active, and in no distress, with normal vital signs.
Height was 76 cm, weight 11.3 kg, and head circumference 46.5
cm. The remainder of the examination was negative, including
the abdomen and anorectal area.

LABORATORY DATA

Hemoglobin:	12.0 gm%
Hematocrit:	36%

White blood cell count: 7,200/mm^3
   PMN's: 44%
   lymphocytes: 54%
   monocytes: 1%
   eosinophiles: 1%
Platelets: 275,000/mm^3
Sedimentation rate: 7 mm/hr
Urinalysis: negative
Serum:
   sodium: 139 meq/L
   potassium: 4.1 meq/L
   chloride: 102 meq/L
   bicarbonate: 22 meq/L
   total protein: 6.2 gm%
   albumin: 4.5 gm%
   calcium: 9.4 mg%
   glucose: 90 mg%
   creatinine: 0.5 mg%
   SGOT: 18 units
   alkaline phosphatase: 180 IU
   carotene: 115 μg%
   folate: 9.0 ng/ml
Stool:
   occult blood: negative
   reducing substances: negative
   culture: negative
   ova and parasites: negative
Barium enema: negative
Upper GI-small bowel series: negative

QUESTIONS

1. Which is the most likely diagnosis of this patient?
   A. Duodenal ulcer
   B. Irritable colon syndrome
   C. Celiac disease
   D. Ulcerative colitis
   E. Regional enteritis

2. Which of the following are the usual clinical features of this condition?
   A. Recurrent dysphagia
   B. Slow growth and development
   C. Chronic diarrhea
   D. Recurrent vomiting
   E. Recurrent abdominal pain ("colic")

Question 3: Answer true (T) or false (F).

3. There is a marked female preponderance in this condition.

4. Which factor(s) have been most implicated in its etiology?
   A. Altered transit time (slowed)
   B. Altered transit time (accelerated)
   C. Exaggerated response to stress
   D. Hormonal imbalance
   E. Allergy

5. Which of the following studies would usually be indicated in the evaluation of such patients?
   A. Complete blood count, urinalysis
   B. Stool pH, reducing substances, and culture
   C. Sigmoidoscopy
   D. Fiberoptic endoscopy
   E. Intravenous pyelography

6. Which of the following measures have been frequently helpful in the treatment of this condition?
   A. Antispasmodics
   B. Antacids
   C. Antihistaminics
   D. Sedatives, tranquilizers
   E. Supportive counseling

ANSWERS AND COMMENTS

1. (B) The irritable colon syndrome (ICS) is the most likely diagnosis of this patient.
   The pattern of pain, specifically without relationship to location, time of day, meals and food types, or to bowel movements, as well as the lack of nausea and vomiting, fever, hematochezia, anorexia, weight loss, and reduced activity, make the possibilities less likely of duodenal ulcer disease, celiac disease, and inflammatory bowel disease.

2. (C,E) The key feature suggesting this condition, and, in fact, the usual clinical feature, is the presence of a well child. Thus, growth and development are normal. The main symptom of this well child is chronic diarrhea. The diarrhea usually consists of less than 6 to 7 bowel movements daily. The bowel movements are usually described as being mushy or loose with variable odor, mainly brown in color, and not floating on top of the water in the toilet bowl. Mucus is frequently noted in the stools,

and undigested food may also be present at times. Blood (red streaks) is infrequent. Melena and occult blood positive stools rarely occur. The diarrhea may be precipitated by stress or any type of infection. The pattern of diarrhea may be continuous, recurrent, or limited to a few weeks or months. In early infancy, this pattern seems to clear spontaneously by 3 1/2 to 4 years of age. (1-5) Recurrent abdominal pain (RAP), colicky in nature, frequently occurs. Its localization may be difficult to ascertain, most commonly being in the periumbilical region. There is usually no relationship to time of day, meals, specific foods, or to bowel movements. Its duration is quite variable usually not interfering significantly with patient activity. Nausea, vomiting, fever, anorexia, pyrosis, and dysphagia essentially do not occur.

3.   (F) There is only a slight male preponderance in this condition. The usual age of onset in infancy is 8 to 18 months of age, although the age range can be 3 months to 30 months. (1-5)

4.   (B,C) The exact cause (or causes) of ICS is unknown. Many associated conditions have been mentioned in conjunction with ICS, including food allergy, constipation, aerophagia, "teething," mittelschmerz, and abdominal "migraine." However, the main etiological factors mentioned have been stress (emotions) and altered transit time (accelerated). (1-13)
   The former has been implicated on the basis of extensive interviews and observations (patient, family) in patients with ICS; and the resultant effect of various stimuli, such as familial interactions, peer relationships, play activity, has been an exaggerated response or summation, expressed in somatic symptomatology, including diarrhea and abdominal pain. (1-13) Whether a generalized disturbance or imbalance of the autonomic nervous system is involved remains unsettled, despite reports of exaggerated responses to stimulation, e.g., pupillary response to cholinergic drugs. (6,7,10) Altered transit time is frequently present, usually 40 to 50% less than age-matched controls, determined by use of a marker system, such as carmine. (8) Mass movements, particularly of the left colon, propel fecal material to the rectosigmoid area. Lower colonic segment tone and pressure have been found to be elevated in some patients subjected to anorectal manometry. This increase could provide a resistance to material moving down, reducing subsequent desiccation due to fluid absorption. (12,13) Additionally, recent studies of basal electrical rhythm by transducers have revealed increased slow wave frequency in ICS. (13) Further correlative studies are obviously needed.

No evidence of malabsorption, e.g., fat, nitrogen, bile acids, reducing substances, parasitic infestation, allergic diathesis, or abnormal electroencephalography have consistently been found in ICS. Finally, a family history of the same or other functional bowel disorders has been found in 20 to 35% of cases. (1-5,11-13) However, a true genetic or ethnic predisposition has not been found.

5. (A,B) It is advisable to restrict the number of studies performed during the initial evaluation unless the history, examination, and/or clinical course suggest otherwise. As previously mentioned, a well child with only chronic diarrhea and normal growth and development suggests this entity. There are no absolute diagnostic studies for confirmation of this condition. Radiological examinations, including barium enema, are nonspecific. The demonstration of an area of spasm in the splenic flexure-proximal descending colon during barium enema examination is not a specific finding. (12,13)

Proctosigmoidoscopic examination usually is of no significant aid. One series emphasized findings, such as patches of hyperemia, dilatation of the rectal lumen, and pallor, as reflecting exaggerated responses to stress, but most authors would agree that these findings are quite common in asymptomatic normals. (9,12,13) Fiberoptic upper endoscopy is obviously of little value unless pathology is expected in the esophagus, stomach, or proximal duodenum. Fiberoptic lower endoscopy will infrequently demonstrate an abnormality in such cases in preschool children, while being more helpful in older children, e.g., inflammatory bowel disease, parasite infestation. (12,13) Therefore, a complete blood count, urinalysis, sedimentation rate, and stool examinations for occult blood, reducing substances and/or pH, and culture are usually sufficient, when normal, to reassure the parents and physician that significant organic disease is not likely. When the history is atypical, appropriate radiological and laboratory studies are indicated.

6. (E) This is one of the more taxing problems in pediatric practice, requiring time, patience, and understanding. The physician must be willing to spend time to explain his findings convincingly to the parents, to provide support and guidance as to dietary and activity management, and to be available in the future for further aid. The physician's thoroughness in initial and subsequent evaluations further reduces anxiety. With reference to diet, between-meal snacks should be avoided. Chilled foods and drinks (trigger mass movements) should be limited or avoided. Adequate caloric intake, however, must be maintained.

The usage of various drugs should be discouraged since they generally do not help, confuse the clinical picture, and, additionally, create unwanted dependence. However, occasional symptomatic relief of severe pain is warranted, e.g., analgesics, such as acetaminophen, 4-6 mg/kg every 4 hours. (12,13) Extreme anxiety may necessitate temporary use of tranquilizers, such as chlorpromazine, 0.5 mg/kg per dose three times daily. (12,13) Antacids, anticholinergics, antispasmodics, and antihistiminic preparations have produced inconsistent results. In summary, a patient, understanding, and available physician to provide guidance and support to the family is the key to successful treatment.

In ICS of infancy, the prognosis is excellent, with spontaneous disappearance occurring in essentially all patients by 3 1/2 to 4 years of age. In older children and adolescents, ICS tends to be more chronic and intermittent, 30 to 60% lasting into adulthood, regardless of treatment or type. (2,14)

REFERENCES

1. Davidson, M. and Wasserman, R.: The irritable colon of childhood. J Pediatr 69:1027, 1966.

2. Apley, J.: The Child with Abdominal Pain, 2nd Edition. Blackwell Scientific Publications, Oxford, 1975.

3. Apley, J.: Psychosomatic illness in children: A modern synthesis. Br Med J 2:756, 1973.

4. Kirsner, J.B. and Palmer, W.C.: The irritable colon. Gastroenterology 34:491, 1958.

5. Lumsden, K., Chaudhary, N., Truelove, S.C.: The irritable colon syndrome. Q J Med 31:123, 1962.

6. Kopel, E., Kim, I., Barbero, G.H.: Comparison of rectosigmoid motility in normal children, children with recurrent abdominal pain, and children with ulcerative colitis. Pediatrics 39:4, 1967.

7. Rubin, L.S., Barbero, G.J., Sibinga, M.S.: Pupillary reactivity in children with recurrent abdominal pain. Psychosom Med 29:111, 1967.

8. Dimson, S.B.: Transit time related to clinical findings in children with recurrent abdominal pain. Pediatrics 47:666, 1971.

9. Stone, R.T. and Barbero, G.J.: Recurrent abdominal pain in childhood. Pediatrics 45:732, 1970.

10. Apley, J., Haslam, D.R., Tulloc, C.G.: Pupillary reaction in children with recurrent abdominal pain. Arch Dis Child 46:447, 1971.

11. Stone, R.T.: Abdominal pain in childhood. Clin Med 80: 27, 1973.

12. Roy, C.C., Silverman, A., Cozzetto, F.J.: Pediatric Clinical Gastroenterology, 2nd Edition. The CV Mosby Co., St. Louis, 1975, p. 195.

13. Liebman, W.M. and Thaler, M.M.: Pediatric considerations of abdominal pain and the acute abdomen. In: Gastrointestinal Disease. Sleisenger, M.H. and Fordtran, J.S. (Eds). WB Saunders Co., Philadelphia, 1978, p. 411.

14. Christensen, M.E. and Mortensen, O.: Long-term prognosis in children with recurrent abdominal pain. Arch Dis Child 50:110, 1975.

Case 48

ABDOMINAL DISTENTION AND FAILURE TO
THRIVE IN A 2-MONTH-OLD GIRL

HISTORY

A 2-month-old white female presented with abdominal enlargement, decreased appetite and activity, and lack of adequate
weight and height gain, of at least 4 weeks' duration. There had
been no associated history of fever, diarrhea, constipation, melena, hematochezia, persistent jaundice, skin lesions, or trauma. The patient was the product of a term pregnancy, birth
weight 7 lbs 4 oz, with normal gestational and delivery history.
The remainder of the past history, developmental history, family history, social history, and review of systems was unremarkable.

EXAMINATION

She was in moderate abdominal distress, with normal vital signs,
head circumference 33.5 cm, length 53 cm, and weight 4.0 kg.
The remainder of the examination was unremarkable except for
moderate abdominal distention, no apparent tenderness to direct
palpation and/or rebound tenderness, and the presence of a definite fluid wave and a shifting dullness. Her spleen and kidneys
were not palpable. A few active bowel sounds were present with
no bruits. No peripheral swelling was noted.

LABORATORY DATA

Hemoglobin:	11.8 gm%
Hematocrit:	35%
White blood cell count:	10,000/mm^3

PMN's:	44%
lymphocytes:	52%
monocytes:	2%
eosinophiles:	2%
Sedimentation rate:	13 mm/hr
Urinalysis:	negative
Serum:	
carotene:	93 μg%
folate:	14 ng/ml
creatinine:	0.4 mg%
total protein:	5.2 gm%
albumin:	2.8 gm%
SGOT:	21 KU
total bilirubin:	0.8 mg%
direct bilirubin:	0.5 mg%
alpha-fetoprotein:	negative
alpha-1-antitrypsin:	260 mg%
VDRL:	negative
sodium:	132 meq/L
potassium:	3.4 meq/L
chloride:	94 meq/L
bicarbonate:	20 meq/L
Cytology:	negative
Stool:	
72 hr ^{51}Cr-albumin:	1.6%

QUESTIONS

1. Which one of the following would be the most appropriate
   step in diagnosis at this time?
   A. Ultrasound examination
   B. Intravenous pyelogram
   C. Barium enema
   D. Sweat test
   E. Recumbent, upright, and lateral films of abdomen

2. Since no peritoneal calcification is present, which one of
   the following would now be the most appropriate step in di-
   agnosis?
   A. Ultrasound examination
   B. Intravenous pyelogram
   C. Barium enema
   D. Sweat test
   E. Electrocardiogram

3. Because the intravenous pyelogram and also the cystoure-
   throgram were normal, which one of the following would
   now be the most appropriate step in diagnosis?
   A. Ultrasound examination
   B. Barium enema
   C. CT scan of abdomen
   D. Sweat test
   E. Electrocardiogram, chest X-ray

4. Since the electrocardiogram and chest X-ray were within
   normal limits, which one of the following would be the most
   appropriate further step in diagnosis?
   A. Ultrasound examination
   B. Sweat test
   C. Serum lysozyme measurement
   D. Liver function tests
   E. Paracentesis

5. Because the fluid is chylous, which of the following would
   be likely causes?
   A. Ovarian cyst
   B. Diffuse lymphangioma
   C. Cryptogenic cirrhosis
   D. Mesenteric cyst
   E. Trauma

6. Which of the following studies would be most helpful at this
   point in this patient's diagnosis?
   A. Ultrasound examination
   B. Upper gastrointestinal-small bowel series
   C. Sweat test
   D. Liver function tests
   E. Electroencephalogram (EEG)

7. Surgery would be indicated in such children under which of
   the following circumstances?
   A. In all cases of chylous ascites
   B. In all cases of chylous ascites under one year of age
   C. Diagnosis of surgically correctable condition
   D. Deterioration of clinical status in patients with undeter-
      mined etiology
   E. Lack of response of chylous ascites to dietary manage-
      ment

ANSWERS AND COMMENTS

1. (E) Plain films of the abdomen are indicated in order to an-
alyze further the patient's abdominal distention with no palpable
masses. Intestinal obstruction, undetected tumors, and ascites
with or without other abnormalities will be demonstrated. (1-12)
Furthermore, serous ascitic fluid will frequently be lucent by
X-ray, while hemorrhagic or chylous fluid will not. (1-5) The
other studies are selective ones and are performed on the basis
of the plain film findings. The only possible change would be
the possible initial use of ultrasound examination, since it is
capable of detecting as little as 100 ml of fluid. (1)
    In this patient, only ascites was visualized. No peritoneal
calcification was noted. A large bladder or myelomeningocele
was not present, either. (If present, is suggestive of urinary
source.)

2. (B) Since this patient is not critically ill, intravenous pyelography and also cystography should be performed. Recent
studies have indicated that urinary abnormalities such as posterior urethral valves, are not as common a cause of neonatal ascites as previously suggested and probably account for only 20
to 25% of cases. (1,4-8) Furthermore, posterior urethral valves
probably account for only 15 to 25% of urinary sources, although
earlier studies had mentioned them as responsible for 50 to 75%.
(4-8) Overall, ureteropelvic obstruction is still the most common cause of neonatal hydronephrosis, despite a few reports de-
tailing only urethral, bladder, or distal ureteral obstruction as
producing hydronephrosis. (7,8) Other urinary causes include
neurogenic bladder, ureterocoele, and urethral stricture. (4-8)
If this patient had been more critically ill, paracentesis would
have been performed next, not only to aid diagnosis but also for
relief of any respiratory compromise. The other studies would
not be as productive as the present choice or are not indicated,
e.g., sweat test (no peritoneal calcification).

3. (E) Since the intravenous pyelogram and cystourethrogram
were normal, the most appropriate test at this point would be
an electrocardiogram and chest X-ray. These studies would be
important in distinguishing possible cardiac causes, could be
accomplished quickly, and would eliminate the possibility of unwarranted time being wasted in further elucidating an analysis
of peritoneal fluid too soon, i.e., paracentesis. The latter would
be the procedure chosen by some authors at this time, but this
author's feeling is that the ECG and chest X-ray do not significantly delay the subsequent performance of a paracentesis and,
as previously mentioned, may save significant time in diagnosis

and treatment in some cases, 5 to 15% in most series. (1) Cardiac causes have included hypoplastic left heart syndrome, paroxysmal supraventricular tachycardia, e.g., Wolff-Parkinson-White phenomenon, erythroblastosis fetalis with hydrops fetalis, and intrauterine cardiac failure. (1, 14)

4. (E) Obviously, at this point, peritoneal fluid analysis (paracentesis) is indicated. This analysis should include gross fluid inspection hematocrit, white blood cell count, protein determinations, amylase determination, culture, and cytology. (1-3, 15, 16) Further determinations, dependent upon appearance and prior studies, may include triglyceride content and bilirubin level.

The author performs paracentesis under sterile conditions by carefully preparing the immediate infra-umbilical region in the midline, with an iodine preparation, then 70% isopropyl alcohol, and then draping with sterile towels. A No. 11 scalpel blade is used to make a small nick, 1.5 to 3.0 cm below the umbilicus in the midline, under local anesthesia (Xylocaine, 1%). A small bore intravenous needle, No. 22 to 26, attached to a sterile syringe, is gently inserted into the "incision" until a popping sensation (peritoneal surface penetration) and flow of fluid are assured. In cases in which the paracentesis is therapeutic, as well as diagnostic, a sterile suction bottle and tubing may be used. However, subsequent ascitic fluid reaccumulation will be augmented (3-4 times), further reducing the intravascular space and "effective" plasma volume. (1, 7, 8, 13) In all cases the patient is maintained in a supine position, or the upper half of the body is elevated slightly.

Paracentesis:
white blood cells:	250/mm^3
lymphocytes:	55%
PMN's:	45%
protein:	3.0 gm%
amylase:	40 units
bilirubin:	0 mg%

5. (B, D, E) Chylous ascites results from the transit of lymphatic fluid from the mesenteric, cisternal, or lower thoracic ductal system into the peritoneal cavity. (16-19) The contents of this lymphatic fluid reflect those nutrients absorbed by the intestinal lacteal system. The chylous fluid is usually alkaline, sterile, milky in nature, with a high lipid content, frequently above 1,000 to 1,500 mg% and with a protein content of about 3 gm%. (16-19) The causes of this problem are lymphatic obstruction due to congenital malformations, inflammation (mesenteric

lymphadenitis, for example), neoplasm (lymphangioma, for example), and traumatic lacteal disruption. (16-19) Symptomatically, increased intraabdominal pressure occurs. (16-19) If more significant ascites develops, scrotal edema or even edema of the lower extremities may result. Frequently, there are no specific physical findings or laboratory data, although mild anemia may be present. (16-19)

6. (A, B) With the finding of chylous ascitic fluid, barium studies, particularly the upper gastrointestinal-small bowel series, and ultrasound examination would be most helpful. (1, 13, 16-19) The former would disclose a malrotation of the small intestine or elsewhere, inflammatory bowel disease, or rare intestinal tumors, while the latter study might disclose a mesenteric cyst, lymphangioma, or other gross lymphatic abnormalities, but usually not mesenteric lymphadenitis unless there was significant enlargement or lymph node aggregation. (16-19)

The other studies, such as sweat test, would not be particularly helpful in the evaluation of chylous ascites. However, special studies, such as lymphangiography, in experienced hands, may be indicated and may be helpful.

7. (C, B, E) If the diagnostic steps previously described do not identify a specific etiology of the chylous ascites, initial treatment consists of supportive measures. If there has been significant caloric deficiency, particularly with associated poor intake, parenteral hyperalimentation, either peripheral or central, may be necessary. Prior attempts at reinfusion of ascitic fluid have been of little or no benefit. (1, 19) Specific shunting, such as venoperitoneal, has been only temporarily beneficial at best. (19) Thus, treatment is aimed at reduction of the formation of chylous fluid, and, therefore, dietary modification is a necessity. (20-22) The core of this treatment is the substitution of short- and medium-chain fatty acids (C_{10-12} or below) for long-chain fatty acids (triglycerides). The latter are absorbed and transported via the lymphatic system (lacteals and lymph ducts) while the former (medium-chain) are transported via the portal system. (20-22) Thus, the amount and concentration of fat and protein in ascitic fluid are markedly reduced. (16-22) The dietary changes could include the use of medium-chain triglyceride oils and/or elemental liquid formulas, containing little or no long-chain triglyceride, e.g., Portagen®, in addition to simplified carbohydrate and protein components. (16-24) Parenteral nutrition would be available as an additional adjunct (calories, essential nutrients) or a substitution for enteral alimentation. (16-25)

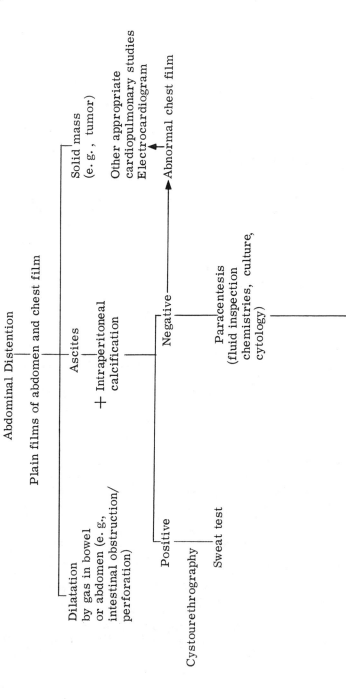

ALGORITHM NEONATAL ASCITES

Abdominal Distention

Plain films of abdomen and chest film

Dilatation by gas in bowel or abdomen (e.g., intestinal obstruction/perforation)

Cystourethrography

Sweat test

Positive

Ascites + Intraperitoneal calcification

Negative

Solid mass (e.g., tumor)

Other appropriate cardiopulmonary studies
Electrocardiogram

Abnormal chest film

Paracentesis (fluid inspection chemistries, culture, cytology)

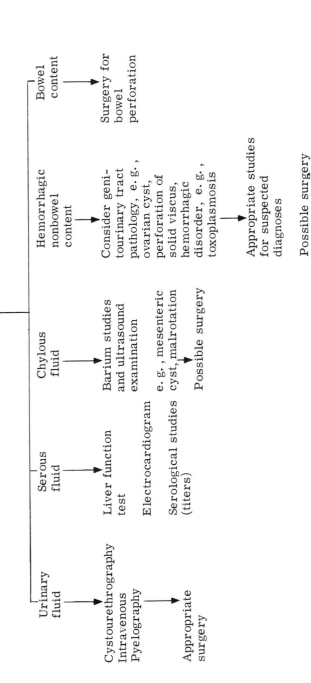

Figure 48.1 Algorithm neonatal ascites. Modified from Griscom, N.T., et al.

Surgical treatment in chylous ascites is indicated in those
cases in which there is an identified surgically-correctable lesion, lack of response to a low-fat (long-chain) diet, or when
there is deterioration of clinical status in patients with undetermined etiology. (26) A relative indication for surgery in some
series, however, has been simply the lack of identification of a
specific etiology, i.e., diagnostic laparotomy. (1-3,16,27) The
author does not recommend such a practice, except very selectively.

REFERENCES

1. Franken, E.A., Jr.: Ascites in infants and children, roentgen diagnosis. Radiology 102; 393, 1972.

2. Winestock, D. and Macpherson, R.I.: Neonatal ascites, a
   case for diagnosis. J Can Assoc Radiol 22:272, 1971.

3. Bughdassarian, O.M., Koehler, P.R., Schultze, G.: Massive neonatal ascites. Radiology 76:586, 1961.

4. Cremin, B.J.: Urinary ascites and obstructive uropathy.
   Br J Radiol 48:113, 1975.

5. Mann, C.M., Leape, L.L., Holder, T.M.: Neonatal urinary ascites: A report of two cases of unusual etiology and
   a review of the literature. J Urol 111:124, 1974.

6. Parker, R.M.: Neonatal urinary ascites: A potentially
   favorable sign in bladder outlet obstruction. Urology 3:589,
   1974.

7. Leonidas, J.C., Leiter, E., Gribetz, D.: Congenital urinary tract obstruction presenting with ascites at birth. Radiology 96:111, 1970.

8. Weller, M.H. and Miller, K.: Unusual aspects of urine
   ascites. Radiology 109:665, 1973.

9. Aziz, E.M.: Fetal ascites secondary to congenital syphilis.
   So Med J 67:81, 1974.

10. Frank, D.J., DeVaux, W.D., Perkins, J.R., et al.: Fetal
    ascites and cytomegalic inclusion disease. Am J Dis Child
    112:604, 1966.

11. Bryan, E.M.: Benign fetal ascites associated with maternal hydramnios. Clin Pediatr 14:88, 1975.

12. Cywes, S. and Cremin, B.J.: Roentgenologic features of hemoperitoneum in the newborn. Am J Roentgenol 106: 193, 1969.

13. Goldberg, B.B., Goodman, G.A., Clearfield, H.R.: Evaluation of ascites by ultrasound. Radiology 96:15, 1970.

14. Leake, R.D., Strimling, B., Emananouilides, G.C.: Intrauterine cardiac failure with hydrops fetalis. Clin Pediatr 12:649, 1973.

15. Birtch, A.G., Coran, A.G., Gross, E.R.: Neonatal peritonitis. Surgery 61:305, 1967.

16. Gribetz, D. and Kanof, A.: Chylous ascites in infancy. Pediatrics 7:632, 1951.

17. Craven, C.E., Goldman, A.S., Larson, D.L., et al.: Congenital chylous ascites: Lymphangiographic demonstration of obstruction into the cisterna chyli and a chylous reflux into the peritoneal space and small intestine. J Pediatr 70:340, 1967.

18. Gross, J.I., Goldenberg, V.E., Humphreys, E.M.: Venous remnants producing neonatal chylous ascites. Pediatrics 27:408, 1961.

19. Sanchez, R.E., Mahour, G.H., Brennan, L.P., et al.: Chylous ascites in children. Surgery 69:183, 1971.

20. Hashim, S.A., Bergen, S.S., Jr., Krell, K., et al.: Intestinal absorption and mode of transport in portal vein of medium chain fatty acids. J Clin Invest 43:1238, 1964.

21. Isselbacher, K.J.: Metabolism and transport of lipid by intestinal mucosa. Fed Proc 24:16, 1965.

22. Hashim, S.A., Roholt, H.B., Babayan, V., et al.: Treatment of chyluria and chylothorax with medium chain triglyceride. N Engl J Med 270:756, 1964.

23. Russell, R.I.: Progress report: Elemental diets. Gut 16:68, 1975.

24. Koretz, R.L. and Meyer, J.H.: Elemental diets. Facts and fantasies. Gastroenterology 78:393, 1980.

25. Coran, A.G.: Parenteral nutrition in infants and children. Surg Clin North Am 61:1089, 1981.

26. Vasko, J.S. and Tapper, R.I.: The surgical significance of chylous ascites. Arch Surg 95:355, 1967.

27. Griscom, N.T., Colodny, A.H., Rosenberg, H.K., et al.: Diagnostic aspects of neonatal ascites: Report of 27 cases. Am J Roentgenol 128:961, 1977.

Case 49

JAUNDICE IN A 7-DAY-OLD MALE

HISTORY

A 7-day-old white male presented with jaundice since birth. The pregnancy was full-term, birth weight 3.7 kg, with no apparent difficulty during gestation or in the immediate postnatal period. His diet consisted of breast milk. There was no history of associated fever, vomiting, diarrhea, constipation, melena, hematochezia, lethargy. The stools were golden yellow in color, soft in consistency, and generally 2 to 3 per day. The baby's appetite and activity were good. The remainder of the past history, family history, social history, and review of systems was unremarkable.

EXAMINATION

He was alert, well-nourished, in no apparent distress, with normal vital signs, weight 3.6 kg, height 53 cm, head circumference 34.5 cm. The remainder of the examination was unremarkable except for (1) scleral and conjunctival icterus and (2) liver, palpable 1.0 cm below the right costal margin in the midclavicular line, not tender or nodular, firm in consistency, total span being 5.0 cm by percussion. No abdominal bruits were noted.

LABORATORY DATA

Hemoglobin:	15.2 gm%
Hematocrit:	45%
White blood cell count:	9,600/mm^3
PMN's:	56%
lymphocytes:	40%

monocytes:	3%
eosinophiles:	1%
Platelet count:	225,000/mm^3
reticulocyte count:	1.3%
Serum:	
SGOT:	28 KU
SGPT:	24 KU
total protein:	6.4 gm%
albumin:	3.8 gm%
total bilirubin:	18.8 mg%
direct bilirubin:	1.1 mg%
alkaline phosphatase:	250 IU
alpha-fetoprotein:	negative
alpha-1-antitrypsin:	325 mg%
prothrombin time:	13.2 seconds (11.5 seconds)
VDRL:	negative
torch titers:	negative
Hb$_S$Ag:	negative
antiHbs:	negative
Hb$_C$Ab:	negative
Urinalysis:	negative
Urine amino acid screen:	negative
Ultrasound, abdomen:	negative

QUESTIONS

Questions 1-3: Answer true (T) or false (F).

1. This patient has an indirect or unconjugated hyperbilirubinemia.

2. Unconjugated hyperbilirubinemia includes physiologic, breast milk, and familial hyperbilirubinemias.

3. Extrahepatic biliary atresia remains a likely diagnosis in this patient.

4. Which of the following studies would be appropriate in this patient?
   A. Direct Coombs test and blood type
   B. Analysis of fractions of serum and bile bilirubin
   C. Ultrasound examination of the abdomen
   D. Pipida nuclear scan
   E. Liver biopsy

5. Which one of the following would be most appropriate in the
    treatment of this patient at this time?
    A. Discontinuation of breast milk
    B. Phenobarbital
    C. Cholestyramine
    D. Steroids
    E. Surgery

6. If breast milk discontinuation is not successful, which of
    the following would be most appropriate in treatment of this
    patient?
    A. Phototherapy
    B. Phenobarbital
    C. Antibiotics
    D. Steroids
    E. Surgery

ANSWERS AND COMMENTS

1. (T) The laboratory studies, i.e., total (18.8) and indirect
fraction (17.7) of bilirubin indicate a hyperbilirubinemia, indirect (unconjugated) in type.
    In the normal full-term infant, maximum bilirubin levels can
reach 8 to 10 mg% by the fourth to sixth days, while premature
infants can have levels of 10 to 18 mg% by the fifth to seventh
days. (1-6) Conjugation reactions, involving the formation of a
glucuronide derivative (water soluble), begin at birth. Localization is in the hepatic microsomes, predominantly in the
smooth endoplasmic reticulum (SER). (1-6) The "toxic" pigment bilirubin (unconjugated) is converted to an excretable product, conjugated bilirubin (mono- or diglucuronide). (1-7) The
conjugation system increases in activity after birth, particularly the first 14 to 21 days. (1-4,6). Factors that can influence hepatic conjugation and excretion include increased breakdown of red blood cells (8ncreased bilirubin), inhibitors of uptake into the hepatocytes and/or conjugation system, e.g., fatty
acids, injury to significant percentage of hepatocytes (hepatitis,
toxins, etc.). (1-8) (Table 49.1)

2. (T) Factors involved in the unconjugated hyperbilirubinemia include (1) augmented red blood cell breakdown and bilirubin
production, including isoimmunization due to Rh or other red
cell antigens, e.g., ABO, red blood cell enzyme deficiencies
(glucose-6-phosphate dehydrogenase, glycolitic pathway deficiencies), hemoglobinopathies, medication; (2) reduced uptake
of bilirubin (receptor) abnormality, reduced hepatocytes; (3)

TABLE 49.1   Unconjugated Hyperbilirubinemia
(Full-Term, Premature)

Genetic
  Crigler-Najjar syndrome
  Gilbert's syndrome
  Familial (transient, persistent)
  Rotor's syndrome?
  Dubin-Johnson syndrome?

Hemolysis
  Red blood cell enzyme deficiency, e.g., G-6-P-D
  Red blood cell isoimmunization, e.g., ABO, Rh
  Hemoglobinopathies
  Infection, e.g., sepsis
  Drugs, e.g., vitamin K

Hepatic
  Extrahepatic biliary atresia
  Hepatitis
  Inborn errors, e.g., galactosemia

Metabolic
  Hypoglycemia
  Hypothyroidism
  Hypoxia
  Respiratory insufficiency

---

binding protein deficiencies (Ligands - Y, Z protein); (4) reduced
or absent conjugation, e.g., Crigler-Najjar syndrome (type I -
no enzyme activity, type II - reduced enzyme activity); (5) altered excretion of bilirubin from the hepatocyte ("reflux" into
plasma); and (6) enhanced enterohepatic shunt activity of unconjugated bilirubin (enhanced beta-glucuronidase activity within
the intestine). (1-9) The latter mechanism, particularly, may
play a role in a so-called physiologic jaundice of the newborn.
(1-4,8,9) (Table 49.1)

3. (F) Extrahepatic biliary atresia (EBA) is an unlikely cause
in this patient, since an unconjugated hyperbilirubinemia has
been noted. Unless there is significant associated intrahepatic
disease along with or resultant from the extrahepatic obstructive
component with or without superimposed infection (cholangitis,

ascending), a conjugated hyperbilirubinemia would be anticipated in EBA. (5,9)

4. (A,B) As the answers in questions 1 and 2 stated, the patient has an unconjugated hyperbilirubinemia. Red blood cell breakdown is one factor contributing to the unconjugated bilirubin pool. The direct Coombs' test and maternal/infant blood type could indicate a red blood cell isoimmunization (hemolysis). In this patient, there is no evidence of anemia, and the reticulocyte count was not elevated, however.

The analysis of serum and bile bilirubin would be performed to confirm the presence or absence of conjugates (mono or di). The conventional method for bilirubin measurement has been a diazo reagent - spectro - photometric determination (blue color). Total and direct-reacting (conjugated) bilirubin are determined. Unfortunately, this method is relatively nonspecific and also the direct-reacting and indirect-reacting fractions are not truly accurate representations of the conjugated and unconjugated fractions. (7,9) More recently, a new, quite specific method has been developed for the determination of unconjugated and conjugated bilirubin. (7) The latter has been noted as either (1) mono or (2) di forms. (7,10). This new method employs high-pressure liquid chromatography (HPLC) and alkaline methanolysis, conversion from water-soluble to methyl ester forms of the mono- and diconjugates. (7,10) The specificity of this new method allows for determination of unconjugated and conjugated hyperbilirubinemias, but also can pinpoint the presence or absence of conjugate, e. g. , no conjugate forms as in Crigler-Najjar syndrome, type I. (7,9,10)

5. (A) Prolonged unconjugated hyperbilirubinemia associated with breast feeding was first noted in the 1960s. (2,3,8,9) The underlying mechanism is inhibition of glucuronyl transferase activity (major conjugating enzyme in the hepatocyte), at least in vitro. (1-4,8,9) The inhibitory factor or factors in breast milk have not been fully characterized, but the fatty acid level in breast milk has been more recently incriminated. (4,5,9) Previously, a steroid, pregnane-3-alpha-20-beta-diol, had been thought to affect bilirubin conjugation, but clinical studies could not confirm this inhibitory activity and resultant unconjugated hyperbilirubinemia. (4,8,9) In vitro confirmation also could not be re-established. (8,9) Genetic or environmental factors could and probably do play a role, too, but further characterization is needed.

Clinically, breast milk jaundice usually occurs by the end of the first or second week of life. (4,9) There is no sex predilection. Total bilirubin levels can reach 25 to 30 mg/100 ml, at least 80 to 90% unconjugated. (4,8,9) There are no other symptoms and the growth pattern remains unaffected. (9) No sequelae have been reported. When the total bilirubin level reaches 18 to 20 mg%, breast-feeding discontinuation should be initiated. Generally, discontinuation for only 3 to 5 days is sufficient to produce a significant decrease in the bilirubin level. Moreover, resumption of breast-feeding usually produces no or minimal increase in the total bilirubin level. (8,9)

The administration of phenobarbital (enhancement of bilirubin conjugation and of bile flow) is certainly not inappropriate at this time, but would be best timed after other factors, e.g., red blood cell breakdown, breast milk, had been eliminated as cause(s) of the unconjugated hyperbilirubinemia. The phenobarbital would then be used to enhance bilirubin conjugation, possibly by an increase of glucuronyl transferase activity via protein synthesis stimulation; if the patient had Crigler-Najjar syndrome, type I, no conjugation is anticipated since there is an apparent genetic inability to conjugate. (1-4,8,9) In type II, there is a partial deficiency, and phenobarbital would produce a positive response, i.e., enzyme induction. (9,14) This is particularly important, since this patient has the Crigler-Najjar syndrome and not another type of unconjugated hyperbilirubinemia.

Cholestyramine, a nonabsorbable anion-exchange resin, is also not inappropriate in the management, but would be best added later, as with phenobarbital. It is effective when bile acids are present in the intestinal lumen (binding) thereby increasing hepatic bile acid synthesis and, subsequently, bile flow. (5,6,9) This drug also can bind bilirubin, unconjugated, and increase fecal bilirubin loss accordingly. Other agents which can affect serum bilirubin levels include agar and charcoal, whether by bilirubin binding or blocking the enterohepatic shunt or by local intestinal irritation and resultant fecal loss. (9)

Steroids and surgery would not be appropriate in this patient.

6. (A,B) As mentioned in question 5, this patient has Crigler-Najjar syndrome, type I. Confirmation of the diagnosis was by alkaline methanolysis high-pressure liquid chromatography of bile, demonstrating no mono- or diconjugates of bilirubin. Liver biopsy with glucuronyl transferase quantitation (enzyme activity) was not performed.

As also mentioned in question 5, phenobarbital administration would be indicated at this point (no effect of breast milk discontinuation), although type I patients would not respond favorably, i.e., lowering of serum bilirubin level and direct (conjugated) bilirubin production. Phenobarbital administration is initiated at a dose of 3 to 5 mg/kg body weight/24 hr, maximum,

10 mg/kg body weight/24 hr. The goal is a lowering of the serum bilirubin level, lack of or minimal side effects, and maintaining the serum phenobarbital level in the therapeutic range, 10 to 40 $\mu g\%$, e.g., seizure activity control. (5,6,9)

The keynote of treatment, however, is phototherapy. Phototherapy, delivered by special lighting fixtures/appliances or with commercial lighting, has been demonstrated to have a marked effect on serum bilirubin levels, i.e., lowering. The bilirubin's photolability results in the production of photoisomers and subsequent passage from peripheral vascular tissues to blood and also biliary excretion. The excretion of photobilirubin is independent of bilirubin, other photodegradation products, and also hepatic function. (9-13) Biliary unconjugated bilirubin excretion is also increased during phototherapy. (9-13) The light source should generally not be more than 45 to 50 cm above the infant, so as to provide 5 to 6 $\mu W/cm^2/nm$ irradiance. (13) Irradiance should not be less than 4 $\mu W/cm^2/nm$, while maximum bilirubin reduction is achieved between 8 to 9 $\mu W/cm^2/nm$. (13) Four daylight and 4 blue 20W lamps will achieve the latter goal. (13) Eye patches should be used during phototherapy, and adequate space should be provided to minimize overheating. Extra fluid must be administered, as well as calories nutritionally, e.g., 10 to 20% increment. (13) In this patient, the goal will be to lower the total bilirubin level (essentially all unconjugated) to less than 15 mg% and to do such with the minimal number of hours of phototherapy and without complications, e.g., eye (retinal) injury. Continuous phototherapy is better than intermittent use (hours on-off-on). (13) In the author's experience, a minimum of 12 to 16 hours of phototherapy will be required during the first 1 to 2 years. Feedings, family visits, and play activity are performed when phototherapy is discontinued. Obviously, a coordinated daily schedule is necessary, and parental patience, understanding, and diligence are paramount. Counseling and support by family, friends, clergy, and medical personnel are important, too. Long-term studies of phototherapy, in general, are minimal in number and duration, but indicate that difficulty in the Crigler-Najjar patients may arise, even in the second or third decade after no morbididy or mortality in the first or second decade. (14,15) Thus, the outlook is rather bleak in the type I patients, because of the necessity for continued phototherapy on an indefinite basis.

Antibiotics, steroids, and surgery are not indicated in this patient.

For further information, see Table 49.1.

REFERENCES

1. Bakken, A.F. and Fog, I.: Bilirubin conjugation in the newborn. Lancet 1:1280, 1967.

2. Gartner, L.N. and Arias, I.M.: Formation, transport, metabolism and excretion of bilirubin. N Engl J Med 280: 1339, 1969.

3. Poland, R.L. and Odell, G.B.: Physiologic jaundice: The enterohepatic circulation of bilirubin. N Engl J Med 284:1, 1971.

4. Irias, I.M.: Inheritable and congenital hyperbilirubinemia. Models for the study of drug metabolism. N Engl J Med 285:1416, 1971.

5. Watson, S. and Giacoia, G.P.: Cholestasis in infancy. A review. Clin Pediatr 22:30, 1983.

6. Van Dyke, P.W., Keefe, E.B., Gollan, J.L., et al.: Hyperbilirubinemia and cholestasis: Current clinical and pathophysiological perspectives. In: Current Hepatology, Vol. 2. Gitnik, G. (ed). John Wiley and Sons, New York, 1982, p. 327.

7. Scharschmidt, B.F.: Cholestasis - Medical Staff Conference. West J Med 138:233, 1983.

8. Cole, A.P. and Hargreaves, T.: Conjugation inhibitors and neonatal hyperbilirubinemia. Arch Dis Child 47:415, 1972.

9. Silverman, A., Roy, C.C.: Pediatric Clinical Gastroenterology, 3rd Edition. The CV Mosby Company, St. Louis, 1983, p. 557.

10. Blanckaert, N., Kabra, P.M., Farina, F.A., et al.: Measurement of bilirubin and its monoconjugates and diconjugates in human serum by alkaline methanolysis and high-performance liquid chromatography. J Lab Clin Med 96:198, 1980.

11. Rubattelli, F.E., Zanardo, V., Granati, B.: Effects of various phototherapy regimens on bilirubin decrement. Pediatrics 61:838, 1978.

12. Brown, A. and Wu P. Y. K. : Efficacy of phototherapy in prevention of hyperbilirubinemia. Pediatr Res 13:277, 1979.

13. Wu P. Y. K. : Phototherapy update. Factors affecting efficiency of phototherapy. Ped N Atr 45, 1981 (Sept. /Oct.)

14. Gollan, J.L., Huang, S.N., Billing, B., et al.: Prolonged survival in three brothers with severe type 2 Crigler-Najjar syndrome: Ultrastructural and metabolic studies. Gastroenterology 68:1543, 1975.

15. Blaschke, T.F., Berk, P.D., Scharschmidt, B.F., et al.: Crigler-Najjar syndrome: An unusual course with development of neurologic damage at age eighteen. Pediatr Res 8:573, 1974.

Case 50

JAUNDICE IN A 2-MONTH-OLD BOY

HISTORY

A 2-month-old white male presented with jaundice since 1 week
of age. The patient was the product of a full-term vaginal delivery with an unremarkable gestational and delivery history,
birth weight 3.0 kg. The presence of jaundice was noted on the
second day of life, possibly disappearing by the 5th to 6th day,
and then reappearing at 1 week of age. The mother thought that
possibly the jaundice never completely cleared, but she was certain of its presence at 1 week of age. Appetite and activity remained unchanged. There was no associated history of fever,
anorexia, constipation, diarrhea, melena, hematochezia, skin
lesions, nasal discharge, trauma, or unusual food, drug, or
plant exposure. The bowel habit pattern consisted initially of
2-3 soft, yellow-brown, now 1-2 lighter yellow, bowel movements daily. The remainder of the past history, developmental
history, family history, social history, and review of systems
was unremarkable.

EXAMINATION

He was apparently active, alert, and in no distress, with normal
vital signs, head circumference 38 cm, weight 4.7 kg, and
length 54.5 cm (birth length, 50 cm). The remainder of the examination was unremarkable except for (1) apparent scleral and
conjunctival icterus; (2) firm, nontender liver, palpable 4.0 cm
below the right costal margin in the midclavicular line, total
span of the liver by percussion being 6.5 cm; (3) spleen palpable
1.0 cm below the left costal margin in the midclavicular line,
firm and nontender in nature; and (4) transverse palmar crease
on the left side.

LABORATORY DATA

Hemoglobin:	11.0 gm%
Hematocrit:	33%
White blood cell count:	6,700/mm^3
PMN's:	42%
lymphocytes:	55%
monocytes:	2%
eosinophiles:	1%
reticulocyte count:	1.8%
Urinalysis:	bile positive
Serum:	
total protein:	6.3 gm%
albumin:	4.4 gm%
SGOT:	220 units
SGPT:	140 units
alkaline phosphatase:	270 IU
total bilirubin:	6.1 mg%
direct bilirubin:	5.6 mg%
prothrombin time:	14.0 seconds (11.5 seconds)
partial thromboplastin time:	37 seconds
alpha-fetoprotein:	negative
alpha-1-antitrypsin:	300 mg%
torch titers:	negative
VDRL:	negative
creatinine:	0.6 mg%
Chest films:	negative

QUESTIONS

1. Which one of the following studies would be most indicated
   in this patient's management at this time?
   A. Intravenous pyelogram
   B. Ultrasonography
   C. CT scan of abdomen
   D. Lipoprotein X determination
   E. Rose Bengal sodium I^{131} excretion test (quantitative)

2. Based on these results (answer 1), which of the following
   studies would be indicated next?
   A. Direct Coombs test
   B. Antimitochondrial antibodies
   C. Quantitative immunoglobulins
   D. Hepatic angiography
   E. Percutaneous biopsy of liver

3. The findings of answer 2 would be most compatible with which one of the following conditions?
   A. Acute viral hepatitis
   B. Chronic persistent hepatitis
   C. Chronic aggressive hepatitis
   D. Alpha-1-antitrypsin deficiency liver disease
   E. Extrahepatic biliary obstruction (biliary atresia)

4. Based on this diagnostic interpretation, which of the following treatments should be recommended?
   A. Gamma globulin injections
   B. Steroids
   C. Exchange transfusion
   D. Surgery
   E. No treatment

Question 5: Answer true (T) or false (F).

5. Newer methods of treatment of this condition have produced significantly higher cure rates.

ANSWERS AND COMMENTS

1. (E) Intravenous pyelography (A) would only be indicated if polycystic (multicystic) disease of the liver and/or congenital hepatic fibrosis were suspected. Ultrasonography (B) and/or CT scan of the abdomen (C) certainly may be helpful for space-occupying lesions of the hepatobiliary system and potentially for obstructive jaundice per se, but their value in children with smaller diameters of the duct system is currently unknown. Hopefully, they will prove to be as valuable as suggested in adults. (1-5) Lipoprotein-X (LP-X), an abnormal low-density lipoprotein, is supposedly an indicator of cholestasis. It has been of limited usefulness, although Poley, et al. (8) utilize this measurement before and after cholestyramine administration in order to provide a better distinction between infection and cholestasis versus obstruction with cholestasis.

In conjugated hyperbilirubinemia, more than 30% of the total bilirubin is direct-reacting; many liver diseases are involved, such as infection (cytomegalic inclusion virus and others), inherited metabolic disorders (galactosemia and others), and biliary malformations. (1-10) At this point in the evaluation of this patient, the main diagnostic problem is to distinguish between an intrahepatic and extrahepatic cause. The absence of bile from the stools is not confirmatory evidence of extrahepatic obstruction, as intrahepatic disease may have a significant associated bile excretory deficit. Thus, a more sensitive test of bile flow to the duodenum is necessary, specifically the quantitative, as well as qualitative, measurement of dye excretion, e.g., Pipida (Iprofenin), a substituted iminodiacetic acid, Rose Bengal. This consists of measuring the amount of radioactivity of labeled ^{99m}Tc-Pipida or (^{131}I) Rose Bengal dye in stools collected for 24 and 72 hours, respectively, reflecting the shorter half-life of the former, 1 rather than 6 days. (2,3,5,6) These measurements are performed in addition to scanning of the liver, 1, 4, 6, 12, 24 hours (Pipida) and also 48 and 72 hours after injection (Rose Bengal). (2,3,5-7) In addition, scanning of the liver should be performed 1 and 4 to 6 hours after injection, as well as 24, 48, and, as necessary, 72 hours after injection. (2, 3,5) Some authors have suggested prescanning treatment with phenobarbital (5-10 mg/kg/day) and/or cholestyramine (4-12 gm/day) administration. More commonly, these drugs are administered for 2 to 3 weeks after a baseline scan and collection. Thereafter, a repeat scan and collection is performed, and the two test results are compared. Less than 5% dye excretion in 72 hours (Rose Bengal) is highly suggestive of extrahepatic biliary obstruction or intrahepatic disease with severe cholestasis, and greater than 10% excretion suggestive of intrahepatic disease with less cholestasis. (3,5,11) The Pipida scan-fecal quantitation has not been correlated yet in controlled studies. The I^{131} Rose Bengal isotope scan result was 11.0% (72 hr stool).

2. (E) Percutaneous liver biopsy would be indicated at this point, since the I^{131} Rose Bengal test demonstrated impaired excretion but not at a level compatible only with extrahepatic biliary obstruction, specifically less than 5% in 72 hours. (3,5) Thus, a biopsy is the most reliable means of establishing diagnosis. Percutaneous liver biopsy can be performed safely without significant morbidity or mortality ($\ll 1\%$). (4,12) In addition, adequate tissue, specifically more than three central veins and portal zones, is almost always obtained in order to sufficiently determine the morphological picture. Several studies have emphasized the morphological criteria for biliary atresia, particularly a significant degree of bile duct proliferation, ductular bile plugging, and hypertrophy of branches of the hepatic artery. (4,12) Additional findings include bile stasis (intracellular and canalicular) and portal and perilobular fibrosis. (3,12) Inflammatory cells (portal and/or focal), variable hepatocellular necrosis, as well as giant cell transformation, extramedullary hematopoiesis, and cholestasis (intracellular and canalicular), can also be present in hepatitis, as well as extrahepatic obstruction. (4,12)

Although percutaneous liver biopsy remains the choice for the vast majority of infants three months of age or younger, some are not candidates for this method. The latter include those with ascites, coagulation defects resistant to vitamin K administration, or with a firm, large-to-shrunken liver, suggestive of cirrhosis. (4,12,13) Open-liver biopsy would usually be used in these cases. Besides the morphological assessment, tissue can be used for culture (bacterial, vital), quantitative chemical study (tissue enzymes, e.g., glucuronyl transferase), and for electron microscopy. Utilizing the previously mentioned criteria, Brough and Bernstein (14) reported a diagnostic error of only 3.5% in histopathologic interpretation of needle and open-liver biopsies. The latter has the theoretical risk of exposing patients with hepatitis to anesthesia and surgery. (3,5,12)

The first three choices are serological tests providing only presumptive evidence for or against the presence of hemolytic causes of jaundice, primary biliary cirrhosis, or, less so, chronic active lung disease and in utero infection, respectively. Hepatic angiography would be helpful if a hepatic neoplasm or abscess were suspected. Otherwise, its value would be minimal. (3,5)

3.   (A) • An acute (neonatal) hepatitis is the most likely diagnosis, based on the histological picture in Fig. 50.1. This biopsy is characterized by the presence of giant cell transformation; hepatocellular necrosis (moderate); inflammatory cells, predominantly mononuclear (in the portal zone and intralobularly); and identifiable bile ductules but no proliferation. The performance of certain laboratory tests (serological) can aid in identifying the specific cause of the hepatitis, such as the rubella syndrome, cytomegalovirus disease, toxoplasmosis, herpes simplex, varicella, Coxsackie virus, hepatitis B, and syphilis, as well as alpha-1-antitrypsin deficiency and cystic fibrosis.

4.   (E) Once the diagnosis of hepatitis is made, medical treatment is in order. This medical treatment is actually supportive in nature, if no specific cause can be ascertained. Nutrition is paramount and may be best served by a formula containing medium-chain triglycerides and/or monosaccharide, such as Pregestimil or Vivonex. (14) Vitamin supplementation is preferable, particularly fat-soluble vitamins (A,D,K,E). For this purpose, Tri-Vi-Sol or Vi-Syneral drops are satisfactory. Aquasol E should also be administered daily. If the prothrombin time is depressed, vitamin K should be supplemented, such as Synkavite 5 mg orally or parenterally. (3,5,16)

If cholestasis is prominent, initiation of treatment with phenobarbital, 5-10 mg/kg day and/or cholestyramine, 4-12 gm/day

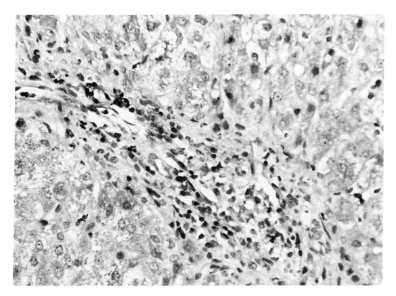

Figure 50.1   Liver. Mild inflammatory reaction (lymphocytes, plasma cells) is present in the portal zone. Hepatocytes contain vacuoles and glycogen; many hepatocytes are undergoing degeneration. Giant cell formation is also seen. The limiting plate can still be delineated (H&E, X250).

should be contemplated. (3,5,6,11) The action of phenobarbital includes an increase in the bile acid-independent fraction of bile flow, enhancement of bile acid synthesis and fecal excretion, possible glucuronyl transferase activity induction as a result of stimulation of protein synthesis in liver cells, and proliferation of smooth endoplasmic reticulum. (3,5,11) Cholestyramine is a nonabsorbable anion-exchange resin which binds bile acids within the intestinal lumen. This results in increased fecal bile acid excretion and hepatic bile acid synthesis. (3,5,11) The bile acid binding is preferential for the dihydroxy-type (chenodeoxycholate). Serum bile acid, cholate:chenodeoxycholate ratio, can be monitored. (10,11) If anemia or bleeding diathesis are prominent, fresh frozen plasma or blood may be necessary, or even exchange transfusion if coagulation disturbances exist.

5. (F) All modalities of treatment have not changed the prognosis of neonatal hepatitis. Only 25 to 30% of affected patients will demonstrate complete recovery. Twenty to 25% will die during the initial phases of the disease process. Fifty to 60%

422 / Case 50

will show variable degrees of residual liver damage. In general, the histological picture does not correlate well with survival, residual liver damage, or death. (14) However, significant necrosis without other findings is a poor prognostic sign. (14) The residual sequelae include intrahepatic biliary hypoplasia, fibrosis, and possible cirrhosis. (14-17) Preventive attempts with gamma globulin and/or hepatitis immune serum are too preliminary.

REFERENCES

1. Danks, D.M.: Prolonged neonatal obstructive jaundice. Clin Pediatr 4:499, 1965.

2. Thaler, M.M.: Neonatal hyperbilirubinemia. Semin Hematol 9:107, 1972.

3. Sass-Kortsak, A.: Management of young infants presenting with direct-reacting hyperbilirubinemia. Pediatr Clin North Am 21:777, 1974.

4. Brough, A.J. and Bernstein, J.: Conjugated hyperbilirubinemia in early infancy: A reassessment of liver biopsy. Hum Pathol 5:507, 1974.

5. Thaler, M.M.: Jaundice in the newborn: Algorithmic diagnosis of conjugated and unconjugated hyperbilirubinemia. J Am Med Assoc 237:58, 1977.

6. Mojel, M., Reba, R.C., Altman, R.P.: Hepatobiliary scintigraphy with 99Tc Pipida in evaluation of neonatal jaundice. Pediatrics 67:140, 1981.

7. Watson, S., Giacoia, G.P.: Cholestasis in infancy. A Review. Clin Pediatr 22:30, 1983.

8. Poley, J.R., Smith, E.J., Boon, D.J., et al.: Lipoprotein-X and the double ^{131}I-Rose Bengal test in the diagnosis of prolonged obstructive jaundice. J Pediatr Surg 7:660, 1972.

9. Porter, C.A., Mowat, A.P., Cook, P.J., et al.: Antitrypsin deficiency and neonatal hepatitis. Br Med J 3:435, 1972.

10. Yeung, C.Y.: Serum 5'-nucleotidase in neonatal hepatitis and biliary atresia: Preliminary observations. Pediatrics 50:812, 1972.

11. Zeltzer, P.M., Neerhout, R.C., Fonkalsrud, E.W., et al.: Differentiation between neonatal hepatitis and biliary atresia by measuring serum alpha-fetoprotein. Lancet 2: 197, 1974.

12. Javitt, N.B., Morrissey, K.P., Seigel, E., et al.: Cholestasis syndromes in infancy: Diagnostic value of serum bile acid pattern and cholestyramine administration. Pediatr Res 7:119, 1974.

13. Javitt, N.B.: Neonatal cholestatic syndromes: A structure-function dilemma. Viewpt Dig Dis 5(1), 1973.

14. Brough, A.J. and Bernstein, J.: Liver biopsy in the diagnosis of infantile obstructive jaundice. Pediatrics 43:519, 1969.

15. Thaler, M.M.: Cryptogenic liver disease in young infants. In: Progress in Liver Disease, Volume 5. Popper, H. and Schaffner, F. (Eds). Grune & Stratton Inc., New York, 1976, p. 476.

16. Silverman, A., Roy, C.C.: Pediatric Clinical Gastroenterology, 3rd edition. The CV Mosby Co., St. Louis, 1983, p. 685.

17. Alagille, D., Odievre, M., Gautier, M., et al.: Hepatic ductular hypoplasia associated with characteristic facies, vertebral malformations, retarded physical, mental, and sexual development, and cardiac murmur. J Pediatr 86: 63, 1975.

Case 51

JAUNDICE AND FAILURE TO THRIVE IN A
14-MONTH-OLD FEMALE INFANT

HISTORY

A 14-month-old white female presented with a 13-month history
of persistent jaundice with associated poor weight gain and feeding. Subsequent evaluation by another physician revealed elevated levels of SGOT, SGPT, alkaline phosphatase, and total
and direct bilirubin levels (maximum total, 6.9 mg/100 ml).
There was no history of vomiting, diarrhea, abdominal pain, constipation, or fever. The past history included a 32-week gestation with birth weight 1,000 grams. There was mild respiratory
distress in the neonatal period and recovery without apparent sequelae. The remainder of the past history, developmental history, family history, and review of systems was unremarkable.

EXAMINATION

She was alert, somewhat irritable, and in no distress, with normal vital signs. Length was 78 cm, weight 9.8 kg, and head circumference was 46 cm. The remainder of the examination was
unremarkable except for the liver which was palpable 3.5 cm below the right costal margin in the midclavicular margin, firm
but not tender or nodular. The total span of the liver by percussion was 6.75 cm. Active bowel sounds were present with no
bruits.

LABORATORY DATA

Hemoglobin:	13.9 gm%
Hematocrit:	39%

White blood cell count:	10,000/mm^3
PMN's:	38%
lymphocytes:	54%
monocytes:	5%
eosinophiles:	3%
Platelet count:	240,000/mm^3
Sedimentation rate:	9 mm/hr
Hemoglobin electrophoresis:	negative
Serum:	
prothrombin time:	11.4 seconds
total bilirubin:	3.8 mg%
direct bilirubin:	3.0 mg%
SGOT:	158 units
SGPT:	112 units
alkaline phosphatase:	278 IU
alpha-fetoprotein:	negative
alpha-1-antitrypsin:	60 mg%
torch titers:	negative
VDRL:	negative
Sweat:	
chloride:	11 meq/L
sodium:	12 meq/L
Urinalysis:	negative
Percutaneous liver biopsy:	(Fig. 51.1)

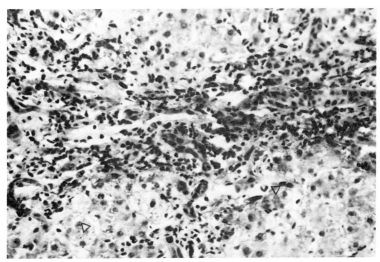

Figure 51.1   Liver. Intense staining of material with periodic acid-Schiff (PAS) stain, diastase-resistant, is seen, prevalent in the periportal zone (arrows) (H&E, X250).

QUESTIONS

1. The liver biopsy of this patient would be expected to show which of the following?
   A. Diastase-fast, intracellular granules and hyaline masses
   B. Intralobular bile stasis
   C. Marked bile duct proliferation
   D. Significant giant cell formation
   E. Variable portal inflammatory reaction

2. What is the frequency of one abnormal gene (heterozygote, Pi^{mz} or otherwise)?
   A. 0.01%
   B. 0.1%
   C. 1%
   D. 5%
   E. 30%

3. What is the frequency of the homozygous state (Pi^{zz})?
   A. 1:1,000
   B. 1:4,000
   C. 1:13,000
   D. 1:25,000
   E. 1:50,000

Question 4: Answer true (T) or false (F).

4. Alpha-1-antitrypsin (Al-AT) deficiency in children is found only with associated liver and/or lung disease.

5. Treatment of this type of liver disease may include which of the following measures?
   A. Cholestyramine
   B. Corticosteroids
   C. Penicillamine
   D. Danazol
   E. Liver transplantation

6. Which of the following statements regarding prognosis are correct?
   A. All develop liver or lung disease
   B. With development of liver disease, there is a significant risk of transition to cirrhosis and probable liver failure
   C. Worse prognosis if liver disease occurs in neonatal period
   D. With liver disease, increased risk of hepatocellular carcinoma
   E. Increase risk of diabetes mellitus

ANSWERS AND COMMENTS

1. (A,B,E) The characteristic finding in the liver is the presence of eosinophilic, intracellular granules (globules) and hyaline masses in sections stained with hematoxylin and eosin. These same granules will stain strongly with the periodic acid-Schiff procedure and be resistant to diastase digestion. These granules are variable in size and in number from cell to cell, with some areas frequently having none. (1-10) These granules are particularly prevalent in cells in periportal zones. (1-10) Less constant features include focal steatosis, glycogen within nuclei, minimal or no portal fibrosis, minimal or no bile duct proliferation, and mild portal inflammation, predominantly round cells. (1-10)

Ultrastructural studies in such cases have demonstrated the accumulation of the granular material (amorphous) in the rough endoplasmic reticulum of hepatocytes. (7,10) The material was single membrane-bound, oval in shape, and moderately electron-dense, homogeneous material. (7,10)

Using fluorescein-conjugated rabbit anti-human Al-AT, immunofluorescent techniques revealed green fluorescence of granules. A membrane-bound cytoplasmic structure is characteristically found. A vesicular form is frequently suggestive, too. (10)

In the neonatal period, intralobular bile stasis, lobular architectural disarray, and variable perilobular fibrosis are usually present. (1-10) Giant cells are minimal or nonexistent, and variable portal inflammatory reaction may also be present.

In later life, cirrhosis, micronodular in type, may develop. Collagen bands surround the regenerating lobules. The previously described granules or globules are present, as are the other findings, such as focal steatosis. (1-10)

Lastly, the characteristic granules are a feature of alpha-1-antitrypsin (A1-AT) deficiency and not of liver disease, per se. In fact, in several of the heterozygous types, these same granules may be found, although less prominently. (1-10)

2. (D) Quantitative levels of A1-AT are controlled by a series of autosomal codominant alleles. (4,6,11) Thirteen or more alleles have been described and most of the possible phenotypes (Pi typing) have been found. (6,10,11) A normal phenotype is Pi[mm] and the most serious deficiency is Pi[zz]. (6,8,11) Certain variants have reduced concentrations of A1-AT, reflected in their activity in serum. (6,9,11) Thus, deficiency represents a reduced concentration. Those with ZZ deficiency usually have 10% or less of normal levels of A1-AT. (6,10,11) Almost 80% of such individuals will develop pulmonary disease, i.e., emphysema, while only 10% will develop liver disease. (6,10,11) The frequency and severity of disease, however, will vary. The frequency of the various alleles is apparently related to ethnicity. (6,10,11) In the United States, the incidence of the heterozygous state has been estimated to be at least 5%. (6,10,11)

Alpha-1-antitrypsin (A1-AT) is protein-carbohydrate in content. The carbohydrate portion, sialic acid, seems to be important in mobility and transport of this protein from hepatocytes. A1-AT is synthesized primarily by the liver. (6,9,11) Its molecular weight is 40 to 50,000 daltons, and it is the major portion (90%) of alpha-1-globulin in the serum. Its serum half-life is 3 to 6 days. It does not cross the placenta. A1-AT is an acute phase reactant. (6,10,11) It is an inhibitor or inactivator of proteases, such as trypsin, chymotrypsin, elastase. (6,9,11) An abnormal A1-AT, as well as reduced synthesis, e.g., enzyme deficiency, may underlie this disease entity. (6,10-12)

3. (B) The ZZ phenotype in Caucasians varies from 1:4,000 to 1:8,000. (6,9,11) Approximate concentrations of A1-AT in the ZZ phenotype is usually 10% or less, but may be as high as 30% of normal. (6,9,11) The MZ phenotype concentration is usually 50 to 60% and MS phenotype 80%. (6,9-11)

The measurement of A1-AT can be accomplished by several tests. The simplest and most frequently used is the radial immunodiffusion method of Mancini, employing agar plates. (6,9-11) Functional assays include the capacity of the serum (patients') to inhibit a trypsin-substrate interaction. Normally, 1 ml of serum inhibits 1.1 to 2.0 mg of trypsin. (6,9-11) The definitive test is phenotyping, the most common procedure being the 2-step immunoelectrophoresis of Laurell and Fagerhol. (6,9-11) The agar strip (acid-starch gel) is placed in agar containing antibody to A1-AT. (6,9-11) The zz molecule migrates more slowly toward the anode than the mm molecule. (6,10,11) Other techniques include isoelectric focusing and an agarose technique. (6,9-11)

4. (F) A1-AT is an acute phase reactant. Therefore, its quantitative measurement will be affected by intercurrent illness, including pneumonia and urinary tract infection, carcinoma, pregnancy, and myocardial infarction. (6,9,10) Their presence could mask an underlying deficiency by raising the levels to normal.

A1-AT deficiency itself has been associated with a number of clinical conditions. The well-documented associations include chronic obstructive pulmonary disease in adults, and less so, in children (genetic), respiratory distress syndrome (nongenetic), cirrhosis in children and adults (genetic), renal homograft rejection (nongenetic). (4,6,10,12,13) Other associations, not as well documented, include chronic pancreatitis, extrahepatic biliary tract disease of infancy, peptic ulcer disease, celiac disease, rheumatoid arthritis, Down's syndrome, and C4 deficiency. (6,10,11) In addition, a recent report from Newark, New Jersey, demonstrated an association between cadmium and A1-AT, in particular, high cadmium and low A1-AT. (14) Whether this association is responsible for the higher incidence of chronic obstructive pulmonary disease in cadmium workers has not been resolved at this time. (14)

5. (A,D,E) There is no specific treatment of A1-AT deficiency. One major aspect of available medical treatment is preventive. Avoidance of exposure to excessive pollutants and cigarette smoke (lung) and to hepatotoxins, such as alcohol, hydrocarbons, blood product transfusion (liver), must be stressed. (6,9,10) Additionally, genetic counseling for the future for homozygotes is obviously necessary but also must be applied to heterozygotes. (6,9,10,15)

For cholestatic liver disease (jaundice), per se, medical management, if applicable, may consist of cholestyramine, 4 to 12 gm daily (divided doses, with meals), phenobarbital, 5-10 mg/kg/day, medium-chain triglycerides (formula, vegetable oil), and water-soluble vitamins. For chronic liver disease, per se, symptomatic therapy is used, such as diuretics (aldactone, lasix), for significant ascites and other measures as previously described. (6,10)

Potential therapeutic agents of A1-AT deficiency, itself, include Danazol, an androgen, which may raise the A1-AT level in homozygotes (4 cases), and tetracycline, (16,17) which has been demonstrated to suppress the secretion of elastase in alveolar macrophages in mice. (17)

A more definitive approach is liver transplantation. Unfortunately, the experience in this approach in A1-AT deficiency is small (few cases) and, so far, discouraging. (6,9,10,17) Hopefully, continued progress in transplantation methodology, including technique, prevention of infection and rejection, will improve this outlook.

6. (B,C,D) Not all individuals with A1-AT deficiency develop liver disease or early emphysema. (6,9,10,18) Approximately 80% of persons with ZZ deficiency will develop emphysema, while only 10% will develop liver disease. (6,9,10,18) The significance of the MZ phenotype remains controversial, although liver disease, chronic, mild to moderate in nature, and, more so, granule deposition intrahepatic, have been reported. (1-10, 19-20) Chronic liver disease has also been associated with the SZ phenotype, too. (19-21) Associations previously described have included chronic obstructive pulmonary disease and chronic liver disease, but these have been rare in occurrence. (6,9,10, 18) However, environmental toxins, plus the MZ phenotype, probably enhance the likelihood of emphysema. (6,9,10,18)

The prognosis appears to be worse if liver disease develops in the neonatal period, cirrhosis being expected in over 60% of survivors. (1-3,6,9,10,18) Regardless, as A1-AT-deficient persons survive into adulthood, the likelihood of chronic liver disease, asymptomatic or otherwise, increases. (6,9,10,18) In patients with A1-AT deficiency, an increased incidence of subsequent development of hepatic carcinoma has been reported. (10,18)

REFERENCES

1. Johnson, A.M. and Alper, C.A.: Deficiency of α-1-antitrypsin in childhood liver disease. Pediatrics 46:921, 1970.

2. Gherardi, G.J.: Alpha$_1$-antitrypsin deficiency and its effect on the liver. Hum Pathol 2:173, 1971.

3. Sharp, H.L., Bridges, R.A., Krurt, W., et al.: Cirrhosis associated with alpha$_1$ antitrypsin deficiency: A previously unrecognized inherited disorder. J Lab Clin Med 73:934, 1969.

4. Tobin, J., Hutchinson, D.C.S.: Alpha-1-antitrypsin deficiency. Current and future therapeutic strategies. Drug Ther 8:105, 1983.

5. Aagenaes, O., Fagerhol, M., Elgjo, K., et al.: Pathology and pathogenesis of liver disease in alpha-1 antitrypsin deficient individuals. Postgrad Med J 50:365, 1974.

6. Talamo, R.C.: Basic and clinical aspects of the alpha$_1$-antitrypsin. Pediatrics 56:91, 1975.

7. Feldmann, G., Bignon, J., Chahinian, P., et al.: Hepatocyte ultrastructural changes in alpha-1-antitrypsin deficiency. Gastroenterology 67:1214, 1971.

8. Morse, J.O., Lebowitz, M.D., Knudson, R.J., et al.: A community study of the relation of alpha$_1$-antitrypsin levels to obstructive lung disease. N Engl J Med 292:278, 1975.

9. Kueppers, F. and Black, L.F.: Alpha 1-antitrypsin and its deficiency. Am Rev Resp Dis 110:176, 1974.

10. Sharp, H.J.: The current status of alpha 1-antitrypsin, a protease inhibitor, in gastrointestinal disease. Gastroenterology 70:611, 1976.

11. Chan, S.K. and Rees, D.C.: Molecular basis for alpha 1-protease inhibitor deficiency. Nature 255:240, 1975.

12. Kane, W.M., Sharp, H.J.: Metabolic liver disease of childhood. Pediatr Ann 6:318, 1977.

13. Fierer, J., Mandl, I., Evans, H.E.: Alpha 1-antitrypsin in the lungs of newborn infants with respiratory distress syndrome. J Pediatr 85:699, 1974.

14. Cottrall, K., Cook, P.J.L., Mowat, A.P.: Neonatal hepatitis syndrome and alpha-1-antitrypsin deficiency: An epidemiological study in South-East England. Postgrad Med J 50:376, 1974.

15. Chowdhury, P. and Louria, D.: Infuence of cadmium and other trace metals on human alpha 1-antitrypsin: An in vitro study. Science 191:480, 1976.

16. Talamo, R.C., Langley, C.E., Levine, B.W., et al.: Genetic vs. quantitative analysis of serum alpha$_1$-antitrypsin. N Engl J Med 287:1067, 1972.

17. Gadek, J., Gelfand, J., Frank, M., et al.: Treatment of homozygous alpha 1-antitrypsin deficiency with danazol, a new anabolic steroid. Clin Res 25:416a, 1977.

18. White, R.R. and Kuhn, C.: Effect of tetracycline on elastase secretion by mouse peritoneal exudate and alveolar macrophages. Am Rev Resp Dis 115:387, 1977.

19. Sharp, H.L.: Alpha-1-antitrypsin deficiency. Hosp Pract 6:83, 1971.

20. Rosenthal, P., Liebman, W.M., Thaler, M.M.: Alpha-1-antitrypsin deficiency and severe liver disease in a young infant with SZ phenotype. Am J Dis Child 133:1195, 1979.

21. Rosenthal, P.R., Liebman, W.M., Thaler, M.M.: Liver disease and alpha-1-antitrypsin deficiency. N Engl J Med 303:1239, 1980.

Case 52

JAUNDICE IN AN 8-YEAR-OLD BOY

HISTORY

A 8-year-old white male presented with jaundice of 4 days' duration. The patient had noted generalized malaise, nausea, upset stomach, and decreased appetite for 5 days prior to the onset of juandice but had no associated fever, vomiting, constipation, diarrhea, melena, hematochezia, skin lesions, dysuria, cough, nasal discharge. There had been no associated history of trauma, unusual food, drug or plant exposure, or recent travel. The bowel habit pattern consisted of 1 to 2 soft, now lighter yellow bowel movements, while the urinary pattern had been unchanged. The remainder of the past history, developmental history, family history, social history, and review of systems was unremarkable.

EXAMINATION

He was alert and in no apparent distress, with normal vital signs, weight 27.2 kg and height 128.5 cm. The remainder of the examination was unremarkable except for (1) apparent scleral and conjunctival icterus and (2) firm, mildly tender liver, palpable 4.5 cm below the right costal margin in the midclavicular line, total span by percussion being 7.25 cm.

LABORATORY DATA

Hemoglobin:	12.7 gm%
Hematrocrit:	38%
White blood cell count:	10,800/mm^3
PMN's:	65%

lymphocytes:	31%
monocytes:	2%
eosinophiles:	2%
reticulocyte count:	1.2%
Urinalysis:	bile positive
Serum:	
total protein:	6.9 gm%
albumin:	4.4 gm%
SGOT:	980 units
SGPT:	875 units
alkaline phosphatase:	320 IU
total bilirubin:	9.3 mg%
direct bilirubin:	7.6 mg%
prothrombin time:	12.5 seconds (12.0 seconds)
ceruloplasmin:	75 mg%
VDRL:	negative
creatinine:	0.5 mg%
Stool:	
occult blood:	negative
culture:	negative
ova and parasites:	negative
Chest films:	negative
Abdomen films:	negative

QUESTIONS

1. Which one of the following studies would be most helpful and indicated in this patient's management at this time?
   A. Intravenous pyelogram
   B. Serum bile acid analysis
   C. Ultrasonography
   D. CT scan of abdomen
   E. Hepatitis virus serology

2. Based on these results (answer 1), which of the following studies would be indicated at this time?
   A. B-cell and T-cell immunological analysis
   B. Antimitochondrial antibodies
   C. Percutaneous liver biopsy
   D. Endoscopic Retrograde Cholangiopancreatography (ERCP)
   E. None of the above

Question 3: Answer true (T) or false (F).

3. The most likely diagnosis is acute viral hepatitis.

4. Based on this diagnosis (answer 3) which of the following
    would be recommended treatment?
    A. Bed rest
    B. Low residue, bland diet
    C. Gamma globulin injections
    D. Steroids
    E. Surgery

Question 5: Answer true (T) or false (F).

5. Newer methods of treatment of this disease have resulted
    in significantly lower morbidity and mortality.

ANSWERS AND COMMENTS

1. (E) An intravenous pyelogram (A) would be indicated only
if renal disease per se or a hepatorenal condition, e.g., congenital hepatic fibrosis, multicystic disease, were suspected.
Serum bile acid analysis (B), either the ratio of trihydroxy
(cholic) to dihydroxy (chenodeoxycholic) bile acids or of sulfated
primary bile acids (cholic, chenodeoxycholic), has been helpful
in differentiating intrahepatic versus extrahepatic cholestasis,
as well as in assessment of liver function (dysfunction) but not
in the actual identification of specific conditions, e.g., intrahepatic. Ultrasonography (C) and/or CT scan of the hepatobiliary system, delineation of causes of obstruction of the hepatobiliary system, i.e., extrahepatic, and assessment of density,
e.g., fat, liver fibrosis.
    Hepatitis A virus (HAV) is immunologically distinct from
hepatitis B virus (HBV), a nonenveloped viral particle, and apparently of RNA type. Hepatitis B virus is apparently of DNA
type, immunologically distinct from hepatitis A virus, and consists of an outer envelope (HBsAG) and an inner core or shell
(HBcAg), containing antigenic specificity and the nuclear material, including DNA polymerase activity. (1-5) Serological
analysis (radioimmunoassay, enzyme-linked immunosorbent assay, ELISA) of HAV is currently confined to antibodies to HAV,
an early type, IgM class, and a delayed type, IgG class, the latter within weeks after the acute illness. (1,6) Serological analysis of HBV (Radioimmunoassay, enzyme-linked immunosorbent
assay, ELISA) includes HBV surface antigen (HBsAg), antibodies
to HBsAg (anti-HBs), antibodies to the inner core material (anti-
HBc), HBV e antigen (exact location - unknown) antibodies to the
e antigen (anti-HBe), as well as assessment of DNA polymerase
activity. (1-5) (Refer to Tables 52.1 and 52.2 for nomenclature
and sequence for HAV and HBV and significance of HAV, HBV
tests).

TABLE 52.1   Hepatitis A and B Viruses Nomenclature

Hepatitis A
  virus, antigen HAVAg
  virus, antibody HAVAb
                IgM (early)
                IgG (late)

Hepatitis B
  virus (Dane particle)   HBV
  surface antigen   HBsAg
  surface antibody   HBsAb
  core antigen   HBcAg
  core antibody   HBcAb
  e antigen   HBeAg
  e antibody   HBeAb
  DNA polymerase activity

The anti-HAV titer was high for IgM type (1:1028) and negative for IgG type.

2.   (E)   The presence of anti-HAV, IgM type (high titer) and absence of IgG antibody titer to HAV is strong presumptive evidence of acute HAV-induced disease.

As mentioned in answer 1, HAV is RNA in type, found as a 27nm particle in fecal matter and blood during the late incubation and acute illness phases. (1,2,4-8) Prevalence increases with age and also lower socioeconomic conditions. Anti-HAV is present in at least 25 to 30% of the adult population. (1,6,8) In the United States, the prevalence rate in children under 14-15 years of age is a minimum of 2 to 3%, regardless of socioeconomic level; the incidence is obviously higher in crowded facilities, e.g., day care centers, schools, mentally retarded residences. (1,2,4,8) It represents the most common etiologic agent of acute viral hepatitis in infants and children over 2 to 3 years of age. (1,4)

Clinical features include an acute onset, minimal or no prodromal symptoms, and possible jaundice (20-70%). Laboratory studies include elevated transaminases, generally more than twofold in magnitude, increased thymol turbidity, variably elevated serum alkaline phosphatase level, and negative hepatitis B serology. (Refer to Table 52.3 for comparison of types of acute viral hepatitis.)

TABLE 52.2   Hepatitis A and B Viruses: Serology

	Test	Initial Appearance	Interpretation
Hepatitis A Virus	HABAb IgM	onset of illness	active or immediate past infection
	IgG	1-4 weeks after illness	past infection
Hepatitis B Virus	HBsAg	before or at onset of illness	acute or chronic infection, variable; carrier state
	HBsAb	within first 8 to 11 weeks of illness	past infection; immunity to HBV
	HBcAb	within first 4 weeks of illness	past infection; high titer, viral replication
	HBeAg	before or at onset of illness	viral replication, infectivity
	HBeAb	within first 4 to 8 weeks of illness	with positive HbsAg, low titer of HBV still present

3. (T) As discussed in answer 2, the most likely diagnosis is acute viral hepatitis, type A. As also mentioned in answer 2, the prodrome may be essentially absent, e.g., lack of significant generalized malaise, fever, abdominal pain, or minimal. However, the appropriate clinical setting, the presence of the usual marked increases in aminotransferases, and the lack of other apparent etiologic agents, e.g., chemical. (1,4,8) (Refer to Tables 52.1, 52.2, 52.3.)

Histologically (liver biopsy), single cell or focal zones of necrosis of hepatocytes are present, as well as mild inflammatory changes, principally round cell (mononuclear) infiltration, with lesser numbers of polymorphonuclear and eosinophilic cells. Less frequently, central vein phlebitis, a "diagnostic" finding, is present. Other findings include balloon cells, prominent

TABLE 52.3   Viral Hepatitis: Types A, B, Non A - Non B
Clinical Features

	Hepatitis A	Hepatitis B	Hepatitis Non A - Non B
Incubation period	10 to 40 days	50 to 180 days	20 to 80 days
Onset	usually acute	usually insidious	either acute or insidious
Prodrome	fever, generalized malaise	fever, generalized malaise, arthralgia	fever, generalized malaise, arthralgia
Jaundice	10 to 50%	10 to 70%	10 to 40%
Laboratory findings	elevated transaminases, alkaline phosphatase, total/direct bilirubin	elevated transaminases, alkaline phosphatase, total/direct bilirubin	elevated transaminases, alkaline phosphatase, total/direct bilirubin
Serology	AntiHAV	HbsAg, antiHBsAb, antiHBcAb, HBeAg, antiHBe Ab-some or all present	none
Immunity	present	present	?
Immunization	gamma globulin	specific immune serum globulin; gamma globulin +; vaccination	gamma globulin
Prognosis	good 1% (morbidity, mortality)	guarded 20 to 40% (morbidity, mortality)	fair to good; 10 to 25% (morbidity, mortality)

Kupffer cells, acidophilic or Councilman bodies. (1,8,9) Ground-glass hepatocytes, as well as cytoplasmic material, orcein or aldehyde fuchsin positive, are typical of hepatitis B viral disease. (1,8)

4. (A) Bed rest or reduced activity is frequently recommended, but there are no conclusive controlled data that absolute, even partial, bed rest will increase the percentage or rate of recovery. Gradated ambulation seems to be a reasonable, sensible approach, but there are no objective data to suggest a bearing on morbidity, mortality, or rate of "healing." (1,10)

With reference to diet (B), there has been frequent adherence to low-fat, moderate to high-carbohydrate content. This diet supposedly is "less aggravating" to patients with symptomatology, such as nausea and decreased appetite. (1,8) However, an unrestricted diet, rich in protein, is a reasonable choice, unless there is a compromise in liver functional capacity, i.e., decompensation (failure). (1,8,11)

Medication has not proven to be of significant value in the treatment of acute viral hepatitis. Symptomatically, drugs which possess antiemetic action, such as Tigan (suppository), Benadryl, can be helpful. The use of cortiodsteroids (D) has been demonstrated not to be of value in the course of acute viral hepatitis. In actuality, some studies have demonstrated a detrimental effect. (1,4,8)

Administration of gamma globulin (C), 0.02 ml/kg, or even immune serum globulin (hepatitis B), 0.06 ml/kg, has had no apparent modifying effect on the course of acute viral hepatitis. (1,8,12) Its role is in prevention of exposed individuals, e.g., household contacts, institution personnel.

Lastly, plasma-derived vaccines (Merck; Pasteur Institute) against hepatitis B have been confirmed as effective in prevention (control) of hepatitis B infection, e.g., homosexual men, hemodialysis units, drug addicts. (1,8,14,15) Minimal side effects have been reported. Optimism is the word regarding its future role and, therefore, markedly reducing or eliminating the need for postexposure immunization with hepatitis B immune serum globulin. (1,8,12-14)

5. (F) Hepatitis A basically runs an acute course, subsiding without incident. Complications, specifically, chronic liver disease and/or acute fulminant disease, occur in less than 1% of cases. Conversely, chronic liver disease and/or acute fulminant disease occur in as many as 50% of cases with hepatitis B infection, most commonly 5 to 15%. (1,4,8) The persistent abnormalities can be those of benign persistent hepatitis (chronic persistent hepatitis) or chronic aggressive hepatitis (chronic active liver disease). The latter should be suspected if transaminase and bilirubin determinations remain abnormal greater than 10 to 12 weeks, especially if transaminases are greater than 5 times normal and/or gamma globulin fraction is above 2 gm%. (1,4,8,16-18) A liver biopsy will be required for diagnosis. Treatment could include steroids. (1,8,18)

REFERENCES

1. Silverman, A., Roy, C.C.: Pediatric Clinical Gastroen-
    terology, 3rd edition. The CV Mosby Company, St. Louis,
    1983, p. 576.

2. Tabor, E., Jones, R., Gerety, R.J., et al.: Asympto-
    matic viral hepatitis type A and B in an adolescent popula-
    tion. Pediatrics 62:1026, 1978.

3. Krugman, S., Overby, L.R., Mushahwar, I.K.: Viral
    hepatitis, type B: Studies on natural history and preven-
    tion re-examined. N Engl J Med 300:101, 1979.

4. Caporaso, N., Coltorti, M., Del Vecchio-Blano, C., et
    al.: Acute viral hepatitis in childhood: Etiology and evo-
    lution. J Ped Gastroenterol Nutr 1:99, 1983.

5. Vittal, S.B.V., Thomas, W., Jr., Clowdus, B.F.: Acute
    viral hepatitis, course and incidence of progression to
    chronic hepatitis. Am J Med 55:757, 1973.

6. Stevens, G.E., Cherubin, C.E., Dienstag, J.L., et al.:
    Antibody to hepatitis A antigen in children. J Pediatr 91:
    436, 1977.

7. Bianchi, L., DeGroote, J., Desmet, V.J., et al.: Acute
    and chronic hepatitis revisited. Lancet 2:914, 1977.

8. Mowat, A.P.: Viral hepatitis in infancy and childhood.
    Clin Gastroenterol 9:191, 1980.

9. Boyer, J.L., Klatskin, G.: Pattern of necrosis in acute
    viral hepatitis: Prognostic value of bridging (subacute hepa-
    tic necrosis). N Engl J Med 283:1063, 1970.

10. Repsher, L.H., Freebern, R.K.: Effects of early and
    vigorous exercise on recovery from infectious hepatitis.
    N Engl J Med 281:1393, 1969.

11. Dienstag, J.L.: Hepatitis B virus infection: More than
    meets the eye. Gastroenterology 75:1172, 1978.

12. Szmuness, W., Stevens, C.E., Oleszko, W.R., et al.:
    Passive-active immunization against hepatitis B: Immuno-
    genicity studies in adult Americans. Lancet 1:575, 1981.

13. Krugman, S., Hollinger, F.B., Mosley, J.W., et al.: Immunoprophylaxis for viral hepatitis: Other views. Gastroenterology 77:186, 1979.

14. Krugman, S.: The newly licensed hepatitis B vaccine. J Am Med Assoc 247:2012, 1982.

15. Fennel, R.S., Andres, J.M., Pfaff, W.W., et al.: Liver dysfunction in children and adolescents during hemodialysis and after renal transplantation. Pediatrics 67:855, 1981.

16. Adler, R., Matinovskia, V., Heuser S., et al.: Fulminant hepatitis. Am J Dis Child 131:870, 1977.

17. Fauerholdt, L., Asnaes, S., Rane, K.L., et al.: Significance of suspected "chronic aggressive hepatitis" in acute hepatitis. Gastroenterology 73:543, 1977.

18. Arasu, T.S., Wyllie, R., Hatch, T.F., et al.: Management of chronic aggressive hepatitis in children and adolescents. Pediatrics 95:514, 1979.

Case 53

JAUNDICE AND GENERALIZED MALAISE
IN AN 8-YEAR-OLD GIRL

HISTORY

An 8-year-old white female presented with a history of persistent jaundice, decreased appetite, easy fatigability, variable darkness of urine, and light bowel movements of 13 weeks' duration. The pertinent prior history included an apparent urinary tract infection with associated fever and **arthralgia,** approximately 8 months prior to this presentation with the subsequent onset of fatigue, decreased appetite, dark urine, and jaundice. A diagnosis of acute viral hepatitis was made at this time, although it was made on the basis of the clinical history and associated increased SGOT, SGPT, and total and direct bilirubin levels. The patient had no history of nausea, vomiting, abdominal pain, constipation, diarrhea, skin rash, ocular difficulty, or trauma. The past history, developmental history, family history, and review of systems were unremarkable.

EXAMINATION

She was alert, active, and in no distress, with normal vital signs. Weight was 24 kg and height was 124.5 cm. The remainder of the examination was unremarkable except for the liver, palpable 4.0 cm below the right costal margin in the midclavicular line, firm, not tender or nodular, total span being 7.5 cm by percussion.

LABORATORY DATA

Hemoglobin:	12.0 gm%
Hematocrit:	36.5%
White blood cell count:	12,000/mm^3
PMN's:	50%
lymphocytes:	47%
monocytes:	2%
eosinophiles:	1%
Platelets:	250,000/mm^3
Sedimentation rate:	22 mm/hr
Direct Coombs' test:	negative
Serum:	
prothrombin time:	14.0 seconds
ceruloplasmin:	60 mg%
alpha-1-antitrypsin:	275 mg%
total bilirubin:	3.0 mg%
direct bilirubin:	2.7 mg%
SGOT:	250 units
SGPT:	220 units
alkaline phosphatase:	225 IU
creatinine:	0.5 mg%
total protein:	8.0 gm%
albumin:	4.0 gm%
HbsAg:	negative
HbcAg:	negative
antiHbs:	negative
antiHbc:	negative
VDRL:	negative
ANA:	negative
Sweat:	
sodium:	18 meq/L
chloride:	20 meq/L
Percutaneous liver biopsy:	(Fig. 53.1)

QUESTIONS

1. The most likely diagnosis is
   A. acute viral hepatitis
   B. chronic persistent hepatitis (benign persistent hepatitis)
   C. alpha-1-antitrypsin deficiency and liver disease
   D. chronic active liver disease (chronic aggressive hepatitis, CALD)
   E. Wilson's disease

444 / Case 53

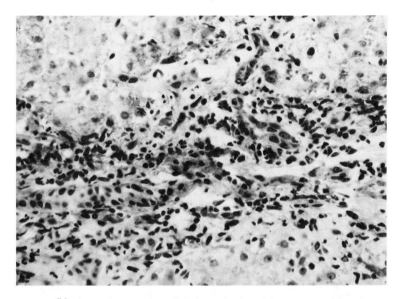

Figure 53.1 Liver. Round cell and, less so, poly infiltration
of the portal zone is present, extending into the lobule itself.
The limiting plate cannot be defined; bile ducts are seen but collapsed in nature. Cholestasis is not evident (H&E, X125).

2.   Potential causes of this condition include
     A. acute hepatitis virus B disease
     B. acute hepatitis virus A disease
     C. ulcerative colitis
     D. diabetes mellitus
     E. none of the above

Question 3: Answer true (T) or false (F).

3.   There is no genetic basis for chronic active liver disease
     (hepatitis).

4.   The predominant clinical manifestations of this condition
     include
     A. fatigue
     B. jaundice
     C. hepatomegaly
     D. arthralgia
     E. ascites

5. The major laboratory features include
   A. elevated transaminases (SGOT, SGPT), over 200-300 units
   B. elevated gamma globulin (over 3.0 gm/100 ml)
   C. reduced serum albumin (less than 2.5 gm/100 ml)
   D. positive hepatitis B surface antigen (Hbs-Ag)
   E. positive antinuclear antibody (ANA)

6. Histological features of chronic active liver disease include
   A. round cell (inflammatory) infiltrate of portal tracts
   B. extension of round cell infiltrate from portal tracts into parenchyma
   C. piecemeal necrosis
   D. intralobular septa
   E. multinucleated giant cells

7. Treatment, as in this patient, should include
   A. salicylazosulfapyridine (Azulfidine)
   B. corticosteroids
   C. azathioprine (Imuran)
   D. D-penicillamine
   E. surgery

8. Prognosis in CALD is characterized by
   A. 60 to 80% five-year survival
   B. reduced survival if initial biopsy demonstrates cirrhosis, subacute hepatic necrosis and/or bridging
   C. reduced survival if colitis is present at onset or develops subsequent to treatment onset
   D. reduced survival if response to steroids only
   E. improved survival if male, antinuclear antibody negative, or lower serum gamma globulin level

ANSWERS AND COMMENTS

1. (D) Chronic active liver disease (CALD), i.e., chronic active (aggressive) hepatitis, implies continuing hepatic inflammation of at least 10 weeks in duration. (1-5) The incriminated factors in its etiology are discussed in answer 2. A myriad of synonyms for CALD have been used over the years in an attempt to depict specific features, clinical, biochemical, histological, or otherwise, such as lupoid hepatitis, plasma cell hepatitis, or active juvenile cirrhosis. (1-5) More recent data suggest that these factors produce an initial injury, the disease itself representing a response to this injury. (1-5) Thus, CALD probably represents a "broad spectrum of diseases," possessing in

common the production of a particular, similar clinicopathological picture.

2. (A, C) As alluded to in answer 1, the precise cause of this clinicopathological picture is unknown. However, several potential factors have been incriminated, possibly by producing an initial injury, the disease being the response to the injury. Obviously, if true, individual susceptibility must play a role. Examples of confirmed factors include drugs, such as alpha-methyldopa, oxyphenisatin, infection (hepatitis B, hepatitis non A-non B), and ulcerative colitis. (1-10)

Several studies have demonstrated the evolution of acute hepatitis virus B disease into chronic active hepatitis. This process can occur in 3 to 4 weeks, e.g., subacute hepatic necrosis, to months or longer. (1-9, 10) The incidence has been estimated to be 10 to 20%. (1-9, 10) Conclusive evidence of such progression with hepatitis A virus disease has been lacking. However, the present ability to detect surface antigen and antibody to the surface antigen of A virus should allow appropriate reevaluation of the question. Patients with chronic hepatitis have had surface antigen (Hbs-Ag) to hepatitis B virus in the serum in as many as 25%. (1-5, 7, 8, 15, 16) At the same time, some have also had antibodies to the B virus core antigen (Hbc-Ag) in hepatocytes by immunofluorescence. (7, 11, 12) In adults, this incidence has been at least 15 to 20%. (7, 13) The presence of e antigen in serum has also been associated with chronic active hepatitis, e.g., as many as 25%, particularly in adults, also DNA polymerase. (12, 13, 14) The difficulty in data interpretation has been the high incidence of Hbs-Ag in certain populations, e.g., Ugandans, Greeks, and Austrians. (1-5, 7, 17)

As previously mentioned, chronic active hepatitis may result from a number of diseases. If this is so, an immunological sequence may be involved. Of course, host susceptibility must be a factor. Host-determined factors may include abnormality of cell-mediated immunity (T-lymphocytes), histocompatibility antigens and one's own antigens, i.e., forbidden-clone concept. (7, 15, 20) With reference to humoral immunity (B-cell), elevation of the three major classes (A, M, G) has been found, particularly IgG. (7, 18, 19) Reduced serum complement levels have been reported, too. (7, 15) In vitro activation of C_3 has also been demonstrated in CALD. (7, 15, 20) In addition, the presence of antinuclear antibody, DNA-binding antibodies, smooth muscle antibodies, and antiglomerular antibodies have been demonstrated in the serum of patients with CALD. (7, 15, 21-23) Antibodies against bovine bile canaliculi and microsomal membranes have been found in serum, the latter particularly in younger patients. (7, 15, 20) Moreover, a number of nonspecific antibody responses to viruses, such as rubella, rubeola, have also been found. (21) Impaired cell-mediated immunity has been suggested because of decreased circulating T-cells (rosette technique), reduced lymphocyte transformation in response to phytohaemagglutinin (PHA), and migration inhibition to biliary proteins, mitochondrial antigens. (20,24,25,26) More recently, in vitro lymphocyte cytotoxicity against homologous or heterologous liver cells has been demonstrated, and this cytotoxicity has been blocked by liver-specific lipoproteins (human, rabbit). (13,27,28) However, caution in interpreting in vitro studies must be exercised because of inadequate controls and the inherent interpretative drawback of in vitro techniques. Thus, the immunological interplay is obvious, but its specific role remains to be defined.

Ulcerative colitis, Sjogren's syndrome, and other disorders have also been associated with CALD. (7,15) However, the incidence of such association is low. Diabetes mellitus has not been associated with CALD·

3. (F) A genetic basis for chronic active disease has been suggested by the increased incidence of certain histocompatibility antigens, e.g., HL-A1 and HL-A8. (9) These HL-A loci are associated with the immune response genes (Ir.). Furthermore, familial CALD has been reported and could be related to such antigens. (9) Another potential genetic basis could be the development of self-antigens via the forbidden-clone concept. (9) This is mainly theoretical at this time.

4. (A,B,C) CALD occurs in children over 2 to 3 years of age, affecting females predominantly (2 to 4:1). (1-5,7,15,28,29) In the early phase, jaundice is the most consistent finding, occurring in 75 to 90% of patients overall. (1-5,7,15,28,29) Fatigue is almost as prevalent as jaundice, i.e., 75 to 90%. (1-5,7,15, 28,29) Other symptomatology includes abdominal pain, usually vague and mild in nature, in 25 to 50%, decreased appetite in 25 to 30%, arthralgia in 25%, altered menstruation in 20 to 30%, fever (low-grade) in 5 to 10%, variable rash in 5 to 10%, and pruritis in 5 to 10%. (1-5,7,15,28,29) The most consistent physical finding is hepatomegaly, 75 to 80%, while splenomegaly is present in 50 to 75% of patients. (1-5,7,15,28,29) The liver is firm and smooth in nature and is usually nontender or mildly so. Other physical findings include acne in 25%; ascites in 10 to 25%; clubbing in 5 to 20%; spider angiomas in 5 to 15%; skin lesions, such as erythema nodosum in 5 to 20%; and endocrine manifestations, almost exclusively in females, including cushingoid facies, and gynecomastia of males in 5 to 25%. (1-5,7,15,28, 29) In addition, urinary symptoms, including hematuria and

proteinuria, have occasionally been found (5 to 10%). (1-5,7,15, 28,29)

5. (A,B) Specific biochemical criteria for the diagnosis of CALD have been suggested: tenfold elevation of SGOT or five-fold elevation of SGOT with twofold elevation of the gamma glob-ulin level. (1-5,7,15) These criteria are applicable after 10 weeks of confirmed hepatic functional abnormality.

The biochemical features of CALD are characterized by per-sistent elevation of serum transaminases (SGOT, SGPT) in 100% of patients, most commonly above 300 IU; elevations of gamma globulin (90 to 95%), usually above 3.0 gm/100 ml, particularly IgG; increased alkaline phosphatase (80 to 90%), usually less than 5.0 mg/100 ml; reduced serum albumin level in 25 to 50%; and prolonged prothrombin time in 25 to 50%, frequently 50% or less activity. (1-5,7,15,28,29) Serological abnormalities have included positive smooth muscle antibody in 50 to 80%, antinu-clear antibody (ANA) in 25 to 50%, elevated antisalmonella anti-body in 25 to 35%, positive rheumatoid factor in 10 to 25%, posi-tive antiglomerular antibody in 5 to 20% and positive direct Coomb's reaction in 5 to 25%. (1-5,7,15,22,23,28,29) Hepatitis B surface antigen (Hb_SAg) was absent in the series of Dubois and Silverman, (31) but has been found in 10 to 60% of patients in other series. (1-5,10-12,15)

With secondary abnormalities, such as portal hypertension and hypersplenism, hematological abnormalities may be present, including anemia, leukopenia, and thrombocytopenia. (1-5,7,15) In advanced liver diseases, acanthocytes or burr cells may be present (peripheral blood smear). (7,15)

6. (B,C,D) By 10 or more weeks, CALD can be strongly sus-pected by clinical and biochemical data, but liver biopsy is in-dicated to provide the definitive answer. Thus, the diagnosis can be confirmed and treatment initiated. Typical histological parameters in chronic active liver disease consist of (1) hepa-tocyte necrosis, patchy and characteristically along the limiting plate of the lobule (piecemeal necrosis), (2) chronic inflamma-tory cell infiltration (lymphocytes, plasma cells) of the portal zones with extension into the parenchyma (toward central zone or adjacent portal zone), and (3) intralobular septa (inflamma-tory and/or fibrous tissue). (1-5,7,15,28,29) At times, por-tions of, or almost all of, lobule(s) may be destroyed. The in-flammatory infiltrate may contain some polymorphonuclear leu-kocytes and eosinophiles. Giant multinucleated cells may be present, too. Fibrous tissue may extend into the lobules from the portal zones as previously mentioned. Thus, architectural disorganization between portal zones and central veins is the

result. Late in the disease, actual cirrhosis may occur. This
cirrhosis may be micronodular or macronodular in type. Normal architectural organization occurs infrequently, 10 to 30%.
(1-5, 7, 15, 28-35)

7. (A, B) Many reports now have confirmed the value of early,
aggressive therapy. These reports have emphasized the significant beneficial effect of prednisone alone (corticosteroids) or in
combination with azathioprine (Imuran), but not of azathioprine
(Imuran) alone. Significant improvement in survival and morbidity have resulted. Clinical, biochemical, and morphological
resolution of CALD have been produced by the use of the previously mentioned agents. Resolution can be expected in 75 to
85% of patients, clinical by 6 months, biochemical by 12 months,
and histological by 18 months, in general. (7, 15, 28-35) If not
treated, the mortality in CALD has been estimated at 40% by 6
months, and 75 to 80% by 5 years of disease. (28-35)
  Prednisone, 1-2 mg/kg/24 hr, is the initial agent of choice
and is continued at that dose for as long as 4 to 6 weeks before
gradual weaning to a maintenance level, 20 mg daily (adults,
older adolescents) or less in younger children. Azathioprine,
1-1.5 mg/kg/24 hr, is added in order to reduce higher steroid
requirements, difficulty in weaning off of steroids, or according
to some authors, because of slightly higher percent resolution
with this combined regimen. Failure of the treatment to suppress clinical and biochemical parameters of activity within 4
weeks should prompt a reevaluation of the diagnosis. Thus,
monitoring of clinical and biochemical parameters of hepatic
function should be performed at least weekly during the initial
4 to 6 weeks of treatment and less often thereafter. (28-35)
  More recently, the above treatment regimen, i.e., immunosuppression, has been questioned with regard to B-positive CAH.
Immunosuppressive therapy has been demonstrated to augment
B virus replication. Although clinical and biochemical improvement had been demonstrated in B-positive CAH under steroid
treatment in the past studies, more recent reports have suggested less effective clinical and biochemical improvement, as
well as increased complication rate and mortality. Further controlled trials in adults, as well, and certainly some (any) in children, are definitely warranted in order to place corticosteroid
therapy in proper perspective in routine therapy for B-positive
CAH. (30-37) Sherlock (37) suggests steroid treatment for a
minimum of 3 to 6 months before potential discontinuation if no
response.
  Side effects, such as cushingoid appearance, are to be expected with steroid use. At times, ascites may occur. Dietary
sodium and fluid intake restriction and judicious use of diuretics,

such as spironolactone (aldactone) will alleviate this effect.
With use of azathioprine, gastrointestinal side effects (upset)
may occur. In addition, white blood count determinations must
be performed in order to identify the presence and magnitude of
leukopenia. Fortunately, significant leukopenia is uncommon.

In the author's experience, maintenance steroid (prednisone)
therapy must be administered daily because alternate day administration has not been as successful in sustaining clinical and biochemical remission. However, Arasu, et al. (38) demonstrated
that high-single-dose prednisone treatment daily, initially and
then on alternate days, would effectively suppress HbₛAg-nega-
tive CAH in children and adolescents. Their mean duration of
treatment was 19 months. (38) The author feels that prednisone
can be administered on alternate days if continuous azathioprine
administration is used. Certainly this approach will alleviate
the major growth-suppressive and cosmetic effects of prednisone
per se.

Once remission has been achieved, continued treatment
should be successful in preventing relapse for as long as 4 to 5
years. If clinical, biochemical, and histologic remission is
achieved and treatment has been administered for at least 12 to
18 months, gradual weaning and ultimate discontinuation of treatment can be contemplated. (1-5, 28-35) However, relapse within
3 to 6 months after treatment discontinuation has occurred in as
many as 50% of patients. If relapse should occur, treatment
should be promptly reinstituted, and the pattern of response
should occur as previously experienced by those patients.
(28-35)

Antacids can be used if gastrointestinal upset should occur
with treatment. Complications of liver disease, e.g., bleeding
from esophageal varices, should be treated by standard measures. Potential hepatotoxic agents should be avoided. Diet and
activity generally should be as desired and tolerated by the patients.

Azulfidine would be applicable in inflammatory bowel disease. D-penicillamine would be applicable in conditions with
excessive copper deposition in organs, such as liver, e.g., Wilson's disease. Surgery is not applicable unless the manifestations of portal hypertension warrant such due to lack of response
to medical treatment and the presence of satisfactory stabilization of the underlying CALD. This is rarely the case. Newer
forms of therapy, e.g., transfer factor, Levamisole, have been
ineffective or insufficiently evaluated. (29-35)

8. (A,B) Definite prolongation of life has been observed in patients receiving appropriate treatment as outlined in answer 7.
The five-year survival rate with treatment has been 60 to 80%.

(28-35) After cessation of treatment initially, long-term remissions have occurred in 30% or more. (28-35) In fact, Dubois and Silverman (31-33) reported less frequent relapses with treatment discontinuation after 18 to 24 months.

In children, in contrast to adults, the prognosis has not been unfavorably affected if the presentation was acute, hepatitis-like. (31,33) In addition, the development of colitis did not seem to unfavorably affect the response to treatment. (31,33) No correlation has been found in those children with high gamma globulin levels, positive antinuclear antibody, or with age, sex, or extraintestinal manifestations. However, the prognosis was worse if the initial histology revealed subacute hepatic necrosis and/or cirrhosis. (28-35) The prognosis in those patients with Hbs-Ag-positive CALD has been reported to be worse by certain authors, while being the same as antigen-negative CALD by others. (29-35) More data are needed.

Occasionally, death occurs early in the disease due to fulminant hepatic failure. However, progressive hepatic failure and coma constitute the more common terminal events. Finally, malignancy, i.e., hepatocarcinoma, has been reported in a few adult patients with CALD. (34,35) This remains to be confirmed in children.

For further information on the repetitive cycles of chronic liver disease or comparison of CALD and CPH, see Tables 53.1 and 53.2.

TABLE 53.1 Characterization of Chronic Active Liver Disease (CALD) and Chronic Persistent Hepatitis (CPH)

Feature	CALD	CPH
Clinical	Significant and progressive symptoms, e.g., jaundice, fatigue, anorexia, nausea, vomiting, fever	Minor symptoms, e.g., fatigue, mild anorexia, nausea
Biochemical	Transaminases: Usually elevated fivefold or more	Transaminases: Normal or mildly elevated (100-200 ku or less)
	Gamma globulin: Usually elevated twofold or more	Gamma globulin: Less than twofold elevation
	Albumin: Frequently reduced less than 3.0 gm%	Albumin: Usually normal, as are alkaline phosphatase, prothrombin time and other studies
	Other serological abnormalities (e.g., ANA, HbsAg)	HbsAg: Positive or negative
Histological	Portal zone inflammatory infiltrate (chronic), extending into parenchyma piecemeal necrosis intralobular septa	Mild portal zone and/or lobular, inflammatory infiltrate (chronic)
Treatment	Steroids with or without azathioprine	None is required
Prognosis	Poor without treatment, good with treatment	Excellent

TABLE 53.2   Chronic Liver Disease: Repetitive Cycles

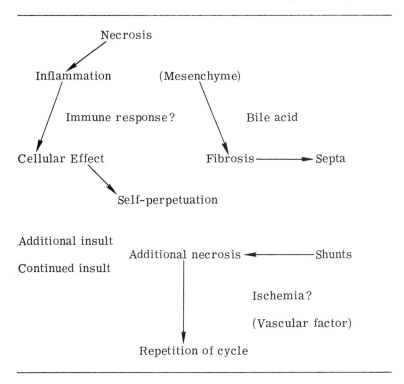

Modified from Appleman, H.D.: Am J Dig Dis 17:436, 1973;
and Roy, C.C., Silverman, A., Cozzetto, F.J. (34)

REFERENCES

1.   Geall, M.G., Schoenfield, L.F., Summerskill, W.H.J.:
     Classification and treatment of chronic active liver disease.
     Gastroenterology 55:724, 1968.

2.   Summerskill, W.H.J.: Chronic active liver disease reex-
     amined: Prognosis hopeful. Gastroenterology 66:450, 1974.

3.   Dubois, R.S., Silverman, A., Slovis, T.L.: Chronic active
     hepatitis in children. Am J Dig Dis 17:575, 1972.

4.   Mistilis, S.P. and Blackburn, C.R.B.: Active chronic hep-
     atitis. Am J Med 48:784, 1970.

5. Becker, M.D., Scheuer, P.J., Baptista, A., et al.: Prognosis of chronic persistent hepatitis. Lancet 1:53, 1970.

6. Boyer, J.L. and Klatskin, G.: Patterns of necrosis in acute viral hepatitis: Prognostic value of bridging (subacute hepatic necrosis). N Engl J Med 283:1063, 1970.

7. Sherlock, S.: Progress report, chronic hepatitis. Gut 15: 655, 1974.

8. Wright, R.: Chronic hepatitis. Br Med Bull 28:120, 1972.

9. Zuckerman, A.J.: Genetic factors in viral hepatitis. In: Human Viral Hepatitis, 2nd Edition. North Holland, Oxford, 1975, p. 254.

10. Hyatt, A.C., Leleiko, N.S.: Autoimmunity in liver and gastrointestinal disorders. Pediatr Ann 11:315, 1982.

11. Fox, R.A., Niazi, S.P., Sherlock, S.: Hepatitis-associated antigen in chronic liver disease. Lancet 2:609, 1969.

12. Edgington, T.S. and Ritt, D.J.: Intrahepatic expression of serum hepatitis virus-associated antigens. J Exp Med 134:871, 1971.

13. Edgington, T.S. and Chisari, F.U.: Immunological aspects of hepatitis B virus infection. Am J Med Sci 270: 213, 1975.

14. Magnius, L.O.: Characterization of a new antigen-antibody system associated with hepatitis B. Clin Exp Immun 20:209, 1975.

15. Elefheriou, N., Thomas, H.C., Heathcote, J., et al.: Incidence and clinical significance of e antigen and antibody in acute and chronic liver disease. Lancet 2:1171, 1975.

16. Almeida, J.D., Gay, F.W., Wreahi, H.T.G.: Pitfalls in the study of hepatitis A. Lancet 2:748, 1974.

17. Gocke, D.J. and McIntosh, R.M.: Cryoprecipitates containing hepatitis B antigen in patients with liver disease. Gastroenterology 65:542, 1973.

18. Anthony, P.P., Vogel, C.I., Sadikali, E., et al.: Hepatitis-associated antigen and antibody in Uganda: Correlation of serological testing with histopathology. Br Med J 1:403, 1972.

19. Feizi, T.: Immunoglobulins in chronic liver disease. Gut 9:193, 1968.

20. Dawkins, R.L. and Joske, R.A.: Immunoglobulin deposition in liver of patients with active chronic hepatitis and antibody against smooth muscle. Br Med J 2:643, 1973.

21. Dehoratius, R.J., Strickland, R.G., Williams, R.C., Jr.: T and B lymphocytes in acute and chronic hepatitis. Clin Immun Immunopath 2:353, 1974.

22. Triger, D.R., Kurtz, J.B., Wright, P.: Viral antibodies and autoantibodies in chronic liver disease. Gut 15:94, 1974.

23. Davis, P. and Read, A.E.: Antibodies to double-stranded (native) DNA in active chronic hepatitis. Gut 16:413, 1975.

24. Levy, R.L. and Hong, R.: Anti-glomerular antibody in chronic active and chronic persistent hepatitis. Pediatrics 85:155, 1974.

25. Dudley, F.J., Fox, R.A., Sherlock, S.: Cellular immunity and hepatitis-associated Australia antigen liver disease. Lancet 1:723, 1972.

26. Gerber, M.J., Phuangsab, A., Vittal, S.B.V., et al.: Cell-mediated immune response to hepatitis B antigen in patients with liver disease. Am J Dig Dis 19:637, 1974.

27. Thomson, A.D., Cochraine, M.A.G., McFarlane, I.G., et al.: Lymphocyte cytotoxicity to isolated hepatocytes in chronic active hepatitis. Nature 252:721, 1974.

28. Paronetto, F., Vernance, S., Gerber, M.: Lymphocyte cytotoxicity in patients with chronic active hepatitis (CAH): Tissue culture studies using autologous liver cells. Gastroenterology 64:889, 1973.

29. Korman, M.G., Hofmann, A.F., Summerskill, W.H.J.: Assessment of activity in chronic active liver disease. N Engl J Med 290:1399, 1974.

30. Soloway, R.D., Summerskill, W.H. J., Baggenstoss, A.H., et al. : Clinical, biochemical and histological remission of severe chronic active liver disease: A controlled study of treatment and early prognosis. Gastroenterology 63:820, 1972.

31. Dubois, R.S. and Silverman, A.: Treatment of chronic active hepatitis in children. Postgrad Med J 50:386, 1974.

32. Cook, G.C., Mulligan, R., Sherlock, S.O.: Controlled prospective trial of corticosteroid therapy in active chronic hepatitis. Q J Med 40:159, 1971.

33. Murray-Lyon, I.M., Stern, R.B., Williams, R.: Controlled trial of prednisone and azathioprine in active chronic hepatitis. Lancet 1:735, 1973.

34. Roy, C.C., Silverman, A., Cozzetto, F.J.: Pediatric Clinical Gastroenterology, 2nd Edition. The CV Mosby Co., St. Louis, 1975, p. 523.

35. Joske, R.A., Laurence, B.H., Matz, L.R.: Familial active chronic hepatitis with hepatocellular carcinoma. Gastroenterology 62:441, 1972.

36. Wright, E.C., Seeff, L.B., Berk, P.D., et al.: Treatment of chronic active hepatitis, an analysis of three controlled trials. Gastroenterology 73:1422, 1977.

37. Sherlock, S.: Chronic active hepatitis. In: Current Pediatric Therapy, 10th edition. Gellis, S.S. and Kagan, B.M. (Eds). WB Saunders Company, Boston, 1982, p. 202.

38. Arasu, T.S., Wyllie, R., Hatch, T.F., et al.: Management of chronic aggressive hepatitis in children and adolescents. Pediatrics 95:514, 1979.

Case 54

HEPATOMEGALY, ABNORMAL LIVER FUNCTION
TESTS IN A 6-YEAR-OLD BOY

HISTORY

A 6-year-old white male presented with a history of apparent
mild hepatomegaly and subsequent discovery of altered hepatic
function tests, discovered by his private physician at the time
of a preschool examination. The patient had no history of fever,
abdominal pain, nausea, vomiting, diarrhea, constipation, jaundice, anorexia, dysuria, skin lesions, fatigue, or trauma. His
activity and appetite had remained unchanged. His school performance was unchanged, as was his performance in many sport-
ing activities. Family history included paternal grandfather
with a history of cirrhosis, type unknown. The remainder of
the past history, developmental history, family history, social
history, and review of systems was unremarkable.

EXAMINATION

He was alert, cooperative, and in no apparent distress, with
normal vital signs, weight 25 kg, height 113 cm. The remainder of the examination was unremarkable except for palpable
liver, 2.0 cm below the right costal margin in the midclavicular line, firm, not tender or nodular, total span by percussion
7.0 cm, and nonpalpable spleen and kidneys. Active bowel
sounds were present with no bruits. Neurological examination
was unremarkable.

LABORATORY DATA

Hemoglobin:	12.4 gm%
Hematocrit:	38%
White blood cell count:	7,200/mm^3
PMN's:	41%
lymphocytes:	56%
monocytes:	1%
eosinophiles:	2%
Sedimentation rate:	11 mm/hr
Alpha-fetoprotein:	negative
Alpha-1-antitrypsin:	300 mg%
Ceruloplasmin:	10 mg%
Urinalysis:	negative
Serum:	
sodium:	138 meq/L
potassium:	4.2 meq/L
chloride:	104 meq/L
bicarbonate:	22 meq/L
creatinine:	0.5 mg%
SGOT:	62 KU
SGPT:	41 KU
alkaline phosphate:	130 IU
total bilirubin:	0.9 mg%
direct bilirubin:	0.6 mg%
total protein:	6.8 gm%
albumin:	4.6 gm%
VDRL:	negative
HbsAg:	negative
antiHbs:	negative
HbcAg:	negative

QUESTIONS

Question 1: Answer true (T) or false (F).

1. This patient's condition is an inborn error of metabolism, inherited as an autosomal dominant trait.

2. The characteristic findings in this condition consist of which of the following?
   A. Ventricular conduction defect
   B. Renal dysfunction
   C. Cirrhosis
   D. Central nervous system degeneration
   E. Proximal arthropathy

Question 3: Answer true (T) or false (F).

3. Of patients with this disease, 25% have symptoms by 15
   years of age.

4. The carrier gene frequency of this condition is estimated
   to be which one of the following?
   A. 0.1%
   B. 0.2%
   C. 0.5%
   D. 1%
   E. 5%

5. The cause(s) of the defect in this condition includes which
   of the following?
   A. Reduced excretion of copper in bile
   B. Abnormal hepatic copper-binding protein
   C. Increased absorption of copper by the small intestine
   D. Increased reabsorption of copper by renal tubules
   E. Enhanced hepatic uptake of copper

Questions 6 and 7: Answer true (T) or false (F).

6. The hemolytic anemia in this disease may be the result of
   release of tissue copper into plasma and the subsequent
   breakdown of red blood cells.

7. At least 50% of pediatric patients will display clinical and/
   or physical manifestations of hepatic involvement in this
   condition.

8. The hepatic manifestations of this condition frequently in-
   clude which of the following?
   A. Acute hepatitis
   B. Fulminant hepatitis
   C. Chronic hepatitis
   D. Cirrhosis
   E. All of the above

9. The diagnosis of Wilson's disease can be strongly suspected
   or confirmed by which of the following?
   A. Presence of Kayser-Fleischer ring(s)
   B. Low serum copper
   C. High serum ceruloplasmin
   D. Elevated urine copper excretion
   E. Markedly elevated hepatic copper content

10. The treatment of this condition, including this patient's, may consist of which of the following measures?
    A. D-penicillamine
    B. Steroids
    C. Triethylene tetramine hydrochloride (TETA)
    D. Azathioprine
    E. Dietary restriction, 1 mg or less of copper intake daily

Question 11: Answer true (T) or false (F).

11. The evaluation of efficacy of treatment should include periodic checks of serum copper and ceruloplasmin.

12. The prognosis and course of this condition are characterized by which of the following?
    A. If untreated, essentially all patients die
    B. Even if cirrhosis is present, therapy can significantly prolong survival
    C. No reversal or neurological sequelae can be accomplished, even with therapy
    D. Orthotopic liver transplantation can be performed in selected patients and will provide elimination of all manifestations
    E. The best prognosis is in affected patients without symptoms on continued therapy

ANSWERS AND COMMENTS

1. (F) This condition, hepatolenticular degeneration (Wilson's disease), is an uncommon inborn error of metabolism which is inherited as an autosomal recessive trait. (1-7) Although Gowers, as well as Kayser and Fleischer, had previously described patients with similar symptomatology, Kinnier Wilson (8) is accorded the credit for first describing this "disease" in 1912. In 1913, Rumpel associated excessive copper content in liver with this disease. In 1921, Hall introduced the concept of hepatolenticular degeneration in this disease. The excessive copper content in liver and in the central nervous system was described with finality by Cumons (4) in 1948, however. Also in 1948, Holmberg and Laurell isolated and characterized the copper-binding protein, ceruloplasmin. (4,7)

2. (B,C,D) Wilson's disease is characterized by cirrhosis, renal dysfunction, and central nervous system degenerative changes. (1-10) The neurologic features in children resemble those in adults. School performance worsens; dysarthria,

intention tremors, ataxia, rigidity, cogwheeling of the limbs, and occasionally spasticity or dystonia, may result. (1-4,7,9, 10) Personality changes and the onset of psychosis may also occur. (1-4,7,9,10)

The renal changes are those suggestive of renal tubular dysfunction. (4,7,11,12) Amino-aciduria, glycosuria, hypercalciuria, uricosuria, and renal tubular acidosis have been described, the latter due to subnormal acidifying ability (urinary concentrating defect) in approximately 25% of patients in response to ammonium chloride loading. (7) Subsequent studies demonstrated proximal and/or distal tubular impairment. The distal variant may be more common. (7)

The hepatic disorders, particularly cirrhosis, will be discussed in answer 8.

3. (F) Diagnosis of Wilson's disease is possible and is made during childhood due to its occurrence in 50% or more by 15 years of age.

The symptomatology is particularly related to hepatic involvement, although neurologic manifestations are also present before adulthood. (4,7,9,10)

4. (B) As previously mentioned (answer 1), Wilson's disease is an autosomal recessive disease. The gene frequency of carriers has been estimated to be about 1:500, but may be more common than previously reported. (1-10)

5. (A,B) The varied manifestations of Wilson's disease have been attributed to the effect of copper deposition in the involved organs. (1-4,7) This involvement would result in the neurological, hepatic, and renal tubular abnormalities, as well as the Kayser-Fleischer rings. (1-10) A number of possible dysfunctions could occur, since copper is an inhibitor of many cell membrane and intracellular enzyme systems. (7,11-14) Recent studies using short half-life copper radioisotopes, ^{64}Cu and $^{67}Cu_3$, particularly the former, have demonstrated decreased excretion of copper in bile but not increased copper absorption. (11,13-15) Small intestinal perfusion with a multilumen tube to determine copper flux across the small intestinal mucosa has revealed no increased absorption. (13) Sternlieb, et al. (6) have further demonstrated reduced copper content in gallbladder bile at surgery. Furthermore, recent studies using ^{64}Cu have revealed a possible lysosomal defect (enzymes) which results in decreased hepatic excretion of biliary copper and the subsequent accumulation of copper in the liver. Hepatic clearance of copper bound to albumin is apparently at a normal rate, certainly earlier on in the disease. Transfer to ceruloplasmin does occur. In

addition, an abnormal protein, copper thionein, has an increased affinity for copper. (16) Supposedly, this protein would be synthesized in homozygous patients, and the copper, predominantly bound to this protein, would reach, enter, and then damage the liver cells. (16) The liver would become progressively saturated and the copper would then become available for deposition in other organs. The exact mechanisms of this extrahepatic deposition are predominantly unknown.

6. (T) Hemolytic anemia occurs in some patients with Wilson's disease. (17) This seems to be the result of rapid release of tissue copper into the plasma. (17) The hemolytic process may recur, jaundice may occur, and eventually gallstones may develop. (17)

7. (T) The major aspect of Wilson's disease in children is the hepatic involvement with its varied manifestations. (1-4,7) Over 50% of pediatric patients will have clinical or physical manifestations of hepatic involvement. Furthermore, some authors have stressed the importance of Wilson's disease as a cause of cirrhosis in children, i.e., next in frequency to chronic aggressive hepatitis. (CAH). (1-5,7)

8. (E) (Refer to answer 7, also) The initial hepatic involvement can be asymptomatic hepatosplenomegaly or a presentation resembling an acute hepatitis, then becoming fulminant or resolving. (1-5,7,18) The subsequent course of survivors is a progressive one, ending in cirrhosis. Portal hypertension will appear and may actually be the presenting sign of the chronic aspects of Wilson's disease. Thus, upper gastrointestinal hemorrhage or ascites or hypersplenism may be the initial manifestations. (1-4,7) Jaundice is an infrequent early manifestation, except when associated with gallstone formation or the fulminant hepatic presentation. (1-5,7) The chronic forms in Wilson's disease are principally chronic aggressive hepatitis and cirrhosis without any degree of activity.

Histologically, certain features may be suspicious for Wilson's disease and include fatty vacuolization in degenerating hepatocytes, glycogenization and cytoplasmic hyaline bodies, so-called Mallory bodies, most typically present in alcoholic liver disease and rare in liver biopsies of children. Other features will be those of the basic hepatic process, i.e., (1) acute hepatitis (focal or spotty necrosis of liver cells, mild inflammatory reaction, principally mononuclear cells, and so forth); (2) fulminant hepatitis (massive necrosis and inflammatory reaction); (3) macrolobular (postnecrotic) cirrhosis; or (4) chronic aggressive hepatitis (predominantly portal zone inflammation, both plasma and mononuclear cells, few polys, necrosis of hepatocytes, particularly periportal with disruption of the limiting plate of the lobule, variable lobular inflammation and deposition of connective tissue, particularly in the portal and periportal zones). (1-5, 7)

9.   (A, D, E)   The presence of a confirmed Kayser-Fleischer ring(s), usually by slit-lamp examination, firmly establishes the diagnosis. (1-5, 7-10)   Copper is deposited along the lateral aspect of the cornea, i.e., Descemet's membrane. (1-5, 7-10)
     A low level (less than 25 mg/100 ml) or absence of serum ceruloplasmin is highly suspicious for the heterozygous or homozygous state of Wilson's disease. (1-4, 7)   Conversely, a normal level does not eliminate the possibility of this disease (4 to 5%). (1-4, 7, 18)   Serum copper levels are the least helpful of measurements, as high, normal, and low levels have been reported in Wilson's disease. (1-4, 7)
     Urine copper excretion is usually significantly elevated in Wilson's disease, i.e., above 50 μg/24 hr. (1-4, 7)   Normal values are usually 30 μg/24 hr or less. (1-4, 7)   False positive results have been reported, such as in biliary tract disease and cirrhosis. (1-4, 7)   In addition, in the early phases of this condition, the urine copper levels may be relatively normal.   However, urine can be collected 6 hours after a single dose of D-penicillamine, 500 mg by mouth.   In Wilson's disease, the levels will almost always be above 50 μg/6 hr, while normals will excrete 300 μg/hr or less. (1-4, 7)
     The most meaningful determination is quantitative hepatic copper.   An abnormal value would be greater than 50 μg/gm of wet weight liver. (1-4, 7)   Obviously, this determination requires liver tissue, adequate in amount, and thus open or closed (percutaneous) biopsy.   Elevated levels of hepatic copper have been reported in cirrhosis, biliary and portal (Laennec's), and in chronic aggressive hepatitis per se, but the age and clinical history and course should eliminate any possible confusion. (1-5, 7)   When available, a definitive test is the lack of incorporation of ^{64}Cu or ^{67}Cu into ceruloplasmin.
     Other studies, such as transaminases, SGOT, and SGPT (elevated), total protein/albumin levels, as well as renal function tests, such as proteinuria, glucosuria, elevated phosphate excretion, are, unfortunately, nonspecific. (1-4, 7)

10.   (A, C, E)   Treatment is initiated in order to restore normal organ function as far as possible and to reverse symptomatology. This is of obvious importance in asymptomatic homozygotes or in the early symptomatic phase.

After the baseline laboratory studies, i.e., urine copper excretion, serum ceruloplasmin, hepatic copper content, and others, the treatment of choice is (1) limitation of dietary copper intake to 1 mg or less daily; (2) D-penicillamine (drug of choice, chelating action), 750 to 1,500 mg/24 hr orally; and (3) vitamin B_6 (pyridoxine), 5 to 10 mg/24 hr, when D-penicillamine is being administered. In addition, potassium sulfide (carbo-resin), 30 to 40 mg t.i.d., may be used in order to promote intestinal copper binding. (7,22,23) If the patient has an untoward reaction to D-penicillamine, or there is a lack of patient response, other medication can be substituted, such as dimercaprol and triethylenetetramine hydrochloride (TETA), 400 mg t.i.d. Their efficacy is reduced in comparison with D-penicillamine. Untoward effects of D-penicillamine include rash, fever, leukopenia, lupus-like syndrome, and nephrotic syndrome. (7,22,23)

11. (F) The physician, patient, and family must be prepared for life-long treatment of this disease. In order to maximize results, periodic clinical and laboratory assessment must be enacted. Therefore, specific schedules should be created, emphasizing basal and, on occasions, post-stimulation (D-penicillamine) urine copper excretion for 24 hr. Liver biopsy and copper content can be and should be reassessed for further confirmatory evidence, although certainly only every few years.

12. (A, E) If untreated, essentially all patients will die within years from hepatic and neurological complications. (1-10) During the initial phases of the disease, a few patients will die due to fulminant hepatic disease, i.e., "hepatitis." (1-4, 7) With disease progression, chronic liver disease will result. In the presence of cirrhosis, therapy, even if prolonged and at effective levels, apparently does not lengthen survival. (1-4, 7) However, some degree of resolution can be accomplished with therapy. (1-4, 7, 23)

Orthotopic hepatic transplantation has only been performed in a very few patients. Liver biopsies have revealed minimal or no histological abnormalities and normal copper content. However, there was variable improvement in neurological manifestations and persistence of Kayser-Fleischer rings, suggesting that extrahepatic sites of copper deposition may not be affected. (24)

Thus, the best prognosis seems to be in those patients without symptomatology, but continued treatment must be maintained. Neurological and hepatic abnormalities can be maintained at the same level, improved, uncommonly reversed, or be progressive. (21) Provided treatment (penicillamine) is initiated before irreversible damage to vital organs has occurred, normal life span can usually be achieved. (18-20) Despite this less than optimistic outlook, the key to management is early diagnosis, prompt family screening, and consistent, vigorous treatment (early; prophylactic) and follow-up. (16,20,22,23,25)

REFERENCES

1. Slovist, L., Dubois, R.S., Rodgerson, D.V., et al.: The varied manifestations of Wilson's disease. J Pediatr 78: 578, 1971.

2. Strickland, G.T. and Leu, M-L.: Wilson's disease: Clinical and laboratory manifestations in 40 patients. Gastroenterology 54:113, 1975.

3. Walshe, J.M.: Wilson's disease: Its diagnosis and management. Br J Hosp Med 4:91, 1970.

4. Scheinberg, I.H. and Sternlieb, I.: Wilson's disease. Ann Rev Med 16:119, 1965.

5. Sternlieb, I. and Scheinberg, I.H.: Chronic hepatitis as a first manifestation of Wilson's disease. Ann Intern Med 76:59, 1972.

6. Sternlieb, I., Van den Hamer, C.J.A., Morell, A.G., et al.: Lysosomal defect of hepatic copper excretion in Wilson's disease (hepatolenticular degeneration). Gastroenterology 64:99, 1973.

7. Roy, C.C., Silverman, A., Cozzetto, F.J.: Pediatric Clinical Gastroenterology, 2nd Edition. The CV Mosby Co., St. Louis, 1975, p. 567.

8. Wilson, S.A.K.: Progressive lenticular degeneration: A familial nervous disease associated with cirrhosis of the liver. Brain 34:295, 1912.

9. Bearn, A.G.: A genetical analysis of thirty families with Wilson's disease (hepatolenticular degeneration). Ann Hum Genet 24:33, 1960.

10. Darley, F.L., Aronson, F.L., Goldstein, N.P.: Dysarthria in Wilson's disease. J Speech Hear Res 17:69, 1974.

11. Wilson, D.M. and Goldstein, N.P.: Bicarbonate excretion in Wilson's disease (hepatolenticular degeneration). Mayo Clin Proc 49:394, 1974.

12. Wilson, D.M. and Goldstein, N.P.: Renal urate excretion in patients with Wilson's disease. Kidney Int 4:331, 1973.

13. Marceau, N., Aspin, N., Sass-Kortsa, K.A.: Absorption of copper-64 from gastrointestinal tract of the rat. Am J Physiol 218:377, 1970.

14. Strickland, G.T., Beckner, W.M., Leu, M-I., et al.: Turnover studies of copper in homozygotes and heterozygotes for Wilson's disease and controls: Isotope tracer studies with 67 CU. Clin Sci 43:605, 1972.

15. Strickland, G.T., Beckner, W.M., Leu, M-L.: Absorption of copper in homozygotes and heterozygotes for Wilson's disease and controls: Isotope tracer studies with 67 CU and 64 CU. Clin Sci 43:617, 1972.

16. Evans, G.W., Dubois, R.S., Hambidge, K.M.: Wilson's disease: Identification of an abnormal copper-binding protein. Science 181:1175, 1973.

17. Iser, J.H., Stevens, B.J., Stening, G.F., et al.: Hemolytic anemia of Wilson's disease. Gastroenterology 67: 290, 1974.

18. Kane, W.J., Sharp, H.L.: Metabolic liver disease of childhood. Pediatr Clin 6:318, 1977.

19. Sass-Kortsak, A.: Wilson's disease: A treatable liver disease in children. Pediatr Clin North Am 22:963, 1975.

20. Danks, D.M.: Hereditary disorders of copper metabolism in Wilson's disease and Menke's disease. In: The Metabolic Basis of Inherited Disease, 5th edition. Stanbury, J.B., Wyngarden, J.B., Fredrickson, D.S., Goldstein, J.L., (Eds). McGraw Hill Book Company, New York, 1982, p. 1251.

21. Steinlieb, I.: Diagnosis of Wilson's disease in 1981. Gastroenterol Clin Biol 5:169, 1981.

22. Goldstein, N.P., Tauxe, W.N., McCall, J.T., et al.: Treatment of Wilson's disease (hepatolenticular degeneration) with penicillamine and low-copper diet. Trans Am Neurol Assoc 94:34, 1969.

23. Falkmer, S., Samuelson, G., Sjolin, S.: Penicillamine-induced normalization of clinical signs and liver morphology and histochemistry in a case of Wilson's disease. Pediatrics 45:260, 1970.

24. Groth, C.G., Dubois, R.S., Corman, J., et al.: Hepatic transplantation in Wilson's disease. Birth Defects 9:106, 1973.

25. Sternlieb, I. and Scheinberg, I.H.: Prevention of Wilson's disease in asymptomatic patients. N Engl J Med 278:352, 1968.

Case 55

ALTERED LIVER FUNCTION TESTS IN A 6-YEAR-OLD BOY
ON MEDICATION FOR ACUTE LYMPHOBLASTIC LEUKEMIA

HISTORY

A 6-year-old white male presented for evaluation of altered liver function tests of at least one year duration. Approximately 18 months prior to this presentation, the patient had been evaluated for persistent fever, generalized malaise, fatigue, and pallor. A subsequent evaluation, including bone marrow examination, revealed the presence of acute lymphoblastic leukemia. The patient's treatment initially consisted of vincristine, steroids (prednisone), 6-mercaptopurine, and methotrexate. After remission was induced, subsequent medication included predominantly 6-mercaptopurine and methotrexate. Blood chemistries were drawn prior to the onset of treatment and were within normal limits, including SGOT, total protein, albumin, prothrombin time, and total and direct bilirubin. Subsequent to the initiation of treatment, blood chemistries, including the previously mentioned studies, were performed no more frequently than every 3 to 6 months. Definite abnormalities were noted at least one year prior to the present evaluation. The patient had had no associated history of fever, nausea, vomiting, abdominal pain, jaundice, anorexia, diarrhea, constipation, melena, hematochezia, or dysuria. His appetite and activity had remained unchanged. Blood chemistries included SGOT, 75 to 250 units, most recently 78 units; SGPT, 52 to 135, most recently 54 units; alkaline phosphatase, 120 to 400 IU, most recently 172 IU; total bilirubin, 0.6 to 2.0 mg/100 ml, most recently 0.9 mg/100 ml (direct fraction predominating). Total protein, albumin, prothrombin time, and partial thromboplastin time had remained within normal limits. The remainder of the past history, developmental history, family history, social history, and review of systems was noncontributory.

468

EXAMINATION

He was alert, active, cooperative, and in no distress, with normal vital signs, height 113 cm, weight 22.5 kg. The remainder
of the examination was unremarkable except for the liver, palpable 2.5 cm below the right costal margin in the midclavicular
line, firm, nontender, and not nodular, with a questionably palpable spleen tip below the left costal margin in the midclavicular line. The total span of the liver by percussion was 7.25 cm.

LABORATORY DATA

Hemoglobin:	12.4 gm%
Hematocrit:	37%
White blood cell count:	6,500/mm³
PMN's:	46%
lymphocytes:	51%
monocytes:	1%
eosinophiles:	2%
Platelet count:	275,000/mm³
Sedimentation rate:	11 mm/hr
Serum:	
SGOT:	76 units
SGPT:	54 units
alkaline phosphatase:	174 IU
isoenzymes:	4+ - liver
total bilirubin:	0.9 mg%
direct bilirubin:	0.6 mg%
prothrombin time:	12.8 sec (11.0 sec)
partial thromboplastin time	38 sec (< 36 sec)
total protein:	6.0 gm%
albumin:	3.7 gm%
uric acid:	3.7 mg%
calcium:	10.1 mg%
cholesterol:	156 mg%
glucose:	88 mg%
amylase:	97 units
HbcAg:	negative
antihb$_S$:	negative
HbsAg:	negative
antiHb$_C$:	negative
VDRL:	negative
ANA:	negative
Liver scan:	
(technetium 99m):	mottled appearance only
Percutaneous liver biopsy:	(Fig. 55.1)

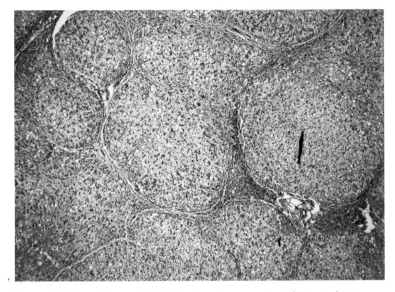

Figure 55.1 Liver. Thin bands of connective (fibrous) tissue surround regenerating nodules of hepatocytes with minimal inflammatory infiltrate (lymphocytes, plasma cells) (H&E, X120).

QUESTIONS

1. Which of this patient's medications (drugs) have been more frequently associated with potential liver injury?
    A. Ampicillin
    B. Prednisone
    C. Vincristine
    D. Methotrexate (amethopterin)
    E. 6-mercaptopurine

2. Which of the following mechanisms are predominant in producing liver injury?
    A. Toxicity (dose-dependent)
    B. Immune complex formation
    C. Idiosyncracy (nondose-dependent)
    D. Interruption of enterohepatic circulation
    E. H_2 receptor antagonism

Question 3: Answer true (T) or false (F).

3. The histological findings in the present case are more compatible with an adverse effect to 6-mercaptopurine than to methotrexate.

4. Treatment of this patient's condition should include which of the following?
   A. Withdrawal of the offending drug(s)
   B. Steroids, e.g., prednisone
   C. Disodium cromoglycate
   D. Cysteamine
   E. Antacids

ANSWERS AND COMMENTS

1. (D, E) The liver plays an important role in drug metabolism, being responsible for the transformation of many drugs into active or inactive compounds, and their subsequent excretion; it can also store or concentrate some agents. (1-3) If liver function is compromised beforehand, drug metabolism may be altered. Adjustment of doses of certain drugs, i.e., decrease, must be enacted. In a few cases, drug administration must be discontinued. Many of the drug reactions seem to result from a common event, activation of stable drugs to alkylating, acylating, or acrylating compounds. (1-9)

   Drug metabolism is mainly a function of the microsomal enzyme system and cytoplasmic cofactors. (1-9) In the microsomal endoplasmic reticulum, two main components are present, NaDPH-cytochrome C reductase and cytochrome P-450. (1-9) Drug metabolism consists of a first step, oxidation reduction or hydrolysis, and a second step, conjugation, such as glucuronidation (glucuronide form).

   Commonly encountered drugs capable of producing hepatic insult include amethopterin (methotrexate), azathioprine (Imuran), chlorpromazine, erythromycin estolate (Ilosone), 6-mercaptopurine, methyltestosterone, oxacillin, para-amino salicylic acid (PAS), salicylates, sulfonamides, tetracyclines, and others. (2,6,7) The main mechanisms of drug effects on the liver will be discussed in answer 2.

2. (A, C) Adverse drug reactions can be separated into two major groups according to the mechanism of insult, i.e., dose-dependent (predictable toxicity) and dose-independent (unpredictable idiosyncracy). (2,6,7) Although these two groups seem to be distinctive, overlap seems frequently to occur, i.e., common

final event(s) before the occurrence of the hepatic insult. (2,6, 7,10) Biotransformation into bioactive products that bind to cellular constituents seems to occur. (2,6,7,10) Thus, hypersensitivity-induced hepatic insult seems to occur less often than previously estimated. (2,6,7,10)

The toxicity type is caused by agents that directly injure the liver. There are two groups of such agents: (1) direct hepatotoxins and (2) indirect hepatotoxins. (2,6,7) The former produce disruption of hepatocytes, resulting in a destruction of the structural integrity for cell function. An example is carbon tetrachloride (CCl₄). (2,6,7) The latter produces hepatic injury by competitive inhibition, essential metabolite diversion, or interference with essential activities of hepatocytes. (2,6,7) Examples include tetracycline, amethopterin, and 6-mercaptopurine. (2,6,7,10,11) The time between exposure and adverse effect is usually short, predictable, and there is a proportionate dose-injury relationship. (2,6,7)

Dose-independent (idiosyncracy) injury is only produced in a very small percentage of patients, thereby being an expression of individual susceptibility. (2,6,7) The common denominator may be the covalent binding to tissue macromolecules, resulting in a subsequent antibody response. (2,6,7) There is a variable, longer "sensitization" period and a high incidence of eosinophilia, rash, and fever. (2,6,7) Other symptoms are frequently present, such as abdominal pain, vomiting, nausea, arthralgia. Jaundice is variable in presence and in intensity. (2,6,7,12) Hepatosplenomegaly is infrequent. (2,6,7,12)

In the toxic type, jaundice and variable hepatic decompensation are present (hepatocellular). Significant elevations of bilirubin, SGOT and SGPT levels, decreased prothrombin time, and a possible increased alkaline phosphatase level are frequently encountered. (2,6,7)

In the idiosyncratic type, the hepatocellular form is characterized by elevation of SGOT and SGPT levels, variable increase in alkaline phosphatase, and/or decrease in prothrombin time, while in the cholestatic form the alkaline level is proportionally more elevated than the SGOT and SGPT levels. (2,6,7,13,14)

3. (F) Methotrexate has been significantly linked to the development of hepatotoxicity. (2,6,7,10,15-19) Various series have reported an incidence of hepatic fibrosis as high as 84%. (2,6, 7,10,15-19) Conversely, 6-mercaptopurine may produce hepatotoxicity after a variable time period. (2,6,7,11,16-19) In acute leukemia, the previously mentioned incidence is usually 10 to 40%. (16-19) The hepatic abnormalities may not return to normal until after cessation of treatment. (16-18)

Histological forms of hepatic injury have consisted of predominantly three: (1) cytotoxic, (2) cholestatic, and (3) mixed
(Table 55.1). (2,6,7) The cytotoxic form is predominantly a
hepatocellular picture with jaundice, variable hepatocyte necrosis, and steatosis. (2,6,7,13) Cholestasis is the predominant
feature of an obstructive-like pattern (cholestatic), also including variable portal inflammation. (2,6,7,13,14,19) The mixed
form has features of "obstruction" and "hepatitis, " such as hepatocyte necrosis, cholestasis, and possible pericholangitis. Examples of drugs producing the hepatocellular (cytotoxic) form
are halothane, isoniazid, and tetracycline. (2,6,7,14,19) Examples of drugs producing the obstructive (cholestatic) form
are chlorpromazine, erythromycin estolate, and anabolic steroids. (2,6,7,14,19) Examples of drugs producing the mixed
form are sulfonamides and phenylbutazone. (2,6,7,14,19)

With reference to this patient's drugs and apparent liver injury, methotrexate more likely produced the portal inflammation, cholestasis, and hepatic fibrosis than 6-mercaptopurine,
which causes a hepatocellular (cytotoxic) or obstructive (cholestatic) form. The latter drug's effect is less frequent and usually not irreversible. (2,6,7,14,19)

4. (A) The treatment of drug-related liver injury should include withdrawal of the offending drug(s). In addition, a high
calorie, high protein and carbohydrate diet should be used, unless hepatic decompensation is present. The latter requires
protein restriction, administration of neomycin orally, 4 to 8
gm/day, or lactulose orally, 15-30 ml t.i.d. or q.i.d., and/or
other measures for hepatic coma, e.g., nasogastric intubation/
suction, intravenous fluid therapy with glucose. (2,6,7,14,19,
20) Special modalities of treatment, including glucocorticoids,
exchange transfusion, and L-dopamine, have not been demonstrated to be of value. (2,6,7,14,19-23) For pruritus and increasing jaundice, phenobarbital, 5-10 mg/kg/day and/or cholestyramine, 4-12 gm/day, may provide symptomatic relief.
(2,6,7,14,19) In acetaminophen poisoning, cysteamine and
other glutathione-like nucleophils may have a preventive effect
against hepatocyte necrosis. (2,6,7,15,20) N-acetylcysteine
(Mucomyst) has been and is currently being used as an adjunct
in treatment of acetaminophen-induced hepatic injury, i. e. ,
oral loading dose, 140 mg/kg, followed by maintenance dosage,
70 mg/kg, every 4 hours for 48 hours. Treatment is particularly effective when administered within 12 hours after ingestion. (21,22)

Prognosis is usually good after elimination of the offending
agent. However, when significant hepatic necrosis occurs, extrahepatic complications can result, and their severity can influence the outcome.

TABLE 55.1 Drug-Induced Hepatic Injury

Clinical	Laboratory		Histology	Examples
	GPT/GOT (KU)	ALK P-TASE (IU)		
Cytotoxic (hepatocellular)	> 100-300	< 100-200	Liver cell necrosis; inflammation steatosis	Halothane, isoniazid
Cholestatic (obstructive)	< 200-300	> 200-300	Portal inflammation, cholestasis	Chlorpromazine, anabolic steroids
Mixed (obstructive, hepatocellular)	> 100-200	> 100-200	Liver cell necrosis, cholestasis, portal inflammation	Sulfonamides, phenylbutazone

Modified from Liebman, W.M. and Thaler, M.M., (2) Zimmerman, H.J. (7)

REFERENCES

1. Williams, R.T.: Progress report. Hepatic metabolism of drugs. Gut 13:579, 1972.

2. Liebman, W. M. and Thaler, M. M. : Drug-induced hepatotoxicity. In: Spanish Textbook of Gastroenterology. Cantor, D.S. (Ed.). McGraw-Hill Co., New York, 1982.

3. Cooksley, W.G.E. and Powell, L.W.: Drug metabolism and interaction with particular reference to the liver. Drugs 2:177, 1971.

4. Jezequel, A.M., Koch, M., Orlandi, F.: A morphometric study of the endoplasmic reticulum human hepatocytes. Correlation between morphological and biochemical data under treatment with some drugs. Gut 15:727, 1974.

5. Mitchell, J.R. and Potter, W.Z.: Drug metabolism in the production of liver injury. Med Clin North Am 59:877, 1975.

6. Berthelot, P.: Mechanisms and prediction of drug-induced liver disease. Gut 13:332, 1973.

7. Zimmerman, H.J.: Liver disease caused by medicinal agents. Med Clin North Am 59:897, 1975.

8. Mitchell, J.R. and Jollow, J.D.: Metabolic activation of drugs to toxic substances. Gastroenterology 9:392, 1975.

9. Remmer, H.: Role of the liver in drug metabolism. Am J Med 49:617, 1970.

10. Dienstag, J.L.: Halothane hepatitis, allergy or idiosyncrasy? N Engl J Med 303:102, 1980.

11. Epstein, E.H., Jr. and Croft, J.D., Jr.: Cirrhosis following methotrexate administration for psoriasis. Arch Derm 100:531, 1969.

12. Einhorn, M. and Davidsohn, I.: Hepatotoxicity of mercaptopurine. J Am Med Assoc 188:802, 1964.

13. Goldfinger, S.E. and Marx, S.: Hypersensitivity hepatitis due to phenazopyridine hydrochloride. N Engl J Med: 286: 1090, 1972.

14. Javitt, N.B.: The cholestatic syndrome. Am J Med 51: 637, 1971.

15. Silverman, A., Roy, C.C.: Pediatric Clinical Gastroen-terology, 3rd Edition. The CV Mosby Co. , St. Louis, 1983, p. 616.

16. Dahl, M.G.C., Gregory, M.M., Scheuer, P.J.: Metho-trexate hepatotoxicity in psoriasis - comparison of differ-ent dose regimens. Br Med J 1:657, 1972.

17. Hutter, R.B.P., Shipkey, F.H., Tan, C.T.C., et al.: Hepatic fibrosis in children with acute leukemia. Cancer 13:288, 1960.

18. Schein, P.S. and Winokur, S.H.: Immunosuppressive and cytotoxic chemotherapy: Long-term complications. Ann Int Med 82:84, 1975.

19. Jaffe, N. : Late side effects of treatment. Skeletal, genetic, central nervous system and oncogenic. Pediatr Clin North Am 23:233, 1976.

20. Sherlock, S.: Diseases of the Liver, 5th Edition. JB Lippincott Co., Philadelphia, 1975, p. 390.

21. Maddrey, W.C. and Boitnott, J.K.: Drug-induced chronic hepatitis and cirrhosis. In: Progress in Liver Diseases, Vol. 6. Popper, H. and Schaffner, F. (Eds). Grune & Stratton, Inc. , New York, 1979, p. 396.

22. Black, M.: Acetaminophen hepatotoxicity. Gastroenter-ology 78:382, 1980.

23. Conn, H.O.: A rational program for the management of hepatic coma. Gastroenterology 57:715, 1969.

Case 56

PROLONGED JAUNDICE IN A 2-MONTH-OLD MALE INFANT

HISTORY

A 2-month-old white male presented with persistent jaundice since the 2nd day of life. The patient was the product of a term pregnancy, unremarkable gestational history, and apparently uncomplicated delivery. Birth weight was 6 lbs 2 oz, length 20 inches. At approximately 36 hours of age, overt jaundice was noted. At that time, total bilirubin level was 16.2 mg/100 ml, direct 1.8 mg/100 ml. Direct Coombs' test was negative at this time. The patient's blood type was 0 Rh positive, and the mother's blood type was 0 Rh positive. The patient continued to remain active and alert with good appetite. The dietary history consisted of formula (Enfamil) feedings every 4 hours. At 3 weeks of age, cereals, initially rice, were added, and at 6 weeks of age, baby foods were added to the diet. The mother stated that the patient's activity and appetite had been good, that he followed light and movement and turned toward sounds with reasonable accuracy, smiled, had begun to coo during the last 1-2 weeks and had begun to intermittently sleep during the night. However, as previously mentioned, the jaundice had persisted and not lessened in visual intensity. Bowel habit pattern had consisted of 3-4 soft, yellow-brown bowel movements daily. There had been no associated history of fever, excessive vomiting (other than occasional regurgitation after feedings), constipation, melena, or hematochezia. The remainder of the past history, developmental history, social and family history, and review of systems was unremarkable.

477

EXAMINATION

He was alert and active, with apparent jaundice, normal vital
signs, head circumference 33 cm, height 53.5 cm, and weight,
3.8 kg. The remainder of the physical examination was unremarkable except for (1) scleral and conjunctival icterus; (2) the
liver palpable 2.5 cm below the right costal margin in the midclavicular line, nontender to palpation and not nodular; and (3)
the spleen tip palpable below the left costal margin the midclavicular line.

LABORATORY DATA

Hemoglobin:	11.9 gm%
Hematocrit:	35%
White blood cell count:	$9,800/mm^3$
PMN's:	44%
lymphocytes:	52%
monocytes:	4%
Reticulocyte count:	1.2%
Direct Coombs' test:	negative
Urinalysis:	bile positive
Serum:	
torch titers:	negative
VDRL:	negative
alpha-fetoprotein:	negative
alpha-1-antitrypsin:	275 mg%
SGOT:	180 units
SGPT:	170 units
alkaline phosphatase:	450 IU
cholesterol:	195 mg%
triglycerides:	180 mg%
total protein:	6.6 gm%
albumin:	4.3 gm%
prothrombin time:	12.0 seconds
Chest film:	negative
I^{131} Rose Bengal Isotope scan:	9% (72-hr stool)
Percutaneous liver biopsy:	(Fig. 56.1)

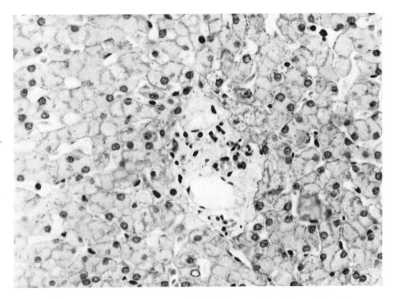

Figure 56.1 Liver. Very mild inflammation (lymphocytes, plasma cells) is present in the portal zone. Bile ducts cannot be definitely identified. Blood vessels in the portal zone can be delineated (H&E, X275).

QUESTIONS

1. The most likely diagnosis of this patient is
    A. acute (neonatal) hepatitis
    B. intrahepatic biliary hypoplasia
    C. extrahepatic biliary atresia
    D. congenital hepatic fibrosis
    E. celiac disease

2. Conditions associated with this disorder include
    A. rubella syndrome
    B. Turner's syndrome
    C. hepatolenticular degeneration (Wilson's disease)
    D. trisomy 13-15 (D)
    E. trisomy 16-18 (E)

3. Usual clinical features include
   A. prolonged neonatal jaundice
   B. fulminant hepatic decompensation
   C. pruritus
   D. coma
   E. diarrhea

4. Laboratory features usually include
   A. minimal or lack of elevation of total bilirubin level (less than 2-3 mg%)
   B. mild to moderate elevation of total bilirubin level (5-15 mg%)
   C. Significant elevation of cholesterol and triglyceride levels
   D. minimal or lack of elevation of alklaine phosphatase level (less than 250-300 IU)
   E. moderate to marked elevation of alkaline phosphatase level (over 250-300 IU)

5. The histological picture usually includes
   A. bile stasis
   B. bile duct proliferation
   C. bile duct paucity
   D. variable fibrosis
   E. piecemeal necrosis

6. Treatment of this condition should include
   A. normal diet
   B. substitution of medium-chain triglycerides in diet
   C. phenobarbital
   D. cholestyramine
   E. corticosteroids (prednisone)

7. The clinical course of this condition frequently includes
   A. complete resolution
   B. peptic ulcer disease
   C. biliary cirrhosis
   D. portal hypertension
   E. hepatocellular carcinoma

ANSWERS AND COMMENTS

1. (B) The presence of prolonged obstructive-like jaundice in a neonate, the lack of intrauterine or antecedent infection, the lack of significant hepatic enlargement, the intermediate stool excretion value of the I^{131} Rose Bengal study, and the biopsy

(see Fig. 56.1) demonstrating paucity of bile ducts makes the most likely diagnosis intrahepatic biliary hypoplasia. Synonyms for this condition include intrahepatic biliary paucity, interlobular biliary atresia, hepatic ductular hypoplasia, and intrahepatic biliary atresia. (1-3) The other answers do not correlate well with the case's features.

2. (A, B, E) Intrahepatic biliary hypoplasia has been postulated to occur usually as a result of inflammatory and/or vascular injury to the biliary system. The injury has been presumed to be in utero, but postnatal occurrence could occur. Other possible causes have been suggested, including placental transport of maternal secondary bile acids, such as lithocholic, and genetic factor(s), such as Byler's disease (cholestasis, reduced number of intrahepatic bile ducts). (1-11) The former has been further suggested by the production of cholestasis, fibrosis, and later loss of intrahepatic bile ducts, as well as an altered common bile duct, in newborn rats by administration of lithocholic acid to pregnant mothers. (1) There is equal sex incidence. Intrahepatic biliary hypoplasia has also been found in association with rubella syndrome, Turner's syndrome, neonatal hepatitis, trisomy 16-18 (E) and alpha-1-antitrypsin deficiency. (1, 8, 11) The latter association has an infrequent occurrence. (1, 8, 11)

3. (A, C) The vast majority of patients present with prolonged, obstructive-like jaundice in the neonatal period. A lesser percentage will demonstrate pruritus with or without associated skin lesions, such as xanthoma. (1-3, 7) The patients usually do not appear ill, are reasonably alert and active, and have a good appetite. There is usually no associated fever, vomiting, or altered bowel habit pattern. The urine may be normal or dark in color, while the stools may be normal or light, e.g., clay-like, in color. Variable growth retardation is usually present. Xanthoma may be found in the palmar creases, nape of the neck, and the extensor surfaces of the arms and legs, although are rarely present early in the disease. (1, 3, 7, 8) The effects of pruritis, evident after 4 to 6 months of age, e.g., excoriations, can be found in many parts of the body. Facial anomalies have been described, e.g., prominent forehead, hypertelorism, straight nose, and small pointed chin. Murmurs, i.e., systolic, have been found in some, secondary to central or peripheral pulmonic stenosis, less so, coarctation of the aorta, in a significant percentage of cases. (1, 3, 8) Hepatosplenomegaly is frequently present, especially in cases with prolonged obstructive-like jaundice. (1-11) Vertebral arch abnormalities, e.g., incomplete fusion of vertebral bodies, renal abnormalities (dysplasia, ectasia), ophthalmoplegia, ataxia, have also been noted

in some children. (10,11) The constellation of abnormal facies, cardiac murmur, growth retardation, as well as vertebral arch defects, and possible mental deficiency in conjunction with intra-hepatic biliary hypoplasia has been characterized by Alagille, et al. (1,8)

4. (B,C,E) The laboratory studies in this entity are not diag-nostic. However, the total bilirubin initially is moderately ele-vated, 8 to 15 mg%, the direct fraction predominating, while the transaminases (SGOT, SGPT) are initially mildly to moderately elevated, 50-200 units. (1-12) The serum cholesterol level and alkaline phosphatase levels are usually moderately to significant-ly elevated, 250 mg% or more and greater than three times nor-mal, respectively. (1-12) In addition, serum lipid (triglyceride) levels are moderately to significantly elevated, 250 mg% or more, as are the serum bile acid levels, the cholic acid (trihy-droxy) fraction being markedly predominant. (1-12) Total pro-tein, albumin, and prothrombin time, especially post-vitamin K administration, are usually within normal limits. The I^{131} Rose Bengal isotope scan, quantitative (72 hr), as well as the Pipida scan (99m-Tc-Pipida), may offer a clue in diagnosis, since the stool excretion values usually fall between those of ex-trahepatic biliary atresia and neonatal hepatitis, i.e., 8 to 20% of injected dose. (1,8,12)

Toward the end of the first year and in the second year of life, the total bilirubin level may decrease to normal or be mild-ly elevated, i.e., 1 to 8 mg%, while serum cholesterol, trigly-cerides, alkaline phosphatase, and bile acids will demonstrate marked elevation. (1-11) The other tests, such as albumin, will usually continue to be normal. (1-11)

Studies measuring alpha-fetoprotein and lipoprotein-X have not been sufficient to confirm present usefulness.

5. (A,C,D) The histological features (liver biopsy) in this con-dition may be variable at any age. The earlier lesion, as in the neonatal period, is bile stasis, present intralobularly, as well as in canaliculi and interlobular bile ducts. (1,8,13) Inflamma-tory reaction in the portal zones may be negligible to marked, consisting of polymorphonuclear cells as well as lymphocytes and plasma cells. The bile ducts in the portal zones are usually free of bile, or, more often, collapsed. The ductule epithelial cells are swollen and irregular, occasionally containing picnotic nuclei. (1-3,8) Usually later in the disease, at times earlier, reduced or absent numbers of bile ducts are found in the portal zones. Terminal branches of the hepatic artery and portal vein are normal. Fibrosis may be absent to marked, even associated with secondary portal hypertension (biliary cirrhosis). (1,8,10)

Serial specimens are very helpful in elucidating the evolution of this disease. (1,8)

6. (B,C,D) Treatment is medical and may be of value in the relief of pruritus and in stabilizing, or even reducing, the amount of fibrosis in the portal zones.

The nutritional consequences can be significant due to reduced bile flow into the duodenum, resulting in malabsorption of fat and fat-soluble vitamins, resulting in caloric deficiency. The substitution of medium-chain (C_6-C_{10}) for long-chain triglycerides can circumvent this problem to a great extent, e.g., elemental formulas. (14,15) Vitamin supplements, especially fat-soluble (A,D,E,K), twice normal daily dose, as well as calcium (1-3 gm/day), may be helpful, too. Recently, a progressive neuromuscular syndrome has been noted in children with long-standing liver disease with cholestasis, including hypo- to areflexia, gait disturbance, gaze paresis. (10,16) Pathological changes were noted neurologically, e.g., posterior columns, and intramuscularly, e.g., basophilic cytoplasmic inclusions. Serum vitamin E concentrations were uniformly low, and the neuromuscular disease improved with high-dose vitamin E administration, oral and/or parenteral, and normalization of serum vitamin E concentrations. (16)

The use of phenobarbital orally has been quite valuable. An increase in bile flow into the duodenum has been reported. The usual dose is 5-10 mg/kg/24 hr. The serum phenobarbital level should be maintained in the usual therapeutic range. (17-19)

Cholestyramine, an anion-binding resin, e.g., bile acids, has been used for the relief of pruritus. The recommended dose is 4 to 20 gm daily. The author has used 4 to 12 gm daily. (20)

7. (C,D) Later in the disease, biliary cirrhosis will develop, as well as portal hypertension. Ascites is not an infrequent finding as a result. Esophageal varices are also found, although they infrequently are a cause of bleeding. (1,8) Conversely, complete resolution is unexpected.

The usual course is one of a slowly, progressive disease with variable portal fibrosis. Thus, the prognosis is good for many years, survival usually being beyond the first decade of life. (1,8)

A high-risk group has been defined by Odievre, Alagille, et al. (22) Prognosis was relatively poor for infants with alpha-1-antitrypsin deficiency, scanty interlobular bile ducts, bile duct proliferation, and "familial hepatitis," as well as for infants with prolonged, severe cholestasis, usually requiring surgery for ultimate diagnosis. (21,23)

Surgery may occasionally be necessary, i.e., shunting (portocaval, splenorenal). The definitive surgical procedure will ultimately be liver transplantation. At this time, however, medical treatment is the choice in management. (1,8,20,23)

Peptic ulcer disease and hepatocellular carcinoma have not been increasingly associated with this condition's natural course.

REFERENCES

1. Alagille, D.: Intrahepatic biliary atresia (hepatic ductular hypoplasia). In: Liver Disease in Infancy and Childhood. Berenberg, S.R. (Ed). Martinus Nijhoff Medical Division, The Hague, 1976, p. 129.

2. Gherardi, G.J. and McMahon, H.E.: Hypoplasia of terminal bile ducts. Am J Dis Child 120:151, 1970.

3. Watson, G.H. and Miller, V.: Arteriohepatic dysplasia: Familial pulmonary arterial stenosis with neonatal liver diseases. Arch Dis Child 48:459, 1973.

4. Calyton, R.J., Iber, F.L., Ruebner, B.H., et al.: Byler's disease: Fatal familial intrahepatic cholestasis in an Amish kindred. J Pediatr 67:1025, 1965.

5. Juberg, R.C., Holland-Moritz, R.M., Henley, K., et al.: Familial intrahepatic cholestasis with mental and growth retardation. Pediatrics 38:819, 1966.

6. Aagenaes, O., Vander Hagen, C.B., Refsum, S.: Hereditary recurrent intrahepatic cholestasis from birth. Arch Dis Child 43:646, 1968.

7. MacMahon, H.E. and Thanhauser, S.J.: Congenital dysplasia of the interlobular bile ducts with extensive skin xanthomatosis: Congenital acholangic biliary cirrhosis. Gastroenterology 21:488, 1952.

8. Alagille, D., Odievre, M., Gautier, M., et al.: Hepatic ductular hypoplasia associated with characteristic facies, vertebral malformations, retarded physical, mental and sexual development, and cardiac murmur. J Pediatr 86: 63, 1975.

9. Sharp, H. and Krivit, W.: Hereditary lymphoedema and obstructive jaundice. J Pediat 78:491, 1971.

10. Silverman, A., Roy, C.C.: Pediatric Clinical Gastroen-
    terology, 3rd edition, CV Mosby Company, St. Louis,
    1983, p. 526.

11. Aagenaes, O., Henriksen, T., Sorland, S.: Hereditary
    neonatal cholestasis combined with vascular malforma-
    tions. In: Liver Disease in Infancy and Childhood. Beren-
    berg, S.R. (Ed). Martinus Nijhoff Medical Division, The
    Hague, 1976, p. 199.

12. Watkins, J.B., Katz, A.J., Grand, R.J.: Neonatal hepa-
    titis: A diagnostic approach. Adv Pediatr 24:399, 1977.

13. Brough, A.J. and Bernstein, J.: Liver biopsy in the diag-
    nosis of infantile obstructive jaundice. Pediatrics 43:519,
    1969.

14. Silverberg, M. and Davidson, M.: Nutritional require-
    ments of infants and children with liver disease. Am J
    Clin Nutr 23:604, 1970.

15. Cohen, M.I. and Gartner, L.M.: The use of medium-
    chain triglycerides in the management of biliary atresia.
    J Pediatr 79:379, 1971.

16. Rosenblum, J.L., Keating, J.P., Prensky, A.L., et al.:
    A progressive neurologic syndrome in children with chron-
    ic liver disease. N Engl J Med 304:503, 1981.

17. Sharp, H.L. and Mirkin, B.L.: Phenobarbital enzyme in-
    duction and bile secretion in intrahepatic cholestasis. Clin
    Res 18:344, 1970.

18. Stiehl, A., Thaler, M., Admirand, W.H.: Effects of phe-
    nobarbital on bile salt metabolism in cholestasis due to in-
    trahepatic bile duct hypoplasia. Pediatrics 51:992, 1973.

19. Sharp, H.L. and Mirkin, B.L.: Effect of phenobarbital on
    hyperbilirubinemia, bile acid metabolism and microsomal
    enzyme activity in chronic intrahepatic cholestasis of child-
    hood. J Pediatr 81:116, 1972.

20. Sharp, H.L., Carey, J.B., White, J.G., et al.: Choles-
    tyramine therapy in patients with a paucity of intrahepatic
    bile ducts. J Pediatr 71:723, 1967.

21. DeLorimier, A.A.: Jaundiced infants: Problems of surgical management. N Engl J Med 288:1284, 1973.

22. Odievre, M., Hadchoud, P., Landrieu, D., et al.: Long-term prognosis for infants with intrahepatic cholestasis and patent extrahepatic biliary tract. Arch Dis Child 56: 373, 1981.

23. Longmire, W.P.: Congenital biliary hypoplasia. Ann Surg 159:335, 1964.

Case 57

HEMATEMESIS IN A 13-MONTH-OLD BOY

HISTORY

A 13-month-old white male presented with a history of hematemesis of more than one day duration, with associated pallor, decreased activity, and appetite. The patient had been well until 5 days prior to the onset of the previously mentioned hematemesis, when he was noted to have increased temperature, up to 102°F rectally, nasal congestion, and cough. These symptoms disappeared after almost 4 days, and approximately one day later his present problem started. The vomitus was characterized as bright red in color and then subsequently darker red and brown-red in color. In addition, he had had two large, dark, odorous stools during the 24 hours of hematemesis. The patient had had no past history of similar episodes. The developmental history included a normal term pregnancy, normal delivery and immediate postnatal period, and normal developmental milestones. The family history included a maternal grandfather with a history of peptic ulcer disease. Otherwise, the remainder of the past history, developmental history, family and social history, and review of systems was noncontributory.

EXAMINATION

He was somewhat pale and drowsy. Blood pressure was 90/40 mmHg, heart rate 160/min, respirations 30/min, weight 10.5 kg, height 82 cm, and head circumference 48 cm. The remainder of the examination was unremarkable except for the liver, palpable 1.5 cm below the right costal margin in the midclavicular line, firm, nontender and not nodular, and total span by percussion, 5.5 cm. Active bowel sounds were present but no bruits. There was no pedal, pretibial, or periorbital edema.

LABORATORY DATA

Hemoglobin:	8.0 gm%
Hematocrit:	25%
White blood cell count:	9,600/mm^3
PMN's:	52%
lymphocytes:	43%
monocytes:	4%
eosinophiles:	1%
Platelets:	130,000/mm^3
Sedimentation rate:	15 mm/hr
Urinalysis:	negative
Serum:	
total bilirubin:	2.0 mg%
direct bilirubin:	1.7 mg%
total protein:	6.0 gm%
albumin:	3.7 gm%
SGOT:	36 units
alkaline phosphatase:	170 IU
creatinine:	0.5 mg%
prothrombin time:	13.5 sec
control:	11.0 sec
partial thromboplastin time:	36.5 sec
control:	36 sec
Upper GI - small bowel series:	(Fig. 57.1)
Fiberoptic upper endoscopy:	confirmed findings of UGI series
Superior mesenteric arteriography/venous phase:	confirmed findings of UGI series
Percutaneous liver biopsy:	normal

QUESTIONS

1. What measures would be most indicated at the initial presentation of this patient?
   A. Complete history and physical examination
   B. Complete blood count and coagulation studies
   C. Proctosigmoidoscopy
   D. Visceral angiography
   E. Fiberoptic upper endoscopy

Questions 2 and 3: Answer true (T) or false (F).

2. Upper gastrointestinal series would be as helpful as fiberoptic upper endoscopy in this patient.

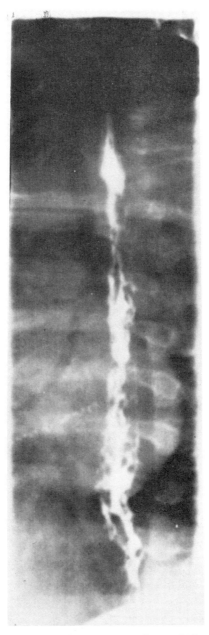

Figure 57.1: Barium Swallow. Irregular cobblestone-like filling defects of the lower esophagus are demonstrated.

3. Visceral angiography could be particularly helpful if the rate of bleeding was less than 0.5 cc/minute at the time of examination.

4. In this patient, if the subsequent performance of visceral angiography is necessary, which one of the following studies would be most important to perform?
   A. Wedged hepatic vein pressure
   B. Splenoportography
   C. Celiac arteriography, including venous phase
   D. Superior mesenteric and splenic arteriography, including venous phase
   E. Inferior mesenteric arteriography, including venous phase

Question 5: Answer true (T) or false (F).

5. Liver biopsy would not be indicated in this patient.

6. In the management of this patient's condition, which of the following measures would be indicated?
   A. Placement of Sengstaken-Blakemore tube or Linton tube
   B. Administration of vasopressin by intravenous or intra-arterial route of infusion
   C. Cimetidine
   D. Splenectomy
   E. Portacaval shunt

Question 7: Answer true (T) or false (F).

7. In extrahepatic portal hypertension, portacaval shunt is the definitive surgical procedure of choice.

ANSWERS AND COMMENTS

1. (A,B,E) A vigorous diagnostic approach should be utilized in order to achieve accurate diagnosis of the site and cause of the hemorrhage as quickly as possible. (1-4) Unless the patient is in shock, the initial management must consist of a complete history and physical examination. The patient's general state of health, past history, and present condition, such as the presence or absence of fever, diarrhea, melena, hematochezia, jaundice, cough, bleeding, diathesis, medication, and trauma must be ascertained. The physical examination should include an assessment of the vital signs immediately, presence or absence of spider angiomas, petecchiae, ecchymoses, ascites, hepatomegaly, splenomegaly, bruits, abdominal veins, or masses.

At this point, venipuncture should be performed for blood for a complete blood count, including absolute platelet count, prothrombin time, partial thromboplastin time, and type and cross matching. At the same time, intravenous infusion is initiated, using normal saline, Ringer's lactate, or plasmanate until normalization of vital signs and/or until blood is available for transfusion. Central venous pressure/fluid monitoring may be necessary.

The next step would be the insertion of a nasogastric or pediatric Ewald tube to determine the presence (or not) and the rate of bleeding. Also, the tube will allow the clearing of the stomach of blood so that the esophagus, stomach, and proximal duodenum can be directly examined by panendoscopy.

The ease, low morbidity, and accuracy of panendoscopy have now been established in children with upper gastrointestinal hemorrhage. Several studies have been published, demonstrating the specificity and high yield of panendoscopy. (1,3,5-8) While radiographic studies have often failed to disclose a demonstrable lesion, i.e., 30 to 70%, endoscopy has disclosed a responsible lesion in 85 to 100%. (1,3,5-8) The most common sources at endoscopy are gastric and duodenal ulcers, hemorrhagic gastritis, esophagitis, and esophageal gastric varices. (1,3,5-8)

Proctosigmoidoscopy would not be indicated in upper gastrointestinal hemorrhage. Visceral angiography would not be indicated as an initial procedure unless bleeding was of a magnitude that would not allow for comprehensive endoscopic examination.

2. (F) As previously described in answer 1, radiographic studies often fail to demonstrate responsible lesions. With reference to esophageal varices, the failure rate ranges from 20 to 70% in various series. (1,3,9,10) Furthermore, a radiographically demonstrated lesion cannot be confirmed as the actual site of bleeding by barium studies.

3. (F) If bleeding is so vigorous that endoscopic examination is not possible, selective visceral angiography may aid in locating the site of bleeding but not the cause. (1,3,9,11,12) Localizing the site of bleeding by angiography, however, is dependent upon the rate of bleeding at the time of examination. This rate must be a minimum of 0.5 cc/minute. Esophageal varices will be visualized on the venous phase of celiac or superior mesenteric angiography, although a significant percentage, 10 to 40%, of bleeding esophageal varices may not be visualized. (1,3,9,11) Barium studies should not be performed if angiography is contemplated since barium will impair the localization of the site of bleeding. Selective angiography in portal hypertension can allow the study of the splenic vein and/or portal vein during the venous

phase of arterial injection into the splenic and superior mesenteric vessels. (1,3,9,11) These procedures are particularly
helpful in children less than 5 years of age when splenoportography is contraindicated. (1,3,9,11,13)

4. (D) As previously described in answer 3, visualization of
the splenic and portal vein during the venous phase of splenic
and superior mesenteric arterial injections is quite valuable in
the management of portal hypertension, especially extrahepatic
in type. (1,3,9,11) It is accurate and has a low morbidity, especially in children less than 5 years of age, when splenoportography is contraindicated. (1,3,13)

Wedged hepatic vein pressure (WHVP) is not particularly
useful in patients with extrahepatic portal hypertension. (1,3,
13-16) The catheter tip is wedged in place and reflects postsinusoidal and probably sinusoidal portal pressures. (1,3,12) This
pressure reflects portal vein pressure in those with cirrhosis.
(12) Pressures above 10 mmHg are abnormal. In addition, a
free hepatic pressure or inferior vena cava pressure can be obtained by withdrawing the catheter (normal, 1 to 5 mmHg). In
extrahepatic portal hypertension, both free and wedged hepatic
pressures are normal. (12) Thus, it is particularly valuable in
intrahepatic portal hypertension.

Splenoportography (percutaneous) allows an assessment of
patency of the portal venous system, size and patency of the
splenic vein, and presence of anastomotic pathways. However,
it has a significant morbidity, at least 5 to 10%, and should be
deferred to the immediate preoperative period. (1,3,13) Especially at risk are children less than 3 to 5 years of age. (13,
14) Blockage of the extrahepatic portal vein may be visualized.

Celiac angiography may demonstrate the bleeding esophageal
varices in the venous phase of the arterial injection. (1,3,9,11)
However, information regarding the portal venous system per se
cannot be obtained due to different vessel origins.

Inferior mesenteric arteriography (venous phase) would not
demonstrate the desired vessels unless by retrograde flow (unlikely). Thus, its performance would not be helpful, although
the presence of internal hemorrhoids could be demonstrated, allowing inferences to be made. (1,3,9,11)

5. (F) Diagnosis, as well as prognosis, can be formulated on
the basis of the microscopic appearance of the liver. Therefore,
some authors prefer an open procedure (wedge biopsy) rather
than the percutaneous method. Entities, such as congenital hepatic fibrosis (CHF), Budd-Chiari syndrome, intrahepatic causes,
can be confirmed. CHF can mimic extrahepatic portal hypertension. (1,3,16-18)

6. (A, B) For acute bleeding episodes, a nasogastric tube should be passed and left in place until bleeding has ceased for 24 hours. Trauma to the varices is minimal. Irrigation with distilled water or saline, cold or warm, is necessary to remove blood. Antacids have frequently been used, although there is no evidence of their efficacy in bleeding esophageal varices. (1, 3, 19) Continued monitoring of vital signs, hemoglobin and hematocrit, and stools for occult blood are enacted.

Fresh whole blood may be necessary. If significant thrombocytopenia exists, platelet transfusions may be indicated.

Vasopressin can be infused intravenously, 0.1-2 unit/ml/min in isotonic saline or 5% dextrose in water (100 ml) over 20 to 30 minutes. (1, 3, 19, 20) This can be repeated every 2 to 3 hours as indicated. Additionally, intra-arterial infusion through the superior mesenteric artery may be of value in a dosage of 0.1 to 0.4 unit/ml/min. (1, 3, 19, 20) Usually there is a gradual increase to the higher dosage in order to control bleeding. (1, 3, 19, 20) The indwelling arterial catheter may be left in place for 72 to 96 hours before its removal. However, most studies have not demonstrated an advantage of intra-arterial infusion over peripheral vein administration. (14) Side effects of vasopressin include elevation of arterial blood pressure, blood flow decrease, and vasoconstriction of coronary arteries. (19, 20)

If other measures fail, the pediatric Sengstaken-Blackemore (S-B) tube (or Linton tube, one balloon only, in older children) may be passed. The gastric balloon is filled to capacity (25 to 100 ml) and is then brought into position against the gastroesophageal junction and gastric fundus. Traction is applied using a helmet or other device. If the hemorrhage is controlled for 24 hours (80 to 90%), the traction is discontinued, and the balloons are deflated. (1, 3, 14, 19)

Cimetidine, an H_2-receptor antagonist, has been shown to be of value in the treatment of gastric and duodenal ulcers. In addition, it has been demonstrated to be of potential value in hemorrhagic gastritis. (1, 3)

Most patients with extrahepatic portal hypertension have a block of the portal vein. Therefore, this vessel cannot be used for shunting procedures. The splenorenal or mesocaval shunt must be the choice. Most series in children less than 10 years of age, especially below 5 years, have reported poor results with shunting procedures. (20-25) However, the results from Bicetre, France, have been particularly good with the splenorenal shunt in children under 10 years of age. (26) Splenectomy must be properly timed, and if performed too soon, at less than 10 years of age, can be detrimental because in shunting, the splenic vein would be "sacrificed." (20-24) In addition, removal of the spleen eliminates collaterals on the splenic capsule as well as perisplenic collaterals and increases the flow into the coronary-esophageal system. (20-24)

7. (F) As mentioned in answer 6, the portal vein is usually blocked in cases of extrahepatic portal hypertension. (1,3,9) Thus portacaval shunting is not possible. The splenorenal shunt, distal (Warren procedure), is one of two shunts realistically possible. (20-24) A satisfactory splenic vessel size is 1 cm in order to insure continued patency; this is usually not present in children less than 10 years of age. (20-24) The second shunt is the mesocaval shunt of Clatworthy-Marion. (20-24) Retroperitoneal edema contraindicates this procedure. Dacron or Teflon grafts have also been used to form interposition mesocaval shunts with variable success. (20-25) (Refer to answer 6.)

With reference to the above-mentioned surgical procedures, selection of patients for such shunts should include (1) recurrent significant hemorrhages due to esophageal varices (proven), (2) rare blood types or difficulty in using transfusions, e.g., reactions, which would lead to earlier surgical intervention, (3) splenectomy (thrombocytopenia), and (4) less so, socioenvironmental considerations in at-risk patients, e.g., geographical location.

Lastly, esophagogastrectomy with or without (Sugiura's procedure) transesophageal variceal ligation, and even endoscopic variceal sclerotherapy (sodium morhuate, ethanolamine oleate) must be considered stop-gap measures at best, e.g., refractory bleeding in poor-risk patient, or short-term benefit only. (14, 27) These comments would also apply to percutaneous transhepatic portal venography or other angiographic techniques and delivery of fibrin or gel foam pellets into the coronary-gastroesophageal vascular system.

REFERENCES

1. Liebman, W.M.: Diagnosis and management of upper gastrointestinal hemorrhage in children. Pediatr Ann 5:688, 1976.

2. Collins, R.E.C.: Some problems of gastrointestinal bleeding in children. Arch Dis Child 46:110, 1971.

3. Berman, W.F. and Holtzapple, P.H.: Gastrointestinal hemorrhages. Pediatr Clin North Am 22:885, 1975.

4. Wagner, M.L.: Acute gastrointestinal bleeding in infants and children. Pediatr Ann 4:663, 1975.

5. Gleason, W.A., Jr., Tedesco, F.J., Keating, J.P., et al.: Fiberoptic endoscopy in infants and children. J Pediatr 85:810, 1974.

6. Tedesco, F.J., Goldstein, P.D., Gleason, W.A., et al.: Fiberoptic gastrointestinal endoscopy in the pediatric patient. Gastroenterology 70:492, 1976.

7. Ament, M.E. and Christie, D.L.: Upper gastrointestinal fiberoptic endoscopy in pediatric patients. Gastroenterology 72:1244, 1977.

8. Liebman, W.M.: Fiberoptic endoscopy of the gastrointestinal tract in infants and children. I. Upper endoscopy in 53 children. Am J Gastroenterol 68:362, 1977.

9. Franken, E.A., Jr.: Gastrointestinal bleeding in infants and children: Radiologic investigation. J Am Med Assoc 229:1339, 1974.

10. Ghaghremani, C.G., Port, R.B., Winans, C.S., et al.: Esophageal varices: Enhanced radiologic visualization by anticholinergic drugs. Am J Dig Dis 17:703, 1972.

11. Baum, S., Nusbaum, M., Clearfield, H.R., et al.: Angiography in the diagnosis of gastrointestinal bleeding. Arch Intern Med 119:16, 1967.

12. Reynolds, T.B., Ito, S., Iwatsuki, S.: Measurement of portal pressure and its clinical application. Am J Med 49:649, 1970.

13. Melhem, R.E. and Rizk, G.K.: Splenoportographic evaluation of portal hypertension in children. J Pediatr Surg 5:522, 1970.

14. Silverman, A., Roy, C.C.: Pediatric Clinical Gastroenterology, 3rd edition. The CV Mosby Company, St. Louis, 1983, p. 770, 776.

15. Shaldon, S. and Sherlock, S.: Obstruction to the extrahepatic portal system in childhood. Lancet 1:63, 1963.

16. Mikkelsen, W.P.: Extrahepatic portal hypertension in children. Am J Surg 111:333, 1966.

17. Voorhees, A.B., Harris, R.C., Britton, R.C., et al.: Portal hypertension in children: 98 cases. Surgery 58: 540, 1965.

18. Kerr, D.N., Harrison, C.V., Sherlock, S., et al.: Congenital hepatic fibrosis. Q J Med 30:91, 1961.

19. Martin, L.W.: Changing concepts of management of portal hypertension in children. J Pediatr Surg 7:559, 1972.

20. Conn, H.O., Ramsby, G.R., Stover, E.H., et al.: Intra-arterial vasopressin in the treatment of upper gastrointestinal hemorrhage: A prospective controlled clinical trial. Gastroenterology 68:211, 1975.

21. Fonkalsrud, E.W. and Longmire, W.P.: Reassessment of operative procedures for portal hypertension in infants and children. Am J Surg 118:148, 1969.

22. Drapanas, T.: Interposition mesocaval shunt for treatment of portal hypertension. Ann Surg 176:435, 1972.

23. Ehrlich, R., Pipatangul, S., Sieber, W.K., et al.: Portal hypertension: Surgical management in infants and children. J Pediatr Surg 9:283, 1974.

24. Burchell, A.R., Moreno, A.H., Panke, W.F., et al.: Hemodynamic variables and prognosis following portacaval shunts. Surg Gynecol Obstet 138:359, 1974.

25. Fonkalsrud, E.W., Myers, N.A., Robinson, M.J.: Management of extrahepatic portal hypertension in children. Ann Surg 180:487, 1974.

26. Bismuth, H., Franco, D.: Portal diversion for portal hypertension in early childhood. Ann Surg 183:439, 1976.

27. Lilly, J.R.: Endoscopic sclerosis of esophageal varices. Surgery 152:513, 1981.

Case 58

VOMITING AND LETHARGY IN A 4-YEAR-OLD GIRL

HISTORY

A 4-year-old white female presented with a history of vomiting
and progressive stupor of 16 hours' duration. The patient had
had nasal congestion, cough, and mildly decreased appetite for
four days, without fever, respiratory distress, diarrhea, skin
lesions, or jaundice, ending approximately 1-1 1/2 days prior
to the onset of the present symptomatic pattern. There had been
no history of unusual food, drug, and/or plant exposure or of
trauma. No other family member was ill during this period of
time. The remainder of the past history, developmental history,
family history, social history, and review of systems was unremarkable.

EXAMINATION

She was lethargic, heart rate 120 per minute, respiration 28 per
minute, temperature 37.7°C, and blood pressure 94/60 mmHg.
The weight was 16.2 kg and the height was 102 cm. The remainder of the examination was unremarkable, except for the liver
palpable 4.0 cm below the right costal margin in the midclavicular line, firm, not tender or nodular, spleen and kidneys not palpable, total span of the liver by percussion 8.75 cm, and occasional active bowel sounds with no bruits. The neurological examination was unremarkable except for hypoactive deep tendon
reflexes.

LABORATORY DATA

Hemoglobin:	12.0 gm%
Hematocrit:	37%
White blood cell count:	10,000/mm^3
PMN's:	41%
lymphocytes:	53%
monocytes:	4%
eosinophiles:	2%
Urinalysis:	negative
Serum:	
sodium	138 meq/L
potassium:	4.6 meq/L
chloride:	106 meq/L
bicarbonate:	28 meq/L
creatinine:	0.5 mg%
SGOT:	340 KU
SGPT:	300 KU
total bilirubin:	0.9 mg%
direct bilirubin:	0.7 mg%
alkaline phosphatase:	150 IU
ammonia:	140 mg%
prothrombin time:	16.4 sec (11 sec)
partial thromboplastin time:	45 sec (< 36 sec)
pH:	7.50
pCO$_2$:	27
pO$_2$:	104
Percutaneous liver biopsy:	(Fig. 58.1)

QUESTIONS

Questions 1-11: Answer true (T) or false (F).

1. The most likely diagnosis of this patient is acute meningo-encephalitis.

2. The cause of this disorder is basically autoimmune.

3. This disorder primarily affects children less than 10 years of age.

4. Most commonly, there is a preceding upper respiratory tract infection.

5. Jaundice is a hallmark of this disorder, but the liver may be normal or mildly enlarged.

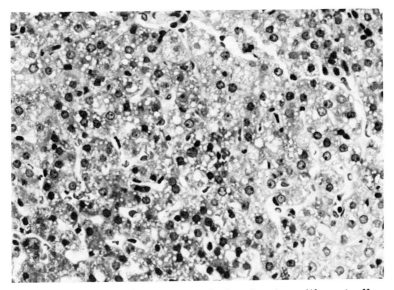

Figure 58.1 Liver. Somewhat pale hepatocytes with centrally located nuclei are shown, containing vacuoles and glycogen/lipid deposits. Significant degenerative change and acute/chronic inflammatory reaction are virtually absent (H&E, X250).

6. The laboratory studies usually detect elevated SGOT and SGPT levels, variable hypoglycemia, prolonged prothrombin time, and hyperammonemia.

7. The electroencephalogram is not diagnostic of this entity but may be helpful in determining the clinical stage of the patient's condition.

8. The pathological examination of the liver is frequently unremarkable.

9. The most important aspects of treatment include glucose homeostasis, reduction of cerebral edema and respiratory system support.

10. Exchange transfusion has been a major advance in treatment of this disorder.

11. Modern management of this disorder has reduced mortality to less than 5% and virtually eliminated sequelae, e.g., neurological (seizures, mental retardation).

ANSWERS AND COMMENTS

1. (F) The most likely diagnosis is Reye's syndrome, first described as an entity in 1963 by Reye, et al. (1) (Refer to answers 2 through 11.)

2. (F) The precise etiology of this disorder remains unknown. (1-4) Despite the relative consistency of clinical presentation, bacterial and viral cultures as well as serological studies have failed to disclose a consistent agent or group of viruses, bacteria or otherwise. Associated agents have included influenza B, varicella, herpes virus (simplex), reoviruses, Coxsackie viruses, echoviruses, mumps virus, Epstein-Barr virus, and streptococci, (1-4) A recent 5-year review of national surveillance for Reye's syndrome concluded that the highest reported incidence occurred during years of primary influenza B and A (HINI) occurrence, and that a higher percentage of cases in blacks occurred in infants under 1 year of age in 3 of the past 4 years. This survey also noted the lower case-fatality ratio in recent years. (5)

Due to the lack of specificity of the antecedent illness, a genetic-metabolic disorder has been suspected. This type of dysfunction could be unmasked by the illness or could act in unison to produce this syndrome. (2-12) The former could result in an endogenous toxin or toxins. Proposed toxins have included proteins, ammonia, short-chain fatty acids, endotoxins, and a "serum factor" disrupting the mitochondrial energy-linked function. (2-13) Exogenous toxins (neurotoxic) include viruses, toxins, e.g., aflatoxins. These exogenous agents could directly affect the brain as well as other organs, such as the liver. (2-13) Other exogenous agents include drugs, e.g., aspirin (refer to later discussion), acetoaminophen. (2-13)

The metabolic defect usually suggested as compatible with Reye's syndrome is a deficiency of the urea cycle, specifically carbamyl phosphate synthetase and/or ornithine transcarbamylase (Fig. 58.2). Both of these enzymes are mitochondrial in location, and such a defect would be compatible with the described ultrastructural abnormalities of mitochondria in Reye's syndrome. (9)

As previously mentioned, excessive free fatty acids (short- and medium-chain) have been implicated in the clinical and pathological course of this syndrome. (2-7) This fatty acidemia is the result of excessive lipolysis, defective fatty acid oxidation, and defective gluconeogenesis. (2-7) The role of these fatty acids still remains unresolved but may be important due to the recent animal model of encephalopathy resulting from excessive short- and medium-chain fatty acids administration, as well as

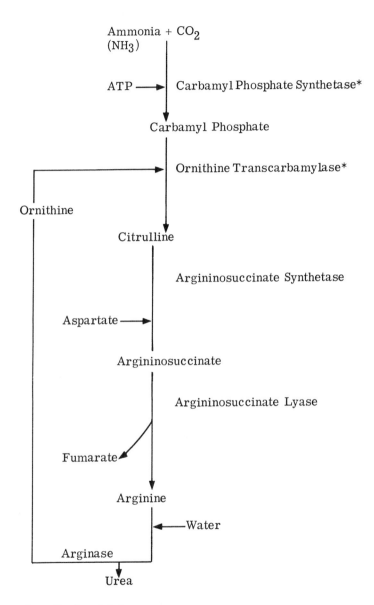

*Intramitochondrial enzymes

Figure 58.2 Urea cycle in man.   Modified from Silverman, A.,
Roy, C.C. (17)

the ability of these fatty acids to produce oxidative phosphorylation, uncoupling and mitochondrial functional disruption. (11)
    Besides the previously mentioned endogenous factors, con-
siderable attention has been directed at identifying potential exogenous toxins. Aflatoxins have been particularly scrutinized,
as has hypoglycin and its active metabolite, methylenecyclopro-
propaneacetic acid. The last two are the agents responsible for
Jamaican vomiting sickness, involving inhibition of long-chain
fatty acid oxidation and uncoupling of oxidative phosphorylation.
(2-7,10) These toxins are produced by Aspergillus flavus, a
fungus, and were suggested as important factors on the basis of
epidemiologic studies in Thailand. (1-4,10) Unfortunately, very
large amounts must be ingested in order to reproduce experimentally compatible hepatic lesions in monkeys or other animals.
(7,10) Another focus of attention has been aspirin. The mechanisms proposed for aspirin have been direct toxicity, i.e., uncoupling of oxidative phosphorylation and thereby, defective ATP
production with its consequent results, including altered membrane integrity and transport function, defective gluconeogenesis,
and/or an idiosyncratic response. (2-7) However, there is considerable doubt as to this effect because of the ability of such patients to tolerate aspirin subsequently and because of the lack of
detectable aspirin levels in many patients. (2-6)

3.   (T) In most series, 60 to 75% of cases are found in children
less than 10 years of age, 30 to 50% being less than 5 years of
age. (14-17) The sex incidence is essentially equal to most
series. (1,14-17)

4.   (T) In the vast majority of patients with this syndrome, an
upper respiratory infection or "flu-like" syndrome is the antecedent illness. This prodomal illness is short, even resolving,
but is then followed by vomiting and disorientation and evolving
coma over hours to a few days. (1,14-17)

5.   (F) Jaundice is a rare feature of Reye's syndrome. Rather,
the lack of jaundice is a characteristic feature. Other clinical
features include vomiting and central nervous system symptomatology, such as lethargy, delirium seizures, and coma. (1,
14-17) Clinical grading has been accomplished by several authors, including Silverman and Roy, (17) i.e., grade (stage 1),
drowsiness, but responsive to verbal commands; grade 2, increasing lethargy, agitated behavior, abnormal respiratory pattern, hyperreflexia, and normal pupillary responses; grade 3,
predominant coma, responsiveness to painful stimuli, sluggish
pupillary responses, hyperreflexia, positive Babinski's reflexes,
and decerebrate-decorticate posturing; and grade 4, deep coma,

fixed and dilated pupils, decerebrate posturing, no response to pain, and absent reflexes. (14,17)

6. (T) The laboratory features of Reye's syndrome, also required for the diagnosis, include (1) variably elevated transaminase levels (SGOT, SGPT), at least twofold, (100%), (2) elevated blood ammonia level, 1 1/2 times normal or greater, (70-90%), (3) prolonged prothrombin time, 50% or less of control time (80-90%), and (4) cerebrospinal fluid, containing less than 10 WBC per mm^3 and normal protein and glucose concentrations. (14, 17) Other laboratory features include normal or slightly elevated total serum bilirubin levels (95-100%), variable hypoglycemia, particularly prominent in children less than 2 years of age (30-70%). Complete blood counts demonstrate normal to decreased hemoglobin and hematocrit levels, dependent upon the stage of the disorder, and elevated white blood cell counts. (1,14-17) Plasma amino acid levels have revealed elevated glutamine, alanine, lysine, and alpha-amino-n-butyrate. (17,18) The specificity of the latter for Reye's syndrome and not other causes of hepatic coma has not been confirmed.

7. (T) The electroencephalogram (EEG) is not diagnostic of Reye's syndrome but is usually abnormal in grades (stages) 2 through 4. (14,17,19) In grade 1, the EEG is usually normal. EEGs can also be graded and correlated with the clinical staging, thereby aiding appropriate classification of patients; they can also be used for comparison with sequential EEGs for the purpose of follow-up and prognosis. (14,17,19) Theta or delta wave predominance (age dependent) occurs in the early stages. Subsequently, the EEG becomes one of high-voltage activity (II), then mainly low-voltage and suppression-burst activity (III), and finally one of isoelectric activity or complete absence of activity (IV). (12,14,17,19)

8. (F) The changes in the liver are essentially diagnostic of and also essential for diagnosis of Reye's syndrome. Macroscopically, the liver is pale, almost white in appearance. Frozen sections, using Giemsa stain, can confirm the typical findings, discussed later, within minutes. Microscopically, steatosis and swelling of the hepatocytes is obvious and prominent. (1, 6,8,15,17,20) Oil-red-O staining particularly will demonstrate the fatty deposition within hepatocytes. The cytoplasm is pale and "fragmented" with significant vacuolization. There is no nuclear displacement, and necrosis and inflammation are usually nonexistent as is glycogen within the hepatocytes. (1,7,8,15,20) Ultrastructurally, the mitochondrial abnormalities are quite prominent, including swelling and loss of intramitochondrial

dense bodies. (8,17,20) Fatty microdroplets are seen in virtually every hepatocyte (neutral fat).

Other organs also are involved, e.g., kidney (swollen proximal tubule cells, fat vacuoles), pancreas (hemorrhagic necrosis, ductal ectasia). (3,17,20) The central nervous system is prominently involved, too, e.g., diffuse neuronal edema, necrosis, especially in the brainstem, periventricular area, and cerebrum. (3,17,20) Mitochondrial alterations are evident under the electron microscope. (3,17,20)

9. (T) Major axiom of treatment should be improvement of glucose homeostasis, reduction of cerebral edema, and adequate attention to respiratory system support, especially in deeper stage (grade) II to stage IV coma. (14,17,24) These are the keynote principles relating to survival.

The basic steps in the treatment of Reye's syndrome include the following: (1) central venous pressure line; (2) intravenous fluid therapy, usually low to 3/4 maintenance in amount, and consisting of 10 to 15% glucose solution; (3) dexamethasone (Decadron) should be administered parenterally every 6 hours, 0.25-0.50 mg/kg; (4) mannitol (alternative, glycerol, 1 to 1.5 mg/kg, every 4 hours), should be administered intravenously, 0.5-1.0 mg/kg, repeating every 4 to 6 hours while patient is comatose; (5) antibiotics, broad spectrum in type, such as ampicillin 150-200 mg/kg/24 hours, are administered parenterally; (6) if gastrointestinal hemorrhage is present, administration of neomycin, 50-100 mg/kg/24 hours, or lactulose, 30 ml 3 times daily, by nasogastric tube, or the former also by retention enema (reduction of ammonia formation); (7) vitamin K, 1-2 mg every 12 hours while coagulation abnormalities exist; (8) in patients with grade (stage) II to IV coma, nasogastric intubation should be performed; (9) phenytoin (Dilantin) is administered if seizures are present (4-8 mg/kg); (10) endotracheal or nasotracheal intubation should be considered in all patients with deep grade II to IV coma; (11) intracranial pressure monitoring (subdural, epidural) has become a "standard" in the management of patients with deep grade II to IV coma and has contributed significantly to the reduced mortality. The reduction of cerebral edema is directed at maintaining inracranial pressure (ICP) below 15 to 20 mmHg and, thereby, cerebral perfusion pressure (mean arterial pressure - intracranial pressure), above 40 mmHg. (3,17,21,22) Other less conventional modalities, including craniectomy, hypothermia, citrulline, 100 mg/kg, nicotinic acid, 0.5 gm every 30 minutes for 3 or 4 doses, pentobarbital, and peritoneal dialysis, cannot be routinely recommended at this time. With reference to pentobarbital use, so-called barbiturate coma, 5 mg/kg over 30 minutes, followed by 2 mg/kg/hr (blood levels, 25 to 40 μg/ml), a multicenter collaborative control study is currently being performed to evaluate its role in management. (17) Exchange transfusion will be covered in answer 10.

10. (F) Exchange transfusion, one to two volumes, although theoretically being particularly beneficial if a toxin were responsible, has not been assessed satisfactorily in a controlled study. Uncontrolled series have reported variable success in improvement in survival, frequently no better than with standard therapy. (17, 24) However, exchange transfusions will correct coagulation abnormalities and thus allow the performance of a percutaneous liver biopsy. In general, exchange transfusions are time-consuming, utilize large amounts of blood, depleting the available blood supply of a hospital, and are not without risk, involving cardiac, metabolic, and infectious problems in particular.

The author's experience with exchange transfusion has been discouraging in that there has been no improvement in survival.

11. (F) Even with the current modalities of therapy as part of a standardized protocol, the mortality rate has been 10 to 35%. (12, 17, 22-25) Lack of progression beyond stage II is associated with a recovery rate of at least 90 to 95%. In children less than 2 years of age, neuropsychological sequelae are more likely, e.g., seizure disorder, developmental delay. Additionally, there has been a significant incidence of sequelae, neurological in particular, such as seizures, mental retardation, and perceptual motor handicaps in patients with deep stage II to IV coma who survive. This incidence has varied from 10 to 40% in various series. (13, 17, 22-25, 26)

REFERENCES

1. Reye, R.D.K., Morgan, G., Baral, J.: Encephalopathy and fatty degeneration of the viscera: A disease entity in childhood. Lancet 2:749, 1963.

2. Thaler, M.M.: Metabolic mechanisms in Reye's syndrome: End of a mystery? Am J Dis Child 130:241, 1976.

3. Pollock, J.D. (Ed): Reye's Syndrome. Grune and Stratton, New York, 1974, p. 179.

4. Glick, T.H., Likosky, W.H., Levitt, L.P., et al.: Reye's syndrome: An epidemiologic approach. Pediatrics 46:371, 1970.

5. Hurwitz, E.S., Nelson, D.B., Davis, C., et al.: National surveillance for Reye's syndrome: A five-year review. Pediatrics 70:895, 1982.

6. DeLong, G.R., Glick, T.H.: Encephalopathy of Reye's syndrome: A review of pathogenetic hypotheses. Pediatrics 69:53, 1982.

7. Brown, R.E. and Madge, G.E.: Fatty acids and mitochondrial injury in Reye's syndrome. N Engl J Med 286:787, 1972.

8. Brown, T., Brown, H., Lansky, L., et al.: Carbamyl phosphate synthetase and ornithine transcarbamylase in liver of Reye's syndrome. N Engl J Med 291:797, 1974.

9. Partin, J.D., Schubert, W.K., Partin, J.S.: Mitochondrial ultrastructure in Reye's syndrome (encephalopathy and fatty degeneration of the viscera). N Engl J Med 285: 1139, 1971.

10. Tanaka, K., Isselbacher, K.J., Shih, V.: Isovaleric and α -methyl-butyric acidemia induced by hypoglycin A: Mechanism of Jamaica vomiting sickness. Science 75:69, 1972.

11. Crocker, J.F.S., Rozee, K.R., Ozere, R.L., et al.: Insecticide and viral interaction as a cause of fatty visceral changes and encephalopathy in the mouse. Lancet 2:22, 1974.

12. Zieve, F.J., Zieve, L., Doizaki, S.M., et al.: Synergism between ammonia and fatty acid in the production of coma: Implications for hepatic coma. J Pharmacol Exp Ther 191:10, 1974.

13. DeLong, G.R., Glick, T.H.: Encephalopathy of Reye's syndrome: A review of pathogenetic hypotheses. Pediatrics 69:53, 1982.

14. Lovejoy, F.H., Jr., Smith, A.L., Bresman, M.J., et al.: Clinical staging in Reye's Syndrome. Am J Dis Child 128:36, 1974.

15. Bourgeois, G.L., Olson, L., Comer, D., et al.: Encephalopathy and fatty degeneration of the viscera: A clinicopathic analysis of 40 cases. Am J Clin Path 56:558, 1971.

16. Berenberg, W. and Kang, E.S.: The congenital hyperammonemic syndrome. Dev Med Child Neurol 13:355, 1971.

17. Silverman, A., Roy, C.C.: Pediatric Clinical Gastroenterology, 3rd edition, The CV Mosby Company, St. Louis, 1983, p. 630

18. Hilty, M.D., Romsche, C.A., Delamater, P.L.: Reye's syndrome and hyperaminoacidemia. J Pediatr 84:362, 1974.

19. Aoki, Y. and Lombroso, C.T.: Prognostic value of electroencephalography in Reye's syndrome. Neurology 23: 333, 1973.

20. Chang, L.W., Gilvert, E.F., Tanner, W., Moffat, H.L.: Reye's syndrome: Light and electron microscope studies. Arch Pathol 96:127, 1973.

21. Liebman, W.M., Thaler, M.M.: Liver failure. In: Pediatric Emergencies. Pascoe, D.J. and Grossman, M. (Eds). JB Lippincott Company, Philadelphia, 1978, p. 226.

22. Caillie, M., Morin, C.L., Roy, C.C., et al.: Reye's syndrome: relapses and neurological sequelae. Pediatrics 59:244, 1977.

23. Corey, L., Rubin, R.J., Hatwick, M.A.W.: Reye's syndrome: Clinical progression and evaluation of therapy. Pediatrics 60:708, 1977.

24. Huttenlocher, P.R.: Reye's syndrome: Relation of outcome to therapy. J Pediatr 80:845, 1972.

25. Shaywitz, B.A., Rothstein, P., Venes, J.L.: Monitoring and management of increased intracranial pressure in Reye's syndrome: Results in 29 children. Pediatrics 66: 198, 1980.

26. Margolis, L.H., Shaywitz, B.A.: The outcome of prolonged coma in childhood. Pediatrics 65:477, 1980.

Case 59

RECURRENT SWELLING AND BURNING OF SKIN IN A 15-YEAR-OLD GIRL

HISTORY

A 15-year-old white female presented with history of recurrent episodes of swelling and associated burning of areas of skin exposed to sunlight for more than 15 minutes. There was no history of fever, abdominal pain, diarrhea, constipation, jaundice, anorexia, melena, hematochezia, dysuria, dyspnea, or of associated trauma. She was an only child and the family milieu was otherwise unremarkable. The remainder of the past history, developmental history, family history, social history, and review of systems was unremarkable.

EXAMINATION

She was alert, cooperative, active, and in no apparent distress, with normal vital signs, height 134 cm, weight 51 kg. The examination was unremarkable except for some fine scarring seen in the malar areas of the cheeks and on the dorsa of the hands, particularly over the knuckle areas.

LABORATORY DATA

Hemoglobin:	12.4 gm%
Hematocrit:	38%
White blood cell count:	7,100/mm^3
PMN's:	61%
lymphocytes:	35%
monocytes:	2%
eosinophiles:	2%

5. The laboratory features of this condition include which of the following?
   A. Positive direct Coombs' test
   B. Positive hepatitis B surface antigen (HbsAg)
   C. Increased urine uroporphyrin
   D. Increased stool coproporphyrin
   E. Increased stool protoporphyrin

6. The specific biochemical defect is which one of the following?
   A. Decreased ALA synthetase
   B. Decreased uroporphyrin I synthetase
   C. Increased hepatic ALA synthetase
   D. Decreased heme synthetase
   E. Decreased fructose-1-phosphate aldolase

7. The treatment of this condition includes which of the following?
   A. Decreased protein intake
   B. Chlorpromazine
   C. Phlebotomy
   D. Intravenous infusion of hematin
   E. β -carotene administration

ANSWERS AND COMMENTS

1. (D) Protoporphyria is the most likely diagnosis in this patient. The presence of skin lesions of this nature and the age and well-being of this patient would make the presence of tyrosinemia, histiocytosis X, and hereditary fructose intolerance unlikely. The lack of associated abdominal pain, organic brain syndrome, or manifestations of autonomic neuropathy, such as tachycardia and labile hypertension, would make the possibility of hereditary coproporphyria less likely.

2. (F) In protoporphyria, the skin manifestations usually begin in the first decade of life. (1-5) These include pruritus, burning sensation, and, subsequently, edema and erythema in areas previously exposed to sunlight. (1-5) Bullous lesions may also occur, although infrequently. (1-5) However, the latter lesions do occur frequently in other forms of porphyria, particularly hereditary coproporphyria, variegate porphyria, and porphyria cutanea tarda. (1-5) These bullae are probably related more to increased fragility of the skin than to the reaction to sun exposure. (1-5) Chronic skin changes may also occur, such as whitish papular lesions on the dorsum of the hands, hirsutism,

and varied pigmentation anywhere. (1-5) The cause of these skin changes is the photosensitizing nature of the porphyrin compounds. (1-5) These compounds absorb sunlight, resulting in an excited state, which then returns to an unexcited state by energy loss. The end result is skin damage. (1-5) In protoporphyria, both the bone marrow and the liver contribute to the excessive production of protoporphyrin (increase in protoporphyrin in red blood cells, feces). (1-6)

3. (E) The listed clinical features are prominent in other forms of porphyria, particularly acute intermittent porphyria, variegate porphyria, and hereditary coproporphyria. (1-5) Whether these manifestations are specifically due to increased Σ-aminolevulinic acid and porphobilinogen (PBG), a finding in these three types, has not been confirmed. (1-5)

4. (D, E) Basically, only two types of porphyria manifest morphological abnormalities of the liver. The two are porphyria cutanea tarda and protoporphyria. (1-5) In the latter, the most characteristic binding is the presence of deposits of protoporphyrin pigment, usually focal in nature. (1-5) Using polarizing microscopy, these deposits display birefringence. (1-5)

With time and increased deposits of protoporphyrin, progressive hepatocellular necrosis with associated cholestasis may result. Fortunately, cirrhosis per se is uncommon in children. (1-5)

In porphyria cutanea tarda, the morphological changes include fatty metamorphosis, siderosis, and hepatocellular necrosis, usually focal in nature. (1-5) The precise etiology of these lesions remains undetermined, although the frequent accompanying alcoholic consumption, as well as iron deposition, may play a role. (1-5)

5. (E) The diagnosis of any type of porphyria is based on the demonstration of increased quantities of porphyrins and/or their precursors in feces, urine, or blood (Table 59.1). These compounds are fluorescent and colored. Their route of excretion is determined mainly by their physiochemical properties, in particular the more water soluble are excreted in urine, e.g., uroporphyrin. Conversely, protoporphyrin is poorly soluble and, therefore, is excreted in stool via bile. (1-5)

The majority of laboratories perform so-called screening tests, since there is considerable technical difficulty in the measurement of porphyrins in feces, urine, and blood. (1-5) The principal screening test used in most laboratories is the Watson-Schwartz test or a variant, which is designed to detect increased PBG in urine. Also it must be remembered that PBG

TABLE 59.1 Hepatic Porphyria

Disease	Main Biochemical Features		
	Red Blood Cells	Urine	Feces
Protoporphyria	Protoporphyrin	-	Protoporphyrin
Acute intermittent porphyria	-	↑PBG, ↑ALA	-
Variegate porphyria	-	↑Coproporphyrin ↑PBG, ↑ALA	↑Protoporphyrin ↑Coproporphyrin
Hereditary coproporphyria	-	↑Coproporphyrin ↑PBG, ↑ALA	Coproporphyrin
Porphyria cutanea tarda	-	↑Uroporphyrin	-
Secondary porphyrinuria	-	↑Coproporphyrin	-

Key: ↑ = increase, ↓ = decrease, - = no abnormality; ALA = delta aminolevulinic acid; PBG = porphobilinogen.
Modified from Bloomer, J.R. (5)

excretion may be too low to give a positive Watson-Schwartz test, particularly during symptom-free intervals of acute intermittent porphyria. (1-5)

With reference to protoporphyria specifically, as previously mentioned, protoporphyrin is poorly soluble and is excreted only in feces. In addition, due to the underlying biochemical defect in this condition (refer to answer 6), increased protoporphyrin (porphyrin precursor) is the compound to be quantitated. Thus, red blood cells or feces must be used for this determination. Similar screening tests of urine can be used, but, obviously, quantitative determination is necessary for absolute confirmation of diagnosis.

6. (D) More recently, several tissues of patients with protoporphyria were analyzed and a deficiency of the enzyme, hemesynthetase, was found. This is the enzyme necessary for the conversion of protoporphyrin III, 9 α , into heme. Iron in the ferrous state is also needed for this conversion (Table 59.2). (1-5)

7. (E) In the management of any type of porphyria, prevention is as important, if not more so, than specific therapy. Factors that can initiate or aggravate clinical symptomatology must be avoided, e.g., porphyrin-stimulating agents, such as chloroquine, griseofulyin. In protoporphyia, underlying liver disease, iron deficiency, alcoholism probably, and drugs possibly (e.g., estrogens), are potential inciting factors.

The specific, current treatment of protoporphyria includes the administration of β-carotene (30 to 150 mg per 24 hours). (7) β-carotene has been shown to be effective in reducing the photosensitivity. (1-5) The treatment of the associated hepatic abnormalities has been less well defined. Recently, the use of cholestyramine has been advocated due to the binding of the protoporphyrin compound in the small intestine interrupting its enterohepatic circulation and thereby decreasing the hepatic load of this compound. (1-5) Further studies, especially long-term, are awaited. In addition, vitamin E administration has been suggested as adjuvant therapy in conjunction with cholestyramine administration for reduction of the protoporphyrin pool (usual dose range, 4 to 12 grams daily). (1-6) Obviously, further study, with reference to therapy, is desirable.

The other choices may be helpful in the treatment of other types of porphyria. These include decreased protein intake in secondary porphyrinurias, chlorpromazine in acute intermittent porphyria, variegate porphyria, and hereditary coproporphyria (pain), phlebotomy in porphyria cutanea tarda, and intravenous hematin infusions in acute intermittent porphyria and variegate porphyria. (1-5)

TABLE 59.2   Heme Biosynthesis

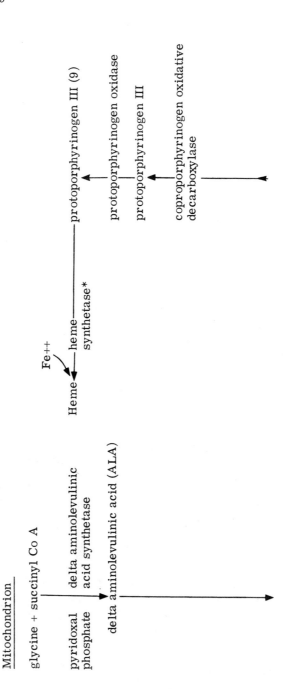

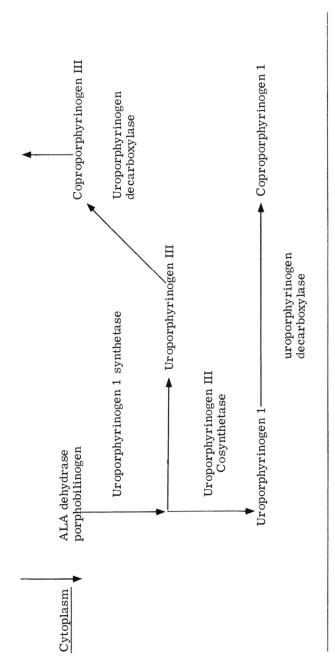

*Defect in protoporphyria. Modified from Bloomer, J. R. (5)

REFERENCES

1. Tschudy, D.P.: Porphyrin metabolism and the porphyrias. In: Duncan's Diseases of Metabolism, 7th Edition. Bondy, P.K.P. and Rosenberg, L.E. (Eds). WB Saunders Co., Philadelphia, 1974, p. 775.

2. Peters, H.A., Cripps, D.J., Reese, H.H.: Porphyria: Theories of etiology and management. Int Rev Neurobiol 16:301, 1974.

3. Meyer, U.A. and Schmid, R.: The porphyrias. In: The Metabolic Basis of Inherited Disease, 4th Edition. Stanbury, J.B., Wyngaarden, J.B., Frederickson, D.S. (Eds). McGraw-Hill Book Co., New York, 1976.

4. Meyer, U.A.: Hepatic porphyrias: New findings on the nature of metabolic defects. In: Progress in Liver Diseases, Volume 5. Popper, H. and Schaffner, F. (Eds). Grune and Stratton, Inc., New York, 1976, p. 280.

5. Bloomer, J.R.: The hepatic porphyrias: Pathogenesis, manifestations and management. Gastroenterology 71:689, 1976.

6. Silverman, A., Roy, C.C.: Pediatric Clinical Gastroenterology, 3rd edition. The CV Mosby Company, St. Louis, 1983, p. 730.

7. Rosenthal, P. and Thaler, M.M.: Disorders of porphyrin, purine and pyrimidine metabolism. In: Current Pediatric Therapy, 10th edition. Gellis, S.S. and Kagan, B.M. (Eds). WB Saunders Company, Boston, 1982, p. 337.

Case 60

RIGHT UPPER QUADRANT FULLNESS IN
AN 18-MONTH-OLD GIRL

HISTORY

An 18-month-old white female presented with a history of fullness in the right upper quadrant of one week duration, detected
at the time of a routine examination by her private physician.
There was no history of fever, nausea, vomiting, diarrhea, constipation, melena, hematochezia, jaundice, anorexia, skin lesions, or trauma. Activity had not significantly changed. The
remainder of the past history, developmental history, family
history, social history, and review of systems was unremarkable.

EXAMINATION

She was relatively alert, active, and in no apparent distress,
with normal vital signs, height 82 cm, weight 11 kg, head circumference 46-1/4 cm. The remainder of the examination was
unremarkable, except for the presence of a firm, nontender
mass in the right upper quadrant within or adjacent to the liver.
The spleen and kidneys were not definitely palpable. There were
active bowel sounds with no bruits.

LABORATORY DATA

Hemoglobin:	12.0 gm%
Hematocrit:	37%
White blood cell count:	9,800/mm^3
PMN's:	40%
lymphocytes:	55%

monocytes:	3%
eosinophiles:	2%
Serum:	
sodium:	138 meq/L
potassium:	4.2 meq/L
chloride:	104 meq/L
bicarbonate:	23 meq/L
creatinine:	0.4 mg%
SGOT:	54 KU
SGPT:	46 KU
total bilirubin:	1.0 mg%
direct bilirubin:	0.6 mg%
alkaline phosphatase:	142 IU
prothrombin time:	12.4 sec (11.5 sec)
partial thromboplastin time:	32 sec (< 36 sec)
HbsAg:	negative
antiHbs:	negative
VDRL:	negative
alpha-fetoprotein:	4+
alpha-1-antitrypsin:	280 mg%
CT scan:	(Fig. 60.1)

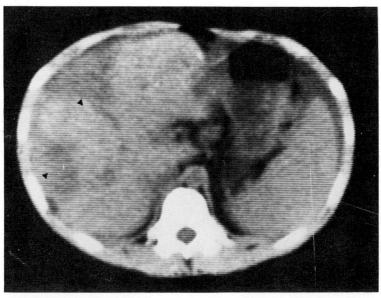

Figure 60.1 CT scan, upper abdomen. Multiple filling defects (arrows) are shown in the right lobe of the liver, filling minimally with contrast material.

QUESTIONS

1. Which of the following studies would be most appropriate in this patient at this time?
   A. Plain X-rays of the abdomen, chest, and bones
   B. Liver scan
   C. Intravenous pyelogram
   D. Upper gastrointestinal series
   E. Visceral angiography (aortography, selective arteriography)

Question 2: Answer true (T) or false (F).

2. Based on the preceding test results, the performance of a needle liver biopsy would be indicated.

3. Which of the following characteristics are usual in this condition?
   A. Predominantly occurs in children less than 3 years of age
   B. Predominant presentation as abdominal distention or mass
   C. Abdominal pain is almost always present
   D. Hepatomegaly or hepatic mass
   E. Negative alpha-fetoprotein

4. Treatment of this patient should include which of the following?
   A. Radiation
   B. Steroids
   C. Azathioprine
   D. Chemotherapy, including vincristine and 5-fluorouracil
   E. Surgical resection

5. The prognosis of this disease, regardless of type of treatment, is characterized by which one of the following?
   A. 5-year survival rate, 66%
   B. 5-year survival rate, 25%
   C. Improved survival rate for the older patient (over 2 years of age)
   D. Improved survival rate for the younger patient (less than 2 years of age)
   E. Determined significantly by histological type

ANSWERS AND COMMENTS

1. (A,B,C,E) The findings of significant hepatomegaly and abdominal distention, weight loss, decreased appetite, and the age of this patient (18 months) suggest an ominous process. In order to evaluate further this patient's condition, plain films of the abdomen, chest, and a bone survey should be done first. The plain films of the abdomen will confirm the hepatomegaly and demonstrate any calcification (usually uncommon in hepatic neoplasms), such as hepatoblastoma. (1-11) Displacement of intra-abdominal structures should be ascertained. Multisystem involvement (vascular, cysts, tumor) can possibly be demonstrated on the other plain films. Intravenous pyelography will aid in differentiating hepatic from renal space-occupying lesions. The normal configuration of the renal pelvis and calyces, as well as normalcy of position, will confirm the impression of a further hepatic lesion. (1-11) The liver scan, Rose Bengal I^{131} or ^{198}Au, may demonstrate a space-occupying lesion, usually "cold" in hepatic neoplasms, and also its size, location, or multiplicity. (11) Ultrasonography is another more recent technique which can demonstrate space-occupying lesions of the kidney, liver, biliary tree, or other areas and can delineate single or multiple lesions, as well as cystic versus solid nature. If an intrahepatic lesion is suspected, then arteriography will be particularly helpful in defining such a lesion. (12) In the preschool age group, aortography is usually used, as well as selective hepatic arteriography, scrutinizing these studies for displacement of vessels around the space-occupying lesions, presence of abnormal vessels, pooling, and tumor stain or "blush." (12) The number, size, and extent of lesions, as well as their benign or malignant nature, may also be ascertained from these studies.

2. (F) Percutaneous liver biopsy can be potentially dangerous in patients with hepatic tumors, due to capsular rupture or hemorrhage. Thus, laparotomy (open biopsy) must be performed for the final diagnosis. In addition, needle biopsy should not be undertaken in patients who have a potentially resectable lesion, since dissemination could result. In other instances, it can be performed cautiously in order to provide histological identification of the type of tumor. (3,4,6,8,10)

3. (A,B,D) Almost 75% of cases of hepatoblastoma occur in children less than 3 years of age, and it is uncommon after 5 years. There is a male predominance, a ratio of 3:2 to 2:1 in most series. (1-11) This tumor usually occurs in the right lobe of the liver (2/3 - 3/4 of cases). (3,4,6,8,10) One explanation is the lower oxygen saturation of blood from the portal vein, the

supplier of the right lobe in utero. (3,4,10) The tumor is usually encapsulated, single in origin, becoming multiple in advanced
cases. (3,4,6,8,10)

The usual modes of presentation are (1) abdominal distention
(enlargement) and/or mass, occurring in almost 65-70%; (2) malaise, including anorexia, weight loss, and lethargy; (3) pathological fracture, uncommonly; and (4) precocious puberty, uncommonly, secondary to gonadotropin secretion and release from
the testes as a result of tumor influence. (3,4,9) During the
clinical course, more commonly encountered symptomatology
and signs include vomiting, abdominal discomfort, irritability,
fever, pallor, hepatomegaly (95-100%), splenomegaly (20-30%),
jaundice (only 5-15%), spider nevi, and palmar erythema. (1-11)

Results of liver function tests are usually within normal limits. (1-11) If significantly abnormal, especially with associated
jaundice, advanced liver disease is to be expected. Alpha-1-
feto-globulin (fetoprotein) is present in sera of 60 to nearly 80%
of children with hepatoblastoma. (13,15) Alpha-1-fetoprotein
is normally synthesized by embryonal liver cells and is detected
in fetal serum and in cord blood. (13,15) Its peak level is at 13
weeks of gestation and then declines. (13,15) After birth, the
decline is rapid, and detectable levels disappear by 2 months of
age under normal conditions. (13,15) Elevated levels have been
reported in neonatal hepatitis while being normal in extrahepatic
biliary atresia. (13,15) Its presence in tumor patients' sera is
supposedly the result of a reversion of the malignant liver cells
to the fetal synthetic state. The qualitative level does not correlate well with tumor size, its growth, or prognosis, but its continued presence after treatment suggests residual tumor or recurrence of tumor. (13,15)

4. (E) Radiation and chemotherapy, in general, apparently
have little or no effect on hepatic tumors in children. (16,17)
Surgical resection remains the only reliable means of treatment
at present. (18-22) Enucleation of tumors is obviously preferred
and certainly does not constitute "radical surgery." If the tumor is small, close to the liver edge or with a pedicle, wedge
resection is performed. However, the location and size in the
majority of cases are such that hepatic lobectomy, hemi-hepa-
tectomy, or even right hepatectomy are the operation of choice.
(20) Resection of up to 80% of liver may be well tolerated. (20)
Regeneration occurs rapidly, with restoration of original weight/
volume within 6 months. (19,21,22) Furthermore, this regenera-
tive response is greater in children than in adults. (19,21)

Medical treatment is not used in solitary, multiple/massive,
and fetal cell liver tumors. (3,5,9,19) Radiation and chemotherapy, therefore, are not indicated. However, in other histological

types of hepatoblastoma, radiotherapy and/or chemotherapy are used postoperatively. Although sensitivity of the liver to radiation and chemotherapeutic agents is greater in children than adults and is further augmented by liver resection, the results have been discouraging. Current studies are in progress, using regimens of adriamycin, vincristine, and cyclophosphamide, and 5-fluorouracil alone or in combination with the other three drugs. Other presently used agents include mitomycin C and methotrexate. Chemotherapy is also used in recurrent (local or otherwise), metastatic, and inoperable cases. (16,19)

Interruption of a branch of the portal vein or hepatic artery has not been used to any extent in children. Early ligation of hepatic veins, hemostasis (inflow, outflow), plasmanate infusions, and other ancillary techniques have not been utilized sufficiently in children to allow definitive conclusions. However, early ligation of hepatic veins would decrease or prevent seeding of the neoplasm during its manipulation. (14) Liver transplantation has been used in a few cases, resulting in longer, temporary survival, but no long-term results. (23) However, future technical and medical control in liver transplantation may provide renewed optimism for this method.

5. (E) In essentially all cases of hepatoblastoma, epithelial cells predominate. (3,4,6,8,10) However, the vast majority of cases are characterized by the presence of several cell types. (3,4,6,8,10) Fetal mesenchyme (almost 50%) and osteoid (25-40%) elements are also commonly found within these tumors. (3, 4,6,8,10) Kasai and Watanabe (10) prepared the following histological tumor typing: (1) fetal cell (resemble fetal/infant liver, usually most common type); (2) embryonal cell (less differentiated); (3) anaplastic cell; (4) hepatocarcinoma; and (5) rhabdomyoblastic (spindle-shaped cells, myofibrils). These tumors can infiltrate into adjacent parenchyma and metastasize via the hepatic veins to the lungs (nodules). (10) Involvement beyond the lungs is uncommon, e.g., bone. (10)

Analysis of results of several series has revealed that the prognosis after more extensive surgery depends chiefly on the histological type, not age or otherwise. (1-11,19) Regardless of the type of treatment, the 5-year survival rate of all types of hepatoblastoma has ranged from 7% to 60%, the higher results generally being associated with series having many fetal cell types and when complete resection has been accomplished. (1-11,18,19) The overall average of these series has been 19%. (1-11,19)

In conclusion, techniques with better identification of early lesions and recurrences/metastases, as well as improved chemotherapeutic agents and regimens, are desperately needed in order to improve survival rate.

TABLE 60.1   Primary Tumors of the Liver

I.   Benign
   A. Hamartoma
   B. Hemangioendothelioma
   C. Hemangioma (capillary cavernous)
   D. Lymphangioma
   E. Cyst (solitary)

II. Malignant
   A. Hepatoblastoma (fetal cell, embryonal cell, anaplastic
      cell, hepatocarcinoma-like cell, rhabdomyoblastic cell)

   B. Hepatocarcinoma

   C. Hemangioendotheliosarcoma

   D. Malignant mesenchymoma

   E. Rhabdomyosarcoma (bile ducts)

REFERENCES

1.   Clatworthy, H.W., Jr., Boles, E.T., Jr., Kottmeier,
     P.K.: Liver tumors in infancy and childhood. Ann Surg
     154:475, 1961.

2.   Fraumeni, J.F., Miller, R.W., Hill, J.A.: Primary car-
     cinoma of the liver in childhood: An epidemiologic study.
     J Natl Cancer Inst 40:1087, 1968.

3.   Ishak, K.G. and Gluntz, P.: Hepatoblastoma and hepato-
     carcinoma in infancy and childhood. Cancer 20:369, 1967.

4.   Keeling, J.W.: Liver tumors in infancy and childhood. J
     Pathol 103:69, 1971.

5.   Linn, T.Y., Chen, C., Lin, W.: Primary carcinoma of
     the liver in infancy and childhood: Report of 21 cases, with
     resection in 6 cases. Surgery 60:1275, 1966.

6. Misugi, K., Okajima, H., Misugi, N., et al.: Classification of primary malignant tumors of liver in infancy and childhood. Cancer 20:1760, 1967.

7. Fish, J.C. and McCary, R.C.: Primary cancer of the liver in childhood. Arch Surg 93:355, 1966.

8. Ito, J. and Johnson, W.W.: Hepatoblastoma and hepatoma in infancy and childhood. Arch Pathol 87:259, 1969.

9. Rickham, P.O. and Artigas, J.L.R.: Tumors of the liver in childhood. Z Kinderchir 7:447, 1969.

10. Kasai, M. and Watanabe, I.: Histologic classification of liver-cell carcinoma in infancy and childhood and its clinical evaluation: A study of 70 cases collected in Japan. Cancer 25:551, 1970.

11. Rosenfield, N., Treves, S.: Liver-spleen scanning in pediatrics. Pediatrics 53:692, 1974.

12. Moss, A.A., Clark, R.E., Palvinskas, A.J., et al.: Angiographic appearance of benign and malignant hepatic tumors in infants and children. Am J Roentgenol 113:61, 1971.

13. Purves, L.R., Bersohn, I., Geddes, E.W.: Serum alpha feto-protein and primary cancer of the liver in man. Cancer 25:1261, 1970.

14. Silverman, A., Roy, C.C.: Pediatric Clinical Gastroenterology, 3rd edition. The CV Mosby Company, St. Louis, 1983, p. 479.

15. Albert, E.: Alpha-1-fetoprotein: Serologic marker of human hepatoma and embryonal carcinoma. Natl Cancer Inst Monogr 35:415, 1972.

16. Filler, R.M., Tefft, M., Vawter, G.F., et al.: Hepatic lobectomy in childhood: Effects of X-ray and chemotherapy. J Pediatr Surg 4:31, 1969.

17. Tefft, M., Mitus, A., Das, L., et al.: Irradiation of the liver in children: Review of experience in the acute and chronic phases, and in the infant. Am J Roentgenol 108:365, 1970.

18. Nixon, H.H.: Hepatic tumors in childhood and their treatment by major hepatic resection. Arch Dis Child 40:169, 1965.

19. Raffuci, F.L. and Ramirez-Schon, G.: Management of tumors of the liver. SGO 130:371, 1970.

20. Taylor, P.H., Fiuer, R.M., Nebesar, R.A., et al.: Experience with hepatic resection in childhood. Am J Surg 117:435, 1969.

21. Samuels, L.P., Grosfeld, J.L., Kartha, M.: Liver scans after primary treatment of tumors in children. SGO 131: 958, 1970.

22. Exelby, P.R., Filler, R.M., Grosfeld, J.L.: Liver tumors in children in the particular reference to hepatoblastoma and hepatocellular carcinoma: American Academy of Pediatrics surgical section survey 1974. J Pediatr Surg 10:329, 1975.

23. Starzl, T.E., Brettschneider, L., Penn, I., et al.: Clinical liver transplantation. Transplant Rev 2:3, 1969.

Case 61

JAUNDICE, FEVER, AND RASH IN A 5-YEAR-OLD MALE

HISTORY

A 5-year-old black male presented with jaundice of 7 days' duration. The patient had had preceding sore throat, fever, nausea, vomiting, diarrhea, and generalized rash 1 week prior to the onset of jaundice. Preceding treatment had included penicillin orally and intramuscularly. The rash was described as exfoliating. There was no associated history of melena, hematochezia, hematemesis, pyrosis, dysphagia, cough, dysuria, arthralgia, oral lesions, or trauma. The remainder of the past history, developmental history, family history, social history, and review of systems, including exposures to ill persons, chemicals, was noncontributory.

EXAMINATION

He was alert, well-nourished, and in no apparent distress, with normal vital signs except temperature of 100.8°F (oral), weight 18.3 kg, height 105 cm. The remainder of the examination was unremarkable except for (1) exfoliation and minimal erythema, including palms and soles; (2) scleral and conjunctival icterus; (3) slight fissuring of the corners of the mouth; (4) liver, palpable 5 cm below the right costal margin in the midclavicular line, mildly tender and not nodular in consistency, total span being 7.5 cm by percussion. No abdominal bruits were noted.

LABORATORY DATA

Hemoglobin:	11.8 gm%
Hematocrit:	33%

White blood cell count:	$11,300/mm^3$
PMN's:	54%
lymphocytes:	38%
monocytes:	5%
eosinophiles:	3%
Platelet count:	$450,000/mm^3$
Sedimentation rate:	26 mm/hr
Serum:	
SGOT:	134 KU
SGPT:	92 KU
total protein:	5.8 gm%
albumin:	3.5 mg%
total bilirubin:	8.6 mg%
direct bilirubin:	6.7 mg%
alkaline phosphatase:	375 IU
ceruloplasmin:	95 mg%
Prothrombin time:	12.0 seconds (11.5 seconds)
VDRL:	negative
HbsAg:	negative
antiHbs:	negative
AntiHAAg:	negative
Urinalysis:	negative
Stool:	
smear:	rare WBC
hemoccult:	negative
culture:	negative
ova and parasites:	negative
Electrocardiogram:	negative
Echocardiogram:	negative

QUESTIONS

Questions 1-3: Answer true (T) or false (F).

1. The likely diagnosis in this patient is hand-foot-mouth disease.

2. This disease/syndrome is more prevalent in children of Japanese ancestry.

3. This disease/syndrome is more prevalent in children over 5 years of age.

4. Principal criteria include which of the following?
   A. Fever, more than 5 days
   B. Abdominal pain
   C. Conjunctival injection
   D. Jaundice
   E. Oral and lip lesions

5. Laboratory abnormalities in this disease/syndrome usually include
   A. increased sedimentation rate (over 20 mm/hr)
   B. increased platelet count (over 400,000/mm^3)
   C. decreased immunoglobulins (IgM, A, G)
   D. decreased platelet counts
   E. electrocardiographic changes (rhythm, voltage)

6. Treatment of this condition should include
   A. aspirin
   B. antacids
   C. antibiotics
   D. steroids
   E. surgery

Question 7: Answer true (T) or false (F).

7. The outcome of patients with this condition is universally good, self-limited, without recurrence, and without apparent progression.

ANSWERS AND COMMENTS

1. (F) The constellation of (1) persistent fever, greater than 5 days; (2) oral lesions, including oropharyngeal erythema and lip fissuring, erythema; (3) rash, induration/erythema of the hands and feet, desquamation, in addition to jaundice, in this patient do not suggest hand-foot-mouth disease per se. Hand-foot-mouth disease is basically a vesicular exanthem and enanthem, involving the oral mucosa, tongue, extremities, apparently associated with Coxsackie A16 virus, in particular. (1, 2) No systemic form per se has been associated with this disease. (1, 2) Other possibilities, particularly Kawasaki syndrome, would be foremost in diagnostic consideration.

2. (T) The syndrome was initially thought to be an intriguing complex of symptoms and signs, one curiously relegated to the Orient. However, in recent years, epidemiological investigations have demonstrated its relative frequency and its worldwide

distribution (all racial groups). (3-11) Regardless, this entity continues to be more prevalent in Japan and children of Japanese ancestry, e.g., in Hawaii. (3,7-11) Japanese studies have not noted any particular geographical or other socioenvironmental factors to date. Additionally, no specific genetic factor, e.g., HLA antigen, has been found, either. (6-8,12) A recent study of Bell, et al. (5) demonstrated a previously unrecognized seasonal variation in the United States, February to May, as well as a prevalence in black children, compared with white children.

No specific agent, e.g., bacterial, viral, has been isolated. (5,9,10,12) Speculation would include many different types of agents, stimulating an abnormal immune response, with a resultant "vasculitis." (12)

3. (F) Kawasaki syndrome is mainly an illness of young children, approximately 50% below 2 years of age, and 75 to 80% below 4 to 5 years of age. (5,10-12) Furthermore, the syndrome has infrequently been noted in children over 8 to 10 years of age. (5,10-12) Also in the recent study of Bell, et al. (5), the median age was 2.3 years. Males are affected more often than females. (3,2) A very small percentage of patients have been found to have an underlying immunodeficiency, cardiac, or other chronic disease. (5,10-12)

4. (A,C,E) Kawasaki syndrome progresses through 3 main clinical phases, acute, subacute, and convalescent, each with relatively predictable features. (3,4,6-8,12) (Table 61.1) However, a positive diagnosis is possible only when a patient fulfills 5 of 6 major diagnostic criteria. (Table 61.2) Obviously, there is some variation in the degree of these symptoms/signs, but their presence and timing seem to be remarkably consistent. (3,4,6-8,12) Over 90% of patients with this disorder have the first 5 criteria, while only 50 to 60% manifest the sixth, i.e., lymph node enlargement. Only strict adherence to the presence of these criteria and also exclusion of diseases mimicking the syndrome can produce a more certain diagnosis.

As previously mentioned (Table 61.1), the course of the disease has 3 main phases. The acute phase is characterized by fever, conjunctival injection, lesions of the lips and mouth, edema of hands and feet, the erythematous rash, and possible lymph node enlargement; diarrhea and hepatic changes may occur during this phase. By the 10th to 14th days, the fever, rash, and lymphadenopathy subside. The subacute phase then begins, characterized by anorexia, fussiness, increasing platelet count, and the desquamative skin changes; associated features, such as arthritis, myocardial abnormalities may occur during this phase. By the 25th day or so, the convalescent phase begins,

TABLE 61.1   Kawasaki Syndrome: Clinical Phases

Acute Phase (1 to 10 days)
  fever
  conjunctival injection
  oral lesions (lips, tongue, oropharyngeal mucosa)
  induration, erythema of hands, feet
  erythematous rash
  lymphadenopathy
  associated features: aseptic meningitis, hepatopathy, gastro-
    intestinal

Subacute Phase (10 to 25 days)
  no fever
  anorexia
  fussiness
  desquamation of rash
  increased platelet count
  associated features: arthropathy, myocardial abnormalities

Convalescent Phase (25 to 60 days)
  disappearance of clinical features
  associated features: residual coronary aneurysm
    electrocardiographic abnormalities (arrhythmias,
    voltage changes)

Modified from Hicks, P.V. (4) and Melish, M.E., et al. (12)

characterized by the abrupt or progressive disappearance of all
clinical signs of disease and a return of the laboratory studies
to normal, e.g., sedimentation rate. (3,4,6-8,12)

5.   (A,B) Unfortunately, laboratory abnormalities associated
with Kawasaki syndrome are not diagnostic. During the acute
phase, the white blood cell count is usually above $20,000/mm^3$,
with a predominance of polymorphonuclear elements. The sedimentation rate and C-reactive protein also increase during the
acute phase with a subsequent decrease over the following 5 to
10 weeks.
    The platelet count is usually within normal limits during the
acute phase but then will increase to levels of 500,000 to
$2,000,000 \ mm^3$ during the subacute phase. The platelet count
will then decrease to normal by the midconvalescent phase. (3,
4,6-8)

TABLE 61.2   Kawasaki Syndrome

Major diagnostic criteria

1. Fever, more than 5 days

2. Conjunctival injection

3. Oral lesions - erythema, fissuring and crusting, oropharyn-
    geal erythema, strawberry tongue

4. Abnormalities of peripheral extremities
    Induration of hands and feet
    Erythema of palms and soles
    Desquamation fingertips and toes, 2 weeks from onset of
        illness
    Transverse grooves across fingernails 2 to 3 months after
        onset of illness

5. Erythematous rash

6. Enlarged lymph node mass

Minor (associated) criteria

   Arthropathy
   Gastrointestinal (diarrhea, abdominal pain)
   Carditis
   Hepatitis
   Hydrops of gallbladder
   Aseptic meningitis
   Thrombocytosis
   Increased sedimentation rate

Modified from Melish, M.E., et al. (12)

   All of the immunoglobulins, including IgE, generally increase
during the acute phase, then falling to normal in the subacute
phase. There has been a suggestion that high IgE levels may occur just before the development of myocardial injury/dysfunc-
tion. (4)
   With reference to the minority of patients who develop associated features, mild elevations of transaminases (SGOT, SGPT)
and total and direct bilirubin may be noted in those with hepatitis

(5 to 20%) and manifestations of acute carditis, 10 to 20 days
after onset, e.g., abnormal ECGs (heart block, arrythmias,
voltage changes, e.g., left ventricular hypertrophy), echocardi-
ograms with aneurysmal dilatations (10 to 30%), have been demonstrated. (4,7,12-14) Ultrasonography of the abdomen has
shown in a small percentage of cases, dilatation of the gallbladder with watery fluid, particularly during the end of the acute
phase, i.e., hydrops of the gallbladder. (4,7,12)

6.   (A) Since the precise etiology of Kawasaki syndrome is unknown, effective treatment must await further investigation regarding pathophysiology. However, supportive therapy can be
offered, including nutritional support.
    Specifically, aspirin has been utilized for its anti-inflamma-
tory and its platelet inhibitory (aggregation) activity. Kawasaki
syndrome does not seem to respond to lower doses, instead requiring major anti-inflammatory doses, i.e., 75-100 mg/kg/
day. This dosage will usually be required for days for the fever
to subside. At this time, the dosage can be reduced rapidly over
24 to 72 hours to 10-20 mg/kg/day or less. (4,7,12) Although
fever is controlled, the real objective would be to reduce or
eliminate the cardiac complications. The reduced aspirin dosage is designed to reduce platelet aggregation and not stimulate
vascular thrombogenic factors. (4,7,12,15)
    Steroids have not been useful in prevention of the cardiac
manifestations, e.g., coronary aneurysms, rather possibly to
increase such. (12)
    Antacids, antibiotics, and surgery have no regular basis in
this entity.

7.   (F) For the vast majority of patients with Kawasaki syndrome, the condition is self-limited, nonrecurrent, and nonpro-
gressive. (6,7,8,12) Concerns regarding progression to collagen-vascular disease, arthritis, have not been well documented. However, cardiac complications during the acute or subacute phase, e.g., cardiac insufficiency, myocardial infarction,
have occurred and can lead to significant sequelae. Melish, et
al. (12) mentioned in a review that a long-term study by their
group noted in several of 85 children residual coronary aneurysms and/or electrocardiographic abnormalities. (12) They
remained very concerned that 51% of this group still had residual
intrinsic vascular disease. (12)
    On an acute basis, the mortality rate is approximately 1 to
2%, usually due to myocardial infarction. Death occurs between
2 to 6 weeks after onset of symptoms. Coronary vasculitis with
coronary thrombosis has been prevalent pathologically at this
time. (12-15)

REFERENCES

1. Tindall, J.R. and Callaway, J.L.: Hand, foot and mouth disease: It's more common than you think. Am J Dis Child 124:372, 1972.

2. Cherry, J.: Newer viral exanthems. Adv Pediatr 16:233, 1969.

3. Kawaski, T., Kosaki, F., Okawa, S., et al.: A new infantile acute febrile muco cutaneous lymph node syndrome (MLNS) prevailing in Japan. Pediatrics 54:271, 1974.

4. Hicks, R.V.: Arthritis as a manifestation of the Kawaski syndrome. In: Arthritis in Children, Report of the Eightieth Ross Conference in Pediatric Research, 1981, p. 26.

5. Bell, D.M., Morens, D.M., Holman, R.C., et al.: Kawaski Syndrome in the United States, 1976 to 1980. Am J Dis Child 137:211, 1983.

6. Melish, M.E., Hicks, R.M., Larson, E.J.: Muco cutaneous lymph node syndrome in the United States. Am J Dis Child 130:599, 1976.

7. Kawasaki, T.: Clinical signs and symptoms of mucocutaneous lymph node syndrome (Kawasaki disease). Jpn J Med Sci Biol 32:237, 1979.

8. Yanagihara, R. and Todd, J.K.: Acute febrile mucocutaneous lymph node syndrome. Am J Dis Child 134:603, 1980.

9. Dean, A.G., Melish, M.E., Hicks, R., et al.: An epidemic of Kawasaki syndrome in Hawaii. J Pediatr 100: 552, 1982.

10. Morens, D.M., Anderson, L.J., Hurwitz, E.S.: National surveillance of Kawasaki disease. Pediatrics 65:21, 1980.

11. Bell, D.M., Brink, E.W., Nitzkin, J.L., et al.: Kawasaki syndrome: Description of two outbreaks in the United States. N Engl J Med 304:1568, 1981.

12. Melish, M.E., Hicks, R.V., Reddy, V.: Kawasaki syndrome: An update. Hosp Pract, March, 1982, p. 99.

13. Landing, B.H. and Larson, E.J.: Are infantile periarteritis nodosa with coronary artery involvement and fatal mucocutaneous lymph node syndrome the same? Comparison of 20 patients from North America with patients from Hawaii and Japan. Pediatrics 59:651, 1976.

14. Fujiwara, H. and Hamashima, Y.: Pathlogy of the heart in Kawasaki disease. Pediatrics 61:100, 1978.

15. Kato, H., Koike, S., Yokoyama, T.: Effect of treatment in coronary artery involvement. Pediatrics 63:175, 1979.

Case 62

FAILURE TO THRIVE AND DIARRHEA IN
A 15-MONTH-OLD BOY

HISTORY

A 15-month-old white male presented with slow height and weight
gain since birth with associated past history of diarrhea, as
many as 10-12 bowel movements daily, now 2-3 soft bowel movements daily. There was no associated history of fever, vomiting, constipation, jaundice, skin lesions, apparent dysuria, anorexia, or respiratory tract infections. Dietary history included
breast feedings only for the first 3 months, addition of cereals,
predominantly rice, at 3 months of age, fruits at 4 months, and
meats and vegetables at 6 months of age (baby foods). The loose
bowel movements were noted between 1-6 months of age; breast
feedings had been discontinued at 3 months of age. Similac, then
Isomil, and finally a soy formula were used without apparent effect. Developmental milestones were felt to be within normal
limits by the private physician. Pertinent family history included maternal grandmother with history of a type of nephritis.
The remainder of the past history, developmental history, family history, social history, and review of systems was noncontributory.

EXAMINATION

He was an active, 15-month-old male in no distress, with normal vital signs; height was 71 cm, weight 7.3 kg, and head circumference was 36.5 cm. The remainder of the examination
was unremarkable, including the abdomen, anorectal area, and
neurological evaluation.

LABORATORY DATA

Hemoglobin:	12.7 gm%
Hematocrit:	36.5%
White blood cell count:	6,200/mm^3
PMN's:	11%
lymphocytes:	79%
monocytes:	8%
eosinophiles:	2%
Platelet count:	205,000/mm^3
Sedimentation rate:	8 mm/hr
Urinalysis:	negative
Serum:	
prothrombin time:	13.0 sec (11.0 sec)
partial thromboplastin time:	27.5 sec
calcium:	10.0 mg%
total bilirubin:	0.7 mg%
direct bilirubin:	0.4 mg%
T$_4$	6 mg%
RT3U:	27%
sodium:	129 meq/L
potassium:	4.1 meq/L
chloride:	103 meq/L
bicarbonate:	26 meq/L
SGOT:	20 units
alkaline phosphatase:	300 IU
amylase:	130 units
lipase:	0.6 units (< 1.0)
IgG:	1,000 mg%
IgA:	65 mg%
IgM:	30 mg%
T-cell rosettes:	81% (> 65%)
d-xylose (1 hr):	38 mg% (> 30)
Urine:	
amylase:	2,800 units
d-xylose:	1.8 gm (> 1.0 gm)
(orally, 5.0 gm)	
Stool:	
occult blood:	negative
reducing substances:	negative
culture:	negative
ova and parasites:	negative
fat (72 hr, quantitative):	34%/24 hr
Sweat chloride:	18:22 meq/L
Chest films:	negative
Skull films:	negative
Bone age:	6 months (chronological age, 15 months)

Upper GI - small bowel series: negative
Barium enema: negative
Small intestinal biopsy:
  histology: negative
  culture (aerobic, anaerobic):   negative
  ova and parasites: negative

QUESTIONS

1. Which of the following studies would be helpful in establish-
   ing the correct diagnosis at this time?
   A. Secretin-pancreozymin stimulation test
   B. Upper gastrointestinal series
   C. Hypotonic duodenography
   D. Bone marrow examination
   E. Serum amylase isoenzyme pattern

2. Which of the following hematological abnormalities have
   been commonly associated with this condition?
   A. Decreased fetal hemoglobin level
   B. Increased fetal hemoglobin level
   C. Neutropenia
   D. Thrombocytopenia
   E. Anemia

3. Which of the following statements are correct with regard
   to the orthopedic features of this condition?
   A. Bone lesions occur in 80 to 90% of patients
   B. Generalized bone abnormalities are found
   C. Serum calcium is elevated and phosphorus decreased
   D. The sites of predilection include the femur, ribs, and
      tibia
   E. Gait is not affected

4. The clinical course is characterized by which of the fol-
   lowing?
   A. Failure to thrive
   B. Diarrhea
   C. Recurrent infections
   D. Diabetes mellitus
   E. Portal hypertension

5. Treatment should consist of which of the following?
   A. Pancreatic enzyme replacement
   B. Dietary changes, including use of medium-chain trigly-
      cerides
   C. Gamma globulin administration
   D. Broad-spectrum antibiotics
   E. Cholestyramine

Questions 6 and 7: Answer true (T) or false (F).

6. Growth is retarded both in height and weight, but pancreatic replacement therapy can significantly alter the rate of
   growth.

7. The mortality rate continues to be high in childhood, 25 to
   45%, and malnutrition seems to be the major factor in this
   outcome.

ANSWERS AND COMMENTS

1. (A, D) Quantitative assessment of pancreatic function must
be performed in order to ascertain the presence or absence of
exocrine insufficiency. For an accurate assessment of exocrine
pancreatic function, the determination of the total volume, bicarbonate concentration, and enzymes secreted during a special
period of time must be performed. These determinations must
be made before (basal) and after a standardized secretory stim-
ulus (secretin-pancreozymin), collections being accomplished
by placement of a duodenal tube (pediatric) in the second portion
of the duodenum. Two 10-minute collection periods serve as
basal values. The usual dosage of secretin is 1-2 units per kg
intravenously (for three 10-minute collection periods), while
the dose of pancreozymin is 1 unit per kg intravenously (for two
10-minute collection periods). The results are then expressed
as ml (volume), meq (bicarbonate), mg (trypsin, chymotrypsin)
or International Units (IU, carboxypeptidase A, B, amylase,
lipase) per kg per 50 minutes. In exocrine pancreatic insufficiency not due to cystic fibrosis, the results usually reveal normal to low volume, low bicarbonate, and low to negligible enzyme levels. (1-7)
   Bone marrow examination is an important diagnostic tool.
The bone marrow will display a maturation arrest of neutrophils,
hypocellularity, increased fatty tissue, and reduced megakaryo-
cytes. (1-7)

Secretin-pancreozymin stimulation test (pancreas):

volume:	1.8 ml/kg/50 min
bicarbonate:	0.06 meq/L
trypsin:	1.9 mg/kg/50 min
amylase:	7.0 IU/kg/50 min
lipase:	0.9 IU/kg/50 min

Newer diagnostic tests, e.g., serum trypsinogen and/or chymotrypsinogen determinations by radioimmunoassay offer promise in establishing a deficiency or absence of exocrine pancreatic function but await additional correlative studies. The precursor zymogens would be decreased or absent secondary to the decrease or lack of formation, i.e., lack of exocrine function (acini). (8)

2. (B,C,D,E) The most consistent laboratory result is a reduced white blood cell count, which is cyclic or continuous. The most affected white blood cell element is the neutrophil, the total count usually being less than $1,500/mm^3$. Other common findings include anemia, usually mild, and usually resistant to treatment with iron, folic acid, and vitamin B_{12}. (1-7) Hemoglobin electrophoresis will reveal an increased fetal hemoglobin level in the majority of patients. (2,3) Thrombocytopenia, i.e., less than $100,000$ platelets/mm^3, is present in some patients. (1-7)

In most series, the hematological abnormalities tend to be less consistent and constant than the pancreatic abnormality and, moreover, may be normal early in the disease course. (9)

3. (D) This disorder does have associated bone lesions in 10 to 15% of patients. (1-7) They are suggestive of metaphysical dysostosis and tend to occur in the femur, tibia, and ribs. If the lesion in the femur is severe, the gait may be disturbed, and a cosa vara deformity may occur. Generalized bone lesions are not present in this disorder, and serum calcium, phosphorus and alkaline phosphatase levels are within normal limits. (1-7)

4. (A,B,C) The vast majority of patients display clinical evidence of pancreatic exocrine insufficiency during the first two years of life. (1-12) Frequent, loose, pungent stools are present, and steatorrhea occurs. (1-12) Eventually, failure to thrive occurs. Both height and weight are affected, although bone age is usually not as delayed as height age. (1-7,9) Interestingly, this symptomatology lessens with increasing age. (1-4)

Increased susceptibility to infections seems to occur in this condition. In fact, overwhelming infections constitute the leading cause of death. (1-4) White blood cell phagocytosis is usually normal, however, and immunological function is also normal in most patients, so the precise etiology of this infectious predisposition remains ill-defined. (1-7,9)

Liver involvement, including chronic liver disease, has been reported in several patients. (13) Portal fibrosis and variable inflammatory activity predominates.

5. (A,B) After the diagnosis has been established, pancreatic replacement therapy, appropriate for age, should be instituted. Choices include pancrelipase (Cotozym), Viokase, and pancreatin (pancreatic granules). Some patients may require smaller amounts, 300 to 600 mg per meal, while others may require 1,800 to 3,000 mg per meal. These extracts can be administered in capsules or packets (powder), 300 mg each. Effectiveness is variable, probably depending on gastric acidity and reduced pancreatic secretion, particularly bicarbonate, the latter being responsible for providing an appropriate duodenal milieu, i.e., pH for the activity of lipase and other enzymes. Therefore, some authors recommend duodenal intubation in order to check the pH and, if low, the addition of bicarbonate, 15 gm/m^2 surface area/day, is recommended. Investigation is now under way to determine the efficacy of cimetidine, H_2-receptor antagonist (gastric acid inhibition), which would be expected in cystic fibrosis. (8,9,15)

After the initiation of appropriate pancreatic enzyme replacement, the diet should be adjusted so as to ensure an adequate caloric intake for appropriate growth. The caloric intake may need to be 150 to 200 cal/kg with adequate protein (3-4 gm/kg/day). In the young infant, medium-chain triglycerides (C6, C8, C10) may be helpful. (1-7,8-12,14-18) Elemental formulas can be used effectively, too. Additionally, low-fat content (long-chain triglycerides) should be considered. Vitamins A, D, E, and K must be administered daily in a water-soluble or miscible form at twice the normal dosage, e.g., Synkayvite, TriViSol. (1-4,14-18) The patient's growth, dietary intake, stool pattern, and repeat laboratory studies, e.g., stool fat content, should be monitored.

The hematological aspects continue to occur despite administration of folic acid, iron, and vitamin B_{12}. In addition, pancreatic replacement treatment does not affect them, either.

Cholestyramine, antibiotics, gamma globulin administration are without benefit.

6. (F) As previously mentioned in answer 5, pancreatic replacement therapy is begun once the diagnosis is established. After replacement therapy is begun, the diarrhea and varying steatorrhea will decrease. As these symptoms decrease, variable weight gain, as well as increased height, occurs. However,

although weight gain may occur, growth does not necessarily follow. (1-4)

7. (F) Despite early diagnosis and subsequent adequate replacement therapy, the prognosis has remained unchanged during the last 10 to 15 years, i.e., mortality rate of 25 to 45%. (1-4) Additionally, as previously described, no form of specific or nonspecific therapy can positively affect the hemotologic aspects of this disorder. (1-4)

TABLE 62.1   Secretin-Pancreozymin Stimulation Test in Normal Children

	Mean	Standard Deviation	Observed Range
Volume (ml/kg/50 min)	3.9	+1.5	1.8 - 8.1
Bicarbonate (meq/kg/50 min)	0.19	+0.08	0.08-0.37
Lipase (IU/kg/50 min)	1,424	+1,100	206-5,095
Amylase (IU/kg/50 min)	476	+350	140-2,050
Trypsin (μg/kg/50 min)	788	+549	215-2,170
Chymotrypsin (μg/kg/50 min)	860	+456	252-1,900
Carboxypeptidase A (IU/kg/50 min)	724	+540	141-2,480

Modified from Hadorn, B., et al. (5)

542 / Case 62

REFERENCES

1. Bodian, M., Sheldon, W., Lightwood, R.: Congenital hypoplasia of the exocrine pancrease. Acta Paediatr Scand 53:282, 1964.

2. Burke, V., Colebath, J.H., Anderson, C.M., et al.: Association of pancreatic insufficiency and chronic neutropenia in childhood. Arch Dis Child 42:147, 1967.

3. Shmerling, D.H., Prader, A., Hitzig, W.H., et al.: The syndrome of exocrine pancreatic insufficiency, neutropenia, metaphyseal dysostosis and dwarfism. Helv Paediatr Acta 24:547, 1969.

4. Shwachman, H., Diamond, L.K., Oski, F.A., et al.: The syndrome of pancreatic insufficiency and bone marrow dysfunction. J Pediatr 65:645, 1964.

5. Hadorn, B., Foppi, G., Shmerling, D.H., et al.: Quantitative assessment of exocrine pancreatic function in infants and children. J Pediatr 73:39, 1968.

6. Brooks, F.: Testing pancreatic function. N Engl J Med 286:300, 1972.

7. Beck, I.T.: The role of pancreatic enzymes in indigestion. Am J Clin Nutr 26:311, 1973.

8. Silverman, A., Roy, C.C.: Pediatric Clinical Gastroenterology, 3rd edition. The CV Mosby Company, St. Louis, 1983, p. 837.

9. Wilson, F.A. and Dietschy, J.M.: Differential diagnostic approach to clinical problems of malabsorption. Gastroenterology 61:911, 1971.

10. DiMagno, E.P., Go, V.L.W., Summerskill, W.H.J.: Relations between pancreatic enzyme outputs and malabsorption in severe pancreatic insufficiency. N Engl J Med 288:813, 1973.

11. Ament, M.E.: Malabsorption syndromes in infancy and childhood. J Pediatr 81:685, 867, 1972.

12. Anderson, C.M.: Intestinal malabsorption in childhood. Arch Dis Child 41:571, 1966.

13. Liebman, W.M., Rosental, E., Hirschberger, M., et al.: Shwachman-Diamond syndrome and chronic liver disease. Clin Pediatr 18:695, 1979.

14. Lebenthal, E. and Shwachman, H.: The pancreas development, adaptation and malfunction in infancy and childhood. Clin Gastroenterol 6:397, 1977.

15. Cox, K.L., Isenberg, J.I., Osher, A.B., et al.: The effect of cimetidine on maldigestion in cystic fibrosis. J Pediatr 94:488, 1979.

16. Klish, W.J., Potts, E., Ferry, G.D., et al.: Modular formula: An approach to management of infants with specific or complex food intolerances. J Pediatr 88:948, 1976.

17. Harkins, R.W. and Sarett, H.P.: Medium-chain triglycerides. J Am Med Assoc 203: 110, 1968.

18. Gracey, M., Burke, V., Anderson, C.M.: Medium-chain triglycerides in pediatric practice. Arch Dis Child 45: 445, 1970.

Case 63

RECURRENT ABDOMINAL PAIN IN A 15-1/2-YEAR-OLD BOY

HISTORY

A 15-1/2 year-old white male presented with a history of abdominal pain of almost 10 days' duration. The pain was located in the epigastric and periumbilical regions without further radiation, could occur in either or both areas, lasted 1 to 3 hours, occurred with eating or just after meals, without association with food types, position, time of day, or bowel movements. There was associated pallor, tiredness, and decreased activity for 2 or more hours after an attack of pain. There was no history of fever, diarrhea, constipation, jaundice, anorexia, melena, hematochezia, skin lesions, dysuria, arthralgia. Bowel habit pattern was once or twice daily, brown in color, firm in nature. Medication, including Donnatal, had been used without apparent relief of this pain. The pertinent prior history included an incident of trauma, hitting a fire hydrant while running, approximately 2 months before the onset of the previously mentioned pain. The pertinent family history included mother and paternal uncle with possible peptic ulcer disease, and paternal great grandmother, maternal grandmother, and uncles (two) and aunt with history of diabetes mellitus. The remainder of the developmental history, social history, and review of systems was noncontributory.

EXAMINATION

He was alert, cooperative, and in no apparent distress, with normal vital signs, weight 20 kg, height 107 cm. The remainder of the examination was unremarkable, including the abdomen.

LABORATORY DATA

Hemoglobin:	12.5 gm%
Hematocrit:	38%
White blood cell count:	10,600/mm^3
PMN's:	50%
lymphocytes:	42%
monocytes:	5%
eosinophiles:	3%
Sedimentation rate:	18 mm/hr
Hemoglobin electrophoresis:	normal
Urinalysis:	negative
Urine amino acid screen:	negative
Serum:	
SGPT:	20 units
SGOT:	22 units
total bilirubin:	0.9 mg%
direct bilirubin:	0.6 mg%
total protein:	6.1 gm%
albumin:	4.4 gm%
prothrombin time:	11.5 sec (11.8 sec)
serum amylase:	100 units
serum lipase:	6.0 units (less than 1.0 units)
Stool:	
occult blood:	negative
reducing substances:	negative
culture:	negative
ova and parasites:	negative
Upper GI - small bowel series:	negative
Urine amylase (diastase):	16,000 units (24 hr)

QUESTIONS

1. The most probable diagnosis of this patient is:
   A. duodenal ulcer
   B. acute viral hepatitis
   C. acute pancreatitis
   D. Meckel's diverticulum
   E. acute ulcerative colitis

2. The most common cause of this condition is
   A. blunt trauma
   B. hepatitis B virus
   C. Giardia lamblia
   D. mumps
   E. steroids

Question 4: Answer true (T) or false (F).

3. Mumps is clinically present in only 25% of cases.

4. The diagnosis of this disorder is strongly suggested or con-
firmed by which of the following studies?
   A. Serum amylase determination
   B. Amylase/creatinine clearance ratio
   C. Intravenous cholangiography
   D. Ultrasonography
   E. Secretin-pancreozymin stimulation test

5. Accepted medical treatment includes which of the following
measures?
   A. Nasogastric suction
   B. Anticholinergics
   C. Antacids
   D. Antibiotics
   E. Aprotinin (Trasylol)

Question 6: Answer true (T) or false (F).

6. Surgery has no significant role in the management of this
condition.

7. Complications of this condition include which of the follow-
ing?
   A. Duodenal ulcer
   B. Abscess of pancreas
   C. Pseudocyst of pancreas
   D. Duodenal diverticulum
   E. Acute cholecystitis

ANSWERS AND COMMENTS

1. (C) The most probable diagnosis of this patient is acute pancreatitis. The character, intensity, and duration of the abdominal pain are most helpful in differentiation from other disorders
such as acute viral hepatitis (minimal or no abdominal pain), peptic ulcer disease (only if penetrates/perforates posteriorly),
Meckel's diverticulum, and ulcerative colitis. Abdominal pain
occurs in at least 75 to 80% of cases (epigastrium, with or without radiation. (1-7) The lack of hematochezia and/or melena
would tend to rule against ulcerative colitis and Meckel's diverticulum. The laboratory findings did not support the diagnosis
of acute viral hepatitis.

2. (A) Over 50% of cases of acute pancreatitis are associated with drug toxicity, blunt trauma of the abdomen, and clinical mumps. (1-7) Other causes include other viruses, such as Coxsackie, hepatitis A and B, drugs/toxins, e.g., steroids, alcohol, and extrapancreatic diseases, e.g., peptic ulcer, systemic lupus erythematosus. (1-9) Despite current, improved diagnostic techniques and increased availability of such, almost 30% of cases are still without specific cause. (1-9)

Once the events of tissue injury are initiated, many factors or agents come into play. Activated pancreatic proteolytic enzymes, such as trypsin, activate other enzymes, including phospholipase A and chymotrypsin (Table 63.1). (1-10) Trypsin digests peri-pancreatic tissue, elastase, the lamina of blood vessels, and phospholipase A converts lecithin into lysolecithin (tissue toxic). (1-9) Additionally, vasoactive agents are released, such as kinins, kallikrein, which alter capillary permeability and have significant cardiovascular effects. (1-9) The role of free fatty acids remains ill-defined.

TABLE 63.1   Proteolytic Enzymes of Pancreas

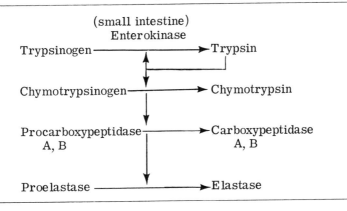

The net result could be a decrease in systemic blood pressure due to reduced intravascular plasma volume and release of vasoactive agents, fat necrosis, and reduced serum calcium level, the latter possibly due to impaired calcium release from bone and/or abnormal parathormone response. Respiratory failure or renal failure may develop in a small percentage of cases. (1-9)

3. (F) Mumps pancreatitis is uncommon in the preschool age period. It is usually mild to moderate in severity. Clinical mumps is present in 50% or more of the cases. (1-6)

4. (A,B) A clinical diagnosis can be suggested by the constellation of symptoms and physical signs, but generally requires more objective, laboratory evidence. The cornerstone of diagnosis has been the serum amylase level, which is abnormally elevated in the vast majority of cases, 70 to 90%. (1-10) Levels over 3 times normal are significant. Amylase is rapidly excreted by the kidneys, can be measured in the urine, too, and the serum level can return to normal within 24 to 72 hours, regardless of the clinical pattern. (1-17) Urine amylase will remain elevated for days to a few weeks, and can be particularly useful in milder cases or later in the disease. (11-15) However, false-positive levels in urine or serum can occur in other conditions, such as penetrating or perforated ulcers, regional enteritis, diabetic ketoacidosis, and renal failure. (11-15,17) Amylase is actually composed of several isozymes (at least seven) and pancreatic types can be identified by electrophoretic techniques, such as agarose and polyacrylamide. (10-17) Isozyme analysis has not been applied to any extent in clinical conditions of children.

A recently developed and more accurate test is the amylase creatinine clearance ratio (% C amylase/C creatinine = 100 X U amylase/S amylase X S creatinine/U creatinine) (S = serum; U = urine; C = clearance). (11-13) Renal amylase clearance rises significantly in acute pancreatitis but usually not in other conditions. (11,12) The accuracy approaches 95%. (11,12)

Other possible helpful studies include the serum lipase level, which has a slow return to normal, usually 2 to 3 weeks, ascitic fluid analysis for amylase (paracentesis), and less frequently, methemalbumin, a heme metabolite attached to albumin in hemorrhagic pancreatitis, in particular. (17,18) Serum calcium levels fall according to the condition. (1-5,17) If quite low, less than 7 mg%, the prognosis is poor. (17) Hypocalcemia can occur early or late in the disease course. (17)

Radiological examination can occasionally be helpful and can show the lack of free intraperitoneal air and presence of sentinel loops on plain films, or irregularity of the antrum and duodenum, particularly the C-loop (second portion). Oral or intravenous cholangiography could demonstrate a stone(s). Ultrasonography and/or computerized axial tomography have been clinically both discouraging and encouraging. Ultrasonography, in particular, has been the most reliable noninvasive technique for diagnosis of pancreatic inflammation, pseudocyst, and/or abscess. (7,13) So-called provocative tests, such as secretin-pancreozymin

stimulation (pancreatic enzymes, volume, bicarbonate) and mor-
phine-prostigmine stimulation (serum amylase level and pain)
have had limited use in children. Moreover, their value is mar-
ginal, since the diagnosis is usually possible with other studies
and definitive interpretation of results is frequently difficult. Endoscopic retrograde pancreatography is technically difficult in infants and younger children, and may not be of particular diagnostic
value. Additional pediatric experience will be necessary to make
any conclusions regarding its relative value.

5. (A, B, D) Treatment will depend to a great extent on the patient's clinical condition and the apparent severity of the disease
process. However, a medical approach is preferable. This
regimen will include (1) discontinuation of oral intake; (2) nasogastric suction; (3) intravenous fluids, such as electrolytes-dex-
trose, at a rate commensurate with clinical need, colloid (plasma, salt-poor albumin, blood) for shock-like states; (4) anticholinergics, e.g., atropine, 0.01-0.02 mg/kg, in order to counter-
act vagal stimulation of pancrease (enzyme volume, bicarbonate);
(5) analgesics, e.g., meperidine, 1 mg/kg intramuscularly,
since morphine and codeine produce more spasm of the sphincter
of Oddi; (6) antibiotics, broad-spectrum, e.g., ampicillin, 150-
200 mg/kg/24 hr, in moderate or severe cases; (7) insulin in
few cases only; and (8) surgery if necessary (refer to answer 6).
Of course, throughout management, close monitoring of vital
signs, intake and output, central venous pressure in moderate
or severe cases, and of serum electrolytes, calcium, glucose,
and other parameters is continued. (1-9, 17-19)

The subsidence or disappearance of pain, return of bowel
sounds, and stabilization of other clinical and laboratory parameters are indications for discontinuation of nasogastric suction
and initiation of oral intake, either clear liquids or a soft, bland,
low-fat diet. (1-9, 17-19) Elemental diets could be utilized effectively at this time, so as to provide minimal pancreatic stimulation and maximal nutrient intake, e.g., calories. (17) In selected cases, total parenteral nutrition (TPN), peripheral/cen-
tral, may be necessary. Anticholinergics are continued, and
antacids may be administered to further buffer acid (reduced secretin release). Evidence of reduced pancreatic functional capacity is an indication for replacement therapy, including Viokase, Cotazym, and Pancreatin granules.

Two controversial measures in treatment have been aprotinin (Trasylol) and glucagon. Trasylol is an inhibitor of proteolytic enzymes, including trypsin, chymotrypsin, and kallikrein,
and has been effective in studies of experimental pancreatitis,

but particularly ineffective in clinical studies. (17,19) The current recommendation is not to use it. Glucagon reduces pancreatic secretion, but has been ineffective in small controlled clinical trials. (17,19) Steroids have no role in management.

6. (F) Surgery has a role in management in certain instances. These include (1) diagnosis, e.g., signs of peritonitis, positive paracentesis; (2) surgical drainage and peritoneal lavage in more fulminant pancreatitis and secondary cardiovascular decompensation; such patients will have enormous losses of plasma volume, as much as fourfold in older children and adolescents (removal of vasoactive substances, reducing colloid requirement); and (3) debridement of necrotic tissue, drainage of abscess(es) or pseudocyst(s), occurring in as many as 40 to 45% of severe (fulminant) cases. (17-23) Surgery, i.e., exploratory laparotomy, does not add to the morbidity or mortality of the disease, provided that unwarranted dissection around the pancreas is avoided. (17-23)

Other, less common indications in children include intestinal perforation and acute cholecystitis without cholelithiasis. (17-23) Operative cholangiography can be attempted, and if indicated, pancreatography can be performed, too.

7. (B,C) Almost 10 to 15% of patients will develop an inflammatory locus in the first two to four weeks after the acute attack. (1-8,17-22) This locus can be (1) a phlegmon or solid area with varying necrosis, usually subsiding spontaneously within 7 to 14 days; (2) abscess (5%) secondary to infection of necrotic areas by colonic flora, occurring predominantly in severe cases (over 90% of such abscesses), multiple in 30% and requiring surgical drainage; and (3) pseudocyst (1 to 5%) formation, having permanence once a capsule is formed and requiring surgical (internal) drainage, e.g., into stomach or defunctionalized jejunum. (17-23)

Fortunately, the overwhelming majority of cases are mild, and the mortality is only 1 to 2% in medically treated patients. With surgically treated cases, other than severe (fulminant) forms, the mortality rises to 5-10%. (1-8,17-22) In fulminant disease, the mortality may be as high as 25% in the medically treated and up to 85% in the surgically treated. (1-9,17-23) Underlying disease elsewhere, such as hepatic or renal, makes the prognosis worse.

Also see Figure 63.1.

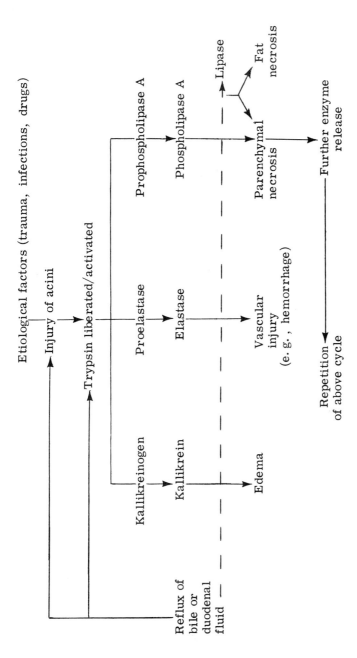

Figure 63.1 Pathogenesis of Pancreatis. Modified from Banks, P. A.: Gastroenterology 61:382, 1971.

REFERENCES

1. Crentzfeldt, W. and Schmidt, H.: Aetiology and pathogenesis of pancreatitis (current concepts). Scand J Gastroenterol (suppl. 6):47, 1970.

2. Hartley, R.C.: Pancreatitis under the age of five years: A report of three cases. J Pediat Surg 2:419, 1967.

3. Frey, C. and Redo, S.F.: Inflammatory lesions of the pancreas in infancy and childhood. Pediatrics 32:93, 1963.

4. Fonkalsrud, G.W. , Hennery, R.P. , Reimenschneider, T.A. , et al. : Management of pancreatitis in infants and children. Am J Surg 116:198, 1968.

5. Hendren, W.H. , Greep, J.M. , Patton, A.S.: Pancreatitis in childhood: Experience with 15 cases. Arch Dis Child 40:132, 1965.

6. Pena, S.D.J. and Medovy, H.: Child abuse and traumatic pseudocyst of the pancreas. J Pediatr 83:1026, 1973.

7. Jordan, S.C. , Ament, M.E.: Pancreatitis in children and adolescents. J Pediatr 91:211, 1977.

8. Geokas, M.C. , Van Lancker, J.L. , Kadell, B.M. , et al.: Acute pancreatitis, Ann Intern Med 76:105, 1972.

9. Wyatt, A.P.: Diagnosis and management of acute pancreatitis. Ann R Coll Surg Engl 54:229, 1974.

10. Webster, P.D. and Zieve, L.: Alteration in serum content of pancreatic enzymes. N Engl J Med 267:604, 654, 1962.

11. Warshaw, A.L. and Fuller, A.F. , Jr.: Specificity of increased renal clearance of amylase in diagnosis of acute pancreatitis. N Engl J Med 292:325, 1975.

12. Johnston, S.G. , Ellis, C.J. , Levitt, M.D.: Mechanism of increased renal clearance of amylase/creatinine in acute pancreatitis. N Engl J Med 295:12, 14, 1976.

13. Cox, K.L. , Ament, M.E. , Sample, W.F. , et al.: The ultrasonic and biochemical diagnosis of pancreatitis in children. J Pediatr 96:407, 1980.

14. Wieme, R.J.: Note on amylase isoenzymes of human serum. Curr Prob Clin Biochem 2:293, 1968.

15. Hobbs, J.R. and Aw, S.E.: Urinary isoamylases. Curr Probl Clin Biochem 2:281, 1968.

16. Lehrner, L.M., Ward, J.C., Harn, R.C., et al.: An evaluation of the usefulness of amylase isozyme differentiation in patients with hyperamylasemia. Am J Clin Pathol 66:576, 1976.

17. Silverman, A., Roy, C.C.: Pediatric Clinical Gastroenterology, 3rd edition. The CV Mosby Company, St. Louis, 1983, p. 843.

18. Ranson, J.H.C., Rifkind, K.M., Turner, J.W.: Prognostic signs and nonoperative peritoneal lavage in acute pancreatitis. Surg Gynecol Obstet 143:209, 1976.

19. Tuzhilin, S.A.: The clinical features of pancreatic inflammation. Am J Gastroenterol 61:97, 1974.

20. Warshaw, A.I., Imbembo, A.L., Civetta, J.M., et al.: Surgical intervention in acute necrotizing pancreatitis. Am J Surg 127:484, 1974.

21. Warshaw, A.L.: Inflammatory masses following acute pancreatitis: Phlegmon, pseudocyst, and abscess. Surg Clin North Am 54:621, 1974.

22. Jacobs, M.L., Daggett, W.M., Civetta, J.M., et al.: Acute pancreatitis: Analysis of factors influencing survival. Ann Surg 185:43, 1977.

23. Buntain, W.L., Wood, J.B., Wooley, M.M.: Pancreatitis in childhood. J Pediatr Surg 13:143, 1978.

Case 64

RIGHT UPPER QUADRANT PAIN AND GENERALIZED MALAISE IN A 14-YEAR-OLD BOY

HISTORY

A 14-year-old white male presented with a history of generalized malaise, nausea, bloating, and upper abdominal aching of 5 days' duration. The pain was located in the right upper quadrant without radiation and was not related to meals, food types, time of day, position, or bowel movements. The bowel habit pattern continued to be 1-2 bowel movements daily, soft to firm in nature. There was no definite history of associated fever, vomiting, diarrhea, constipation, melena, hematochezia, skin lesions, arthralgia, ocular difficulties, or trauma. There was a history of a 10-year-old sister with a similar clinical pattern approximately 2 weeks prior to onset of the patient's clinical pattern, disappearing shortly thereafter. In addition, the mother had had a prior history of possible serum hepatitis 19 years before without sequelae. The remainder of the past history, developmental history, family history, social history, and review of systems was unremarkable.

EXAMINATION

He was alert, cooperative, and in no apparent distress, with normal vital signs, weight 51 kg, and height 139 cm. The remainder of the examination was unremarkable except for a palpable liver, 2.0 cm below the right costal margin in the midclavicular line, mildly tender to palpation, firm in nature, and not nodular. The total span by percussion was 7.5 cm. The spleen and kidneys were not palpable. Active bowel sounds were present, but no bruits.

LABORATORY DATA

Hemoglobin:	12.8 gm%
Hematocrit:	38%
White blood cell count:	8,900/mm^3
PMN's:	54%
lymphocytes:	40%
monocytes:	4%
eosinophiles:	2%
Sedimentation rate:	15 mm/hr (< 20)
Urinalysis:	negative
Urine amylase:	3,400 units
Serum:	
total protein:	7.1 gm%
albumin:	4.9 gm%
SGOT:	75 units
SGPT:	85 units
total bilirubin:	1.8 mg%
direct bilirubin:	1.4 mg%
alkaline phosphatase:	140 IU
amylase:	100 units
lipase:	0.8 units
prothrombin time:	11.0 sec
control:	12.0 sec
rheumatoid factor:	negative
ANA:	negative
monospot:	negative
HbsAg:	negative
antiHbs:	negative
HbcAg:	negative
antiHbc:	negative
Plain films - abdomen:	negative
Oral cholecystogram:	no visualization

QUESTIONS

Question 1: Answer true (T) or false (F).

1. Acute cholecystitis in children almost always occurs in the presence of stones.

2. Which of the following associated conditions have been found with acute cholecystitis in children?
   A. Typhoid fever
   B. Parasites (G. lamblia, ascaris)
   C. Peptic ulcer disease
   D. Hiatus hernia
   E. Hemoglobinopathies (sickle cell disease, thalassemia)

Questions 3-7: Answer true (T) or false (F).

3. This disorder occurs particularly in males, 4:1.

4. The most frequent presentation of this condition is right-sided abdominal pain.

5. Fatty food intolerance is frequent in children.

6. Laboratory studies, including the white blood cell count, total bilirubin, and amylase levels, may be diagnostic in the acute condition.

7. Oral cholecystography (nonfilling) is not as helpful in diagnosis in children as in adults.

8. Stones, when found, contain which of the following?
   A. Bilirubin
   B. Cystine
   C. Cholesterol
   D. Oxalate
   E. Chenodeoxycholate

9. The treatment of choice is which of the following?
   A. Antibiotics
   B. Cholecystokinin
   C. Low-fat diet
   D. Metoclopramide
   E. Cholecystectomy

ANSWERS AND COMMENTS

1. (F) Acute cholecystitis remains an uncommon disease in the pediatric age, being 1:1,000 as common as in adults. (1-7) It occurs more frequently in the absence of stones than in their presence. (1-7) There has been an association with intercurrent illnesses, e.g., pneumonitis, bacterial entercolitis. (1-8) A unifying concept has been postulated in the absence of stones,

i.e., biliary stagnation. (1-8) The end result is biliary stasis, concentration, and possible stone formation. (1-7) The latter is a result of an alteration of the ratio of the components of bile, notably cholesterol, bile salts, and phospholipid, (lecithin). (4, 6) Stones within the cystic or common bile ducts are not commonly discovered. Hydrops of the gallbladder is uncommon. (1-8) At times, common duct stones may actually lodge in the ampulla of Vater, simulating acute or relapses of hepatitis.

2. (A,B,E) As mentioned in answer 1, there are a number of systemic diseases implicated as causes of biliary stagnation. Intestinal bacterial infections, such as typhoid fever, shigellosis, gastroenteritis, scarlet fever, pneumonia, and parasitic infection (such as giardiasis and ascariasis) have been associated with acute cholecystitis. Biliary stagnation within the gallbladder ("obstruction") could then predispose to secondary bacterial or viral invasion. Cultures of the gallbladder or of bile have disclosed positive bacterial cultures in as many as 50 to 60%. The most common organisms have been E. coli, Klebsiella-enterobacter, enterococci, Clostridia (perfringens), and staphylococci. (1-7) Hereditary red blood cell disorders (such as spherocytosis) and hemoglobinopathies (such as sickle cell disease, thalassemia) have been well-known causes of gallbladder disease in pediatric patients. (1-12) In addition, congenital anomalies can lead to biliary stagnation, especially intrabiliary. (1-7) Mechanical causes include choledochal cysts and biliary atresia. However, these causes seem to play a small role in pathogenesis (small number of patients with cholecystitis). (1-7)

3. (F) The incidence in females is quite striking, and this female preponderance is more prominent in calculous than a calculous disease. (1-7) The usual female:male ratio is 4:1. (1-7)

4. (T) The acute onset of right upper quadrant pain, colicky or steady, is present in essentially all patients. (1-7) In infants or toddlers, localization of pain may be difficult, but the intensity is usually maximum in the right upper quadrant. (1-13) However, in the early phase of this condition, the pain may be maximum in the epigastrium or in the periumbilical region. In 2/3 to 3/4 of cases, nausea and vomiting are present. (1-7) Jaundice is present in only 20 to 25%. (1-7) Fever is present in only a small percentage. (1-7)

The physical examination may reveal variable tenderness in the right upper quadrant or elsewhere, voluntary guarding, and, less commonly, rebound tenderness or a mass. (1-7) Tenderness in the back or provocative maneuvers, e.g., "punch," is usually negative. (1-7)

5. (F) A history of fatty food intolerance is quite uncommon in children. (1-7) However, in one series, in cases with symptoms less than 6 months in duration, fat intolerance was present in 12.5%. (1-7)

6. (F) Laboratory studies are not particularly helpful. The white blood cell count may be elevated, with a polymorphonuclear predominance. However, this is obviously a nonspecific finding. Total bilirubin, serum enzymes (SGOT, SGPT), and serum amylase may be elevated, but, once again, they are nonspecific. Additionally, the sedimentation rate may be increased, suggesting an inflammatory condition, but more commonly the elevation is slight and thus not of significant aid. (1-7)

7. (T) Absolute diagnosis of acute cholecystitis is frequently not possible by oral cholecystography, since a lack of visualization is frequent. This nonfilling is not as helpful as in adults, i.e., correlative with the finding of inflammation within. Potentially helpful is the lack of emptying of contrast material from the gallbladder after stimulation with cholecystokinin or a fatty meal. This finding is indicative of an obstruction of the cystic or common bile duct. (1-8) The role of ultrasonography, grey scale or otherwise, has not been adequately evaluated in children, but can be useful to separate calculous cholecystitis from acute noncalculous cholecystitis and/or acute hydrops of the gallbladder. (1-8, 14) Nuclear medicine techniques (scanning), i.e., HIDA 99m TC, has been helpful in the diagnosis of acute cholecystitis (filling-poor to absent), less so chronic cholecystitis (wall thickening; decreased visualization) in adults, but has not been adequately studied in children. Computed tomography (CT scan) has not been assessed in children but in adults offers no advantage to ultrasonography. (1-8) Transhepatic cholangiography, percutaneous, and endoscopic retrograde cholangiopancreatography (ERCP) have been helpful in occasional pediatric patients, but additional pediatric experience will be necessary before a conclusion regarding its potential role can be reached. These two procedures are particularly directed toward evaluation of obstructive lesions. (1-8) Intravenous cholangiography is seldom indicated.

8. (A, C) Gallstones are not common in the cystic or common bile ducts, occurring in only 3 to 15% in most series. (1-7, 13) However, the incidence has been as high as 67%. (1-7, 13) Furthermore, cholelithiasis is proportionately more frequent in adolescence. (1-7, 13) These stones are composed of bilirubin or cholesterol. (1-7, 13) Certain conditions predispose to stone formation, including hemolytic states, such as sickle cell anemia

(10%), obesity, malformations of cystic or common bile ducts, parasites, cystic fibrosis, and metachromatic leukodystrophy. (1-7,13) Stones are uncommon before 8 to 10 years of age. (1-13) Other potentially lithogenic factors include pH, protein and mucus content, drugs, e.g., oral contraceptives. (6,8)

9. (E) Cholecystectomy (early; delayed) is the treatment of choice. (1-13,15) Occasionally, severe inflammation may necessitate cholecystostomy with or without later removal of the gallbladder. Common duct exploration should be undertaken if it is dilated or thick-walled, if there are palpable stones, or if there has been a prior history of pancreatitis or jaundice. Operative cholangiography may be in order. The prognosis is excellent with very low morbidity or mortality, unless there is an underlying hemolytic disease. (1-13)

The chemical dissolution (bile acid use) of stone(s) in the gallbladder has not been evaluated in children. Its potential role in treatment would and should certainly be limited. (8)

REFERENCES

1. Crystal, R.J. and Fink, R.L.: Acute acalculous cholecystitis in childhood: A report of two cases. Clin Pediatr 10: 423, 1971.

2. Gravier, L., Porman, G.W., Vitteler, T.P.: Gallbladder disease in infants and children. Surgery 63:690, 1968.

3. Morales, L., Taboada, E., Toledo, L., et al.: Cholecystitis and cholelithiasis in children. J Pediatr Surg 2:565, 1967.

4. Sears, H.F., Golden, G.T., Horsley, J.S., III: Cholecystitis in childhood and adolescence. Arch Surg 106:651, 1973.

5. Strauss, R.G.: Cholelithiasis in childhood. Am J Dis Child 117:689, 1969.

6. Calabrese, C. and Pearlman, D.M.: Gallbladder disease below the age of 21 years. Surgery 70:413, 1971.

7. Murgas, I.: Inflammation of the gallbladder in children. I Rozhl Chir 44:103, 1965.

8. Silverman, A., Roy, C.C.: Pediatric Clinical Gastroen-
    terology, 3rd edition. The CV Mosby Company, St. Louis,
    1983, p. 798.

9. Chamberlain, J.W. and Hight, D.W.: Acute hydrops of
    the gallbladder in childhood. Surgery 68:899, 1970.

10. Dewey, K.W. , Grossman, H. , Canale, V.C. : Cholelithi-
    asis in thalassemia major. Radiology 96:385, 1970.

11. Flye, M.W. and Silver, D.: Biliary tract disorders and
    sickle cell disease. Surgery 72:361, 1972.

12. Cameron, J.L., Maddrey, W.C., Zuidema, G.D.: Bili-
    ary tract disease in sickle cell anemia: Surgical consid-
    erations. Ann Surg 174:702, 1971.

13. Whitaker, J.A., Windmiller, J., Viett, T., et al.: He-
    reditary spherocytosis associated with sickle trait and
    cholelithiasis. J Pediatr 63:65, 1963.

14. Holt, R.W., Wagner, R., Homa, M.: Ultrasonic diagno-
    sis of cholelithiasis. J Pediatr 92:418, 1978.

15. Mitchell, A., Morris, P.J.: Trends in management of
    acute cholecystitis. Br Med J 284:27, 1982.

INDEX

566 / Index

Folic acid
  deficiency of, 206, 242
Foramina of Bochdalek and Morgagni, 2, 4, 5, 7
Foreign bodies
  in alimentary tract. See Esophagus
Formulas
  caloric intake and, 156-159
  composition of, 156-159, 204
  in diarrhea, 156-159, 185, 193,
    204, 217
  failure to thrive diagnosis and, 204
  for gavage feedings, 159, 204
  low-fat, 482
Fructose, 183
Functional intestinal obstruction, 310
Fundoplication, 113, 114
Fungal disease. See Parasitic and
  fungal disease

Galactose. See also Galactosemia
  absorption of, 183, 184, 191
Galactosemia
  jaundice and, 418
  neonatal hepatitis and, 418
  tests for, 418
Gallbladder
  cystic fibrosis and, 558
  jaundice and, 557
  noncalculous distention of, 557
  radiologic procedures and, 557,
    558
  recurrent abdominal pain and, 557
Gallstones, 461, 556, 558
Gamma globulin
  hepatitis and, 421
    chronic active, 446, 450
  intestinal lymphangiectasis and,
    213-215
Ganglion cells
  Hirschsprung's disease and, 311. See
    also Hirschsprung's disease
  in myenteric plexus, 100, 311
Gastric acid. See also Hydrochloric
    acid
  measurement of, 124-127
  peptic ulcer and, 134-135
  Zollinger-Ellison syndrome and, 158
Gastric burns, 94
Gastric emptying time, 262
Gastric hypersecretion, 144
Gastric lavage, bleeding and, 490
Gastric suction. See Nasogastric suc-
  tion
Gastric ulcer. See Peptic disease
Gastric varices, 144-146

Gastrin
  assays of, 134, 135, 144, 145
  Zollinger-Ellison syndrome and,
    144, 145, 147
Gastritis. See also Gastroenteritis
  corrosive, 94
  hematemesis and, 490
  panendoscopy and, 490
  rectal bleeding and, 490
  vomiting and, 489
Gastrocolic reflex, 263
Gastroenteritis. See also Enteritis;
    Gastritis
  acute, 489
    nonspecific, 153-159, 555
    vomiting and, 164-166
  bacterial, 163-169, 223, 225, 556
  diarrhea and, 153-155
  eosinophilic, 174-176
  Hirschsprung's disease and, 309, 310
  infectious, 163-169, 223-225
  lactose and, 156, 176
  malnutrition and, 156
  viral, 153-161
  pain and, 153, 154
Gastroenteropathy
  allergic
    ulcerative colitis and, 279
  diarrhea and, 153-155
Gastroesophageal reflux. See Reflux,
    gastroesophageal
Gastrointestinal emergencies of neo-
    nate
  diaphragmatic hernia and, 4-6
  intestinal obstruction and. See Intes-
    tinal obstruction
  meconium plug syndrome and, 32, 33
  necrotizing enterocolitis and, 309,
    310
  perforations and, 309
  peritonitis and, 309
Gastrointestinal immunocyte complex,
    241, 242
Gastrointestinal tract
  bleeding from. See Bleeding, gastro-
    intestinal
  diseases of. See specific disease
  immune competence and, 201, 202
  injury to. See Duodenum hematoma
    of
  obstruction in. See Intestinal ob-
    sturction
  small bowel biopsy and. See Celi-
    ac disease
  tumors of. See Tumors
Gastrostomy

Ileocecal valve, 240, 291
Ileocolitis, granulomatous, 240-246
Ileostomy
  Hirschsprung's disease and, 312,
    313
  inflammatory bowel disease, 293
  meconium ileus and, 33, 34
Ileum
  atresia of, 27
  obstruction of, 30-34, 245, 246
  perforation of, 30-34, 245, 246
  stenosis of, 27
Ileus
  adynamic, 230-233
  functional, 230-233
  meconium. See Meconium ileus
Immune competence, 125, 126
Immune deficiencies. See also Immuno-
    globulins
  celiac disease and, 201, 202
  Crohn's disease and, 241, 242
  diarrhea and, 334, 335
  malabsorption and, 206
  milk allergy and, 175, 176
  thymic alymphoplasia and, 124, 125
  thymic dysplasia and, 124, 125
  ulcerative colitis and, 278-280
Immune homeostasis
  gastrointestinal diseases and, 124-
    126, 175, 176, 200-205, 270
  immune competence and, 124-126
  primary immune deficiencies and,
    124, 125
Immune responses, abnormal, 124-
    126, 201, 202
Immunity
  cellular, 201-202, 241, 242, 270,
    446, 447
  humoral, 124-126, 201, 202, 241,
    242, 270, 446, 447
Immunization
  in virus hepatitis, 421
Immunocyte complex, gastrointes-
    tinal, 124-126
Immunoelectrophoresis, 446
Immunoglobulins. See also Immune
    deficiencies
  celiac disease and, 201, 202, 241,
    242
  deficiency of
    giardiasis and, 270, 334, 335
    IgA, 201, 202, 241, 242, 270, 446
    lymphoid polyposis and, 270
  IgA
    isolated deficiency of, 270
    tests for, 201, 202, 241, 242

IgE, 176, 201, 202, 241, 242, 279
IgG, 201, 202, 241, 242, 446
IgM, 201, 202, 241, 242, 446
  elevation of, 202, 446
  tests for, 201, 202
  viral hepatitis and, 446
Immunologic disorders. See Immune
    deficiencies
Immunologic reactivity, hepatitis and,
    446, 447
Immunosuppressives
  in Crohn's disease, 244
  hepatitis and,
    chronic, 449, 450
    chronic active, 449, 450
  liver transplantation of, 464
  ulcerative colitis and, 292
Impactions, fecal. See Fecal impac-
    tions
Imperforate anus. See Anus, imper-
    forate
Imuran. See Azathioprine
Inborn errors of metabolism
  liver and, 500, 501
  malabsorption and, 158
Incontinence, fecal
  anorectal anomalies and, 67, 68
Indirect hemagglutination test, 362
Infants
  formulas for. See Formulas
  intractable diarrhea of, 158, 159
Infection. See also Inflammation;
    Sepsis
  appendicitis and, 254, 255
  ascites and, 402
  bacterial. See Bacteria
  biliary atresia and, 77
  cholecystitis and, 556-558
  cirrhosis and, 77
  Crohn's disease and, 240, 241
  cryptitis and, 318
  diarrhea and, 153-155, 166-168
  enterocolitis and
    necrotizing, 309, 310
    neonatal, 309, 310
  fungal. See Parasitic and fungal
    disease
  jaundice and, 78
  parasitic. See Parasitic and fun-
    gal disease
  perianal, 243
  protein-losing enteropathy and, 214
  ulcerative colitis and, 278, 290
  of urinary tract. See Urinary tract
    infection
Inferior vena cava, 522

radioactive. See Rose bengal
^{131}I test
Iproniazid, 473, 474
Iron. See Iron-deficiency anemia
Iron-binding capacity, 201, 202
Iron-deficiency anemia
  celiac disease and, 201, 202
  Crohn's disease and, 243
  milk allergy and, 175
Irritable colon syndrome
  diarrhea and, 262, 263
  recurrent abdominal pain and, 262,
    263
Ischemia of bowel, enterocolitis and.
    See Necrosis
Islet cell tumors, 144
Isoimmunization. See Autoimmune
    phenomenon
  jaundice and, 78
  neonatal hepatitis and, 78
  RH. See Erythroblastosis
Isomaltase
  deficiency of, 156-159, 189-196
Isomaltase-sucrase deficiencies,
    156-159, 189-196
Isoniazid, 474

Jaundice
  alpha-1-antitrypsin deficiency and,
    424
  cholecystitis and, 557
  cholelithiasis and, 557
  in cirrhosis, 448
  Coombs' test and, 281, 417
  evaluation of, 445-448
  hepatitis and
    acute viral, 416
    chronic, 445-448
    chronic active, 445-448
    drug-induced, 472, 473
    fulminating, 453, 464
    toxin-induced, 472, 473
  hyperbilirubinemia and. See Hyper-
    bilirubinemia
  liver abscess and, 361, 362, 364
  obstructive
    biliary atresia in. See Biliary
      atresia
    cystic fibrosis and, 421
    neonatal hepatitis in. See Hepatitis,
      neonatal
  physiologic, of newborn, 78
  Wilson's disease and, 461, 462
Jejunum
  atresia of, 27

biopsy of
  celiac disease and, 203
  giardiasis and, 335
obstruction of
  congenital, 26, 27
Juvenile polyps, 301-304

Kasai procedure, 76, 77
Kayser-Fleischer rings, 460-462, 464
Kernicterus. See Jaundice
Kidneys
  ascites and, 398, 399

L-dopamine, 473
Laboratory studies. See Tests
Lactase
  deficiency of, 156-159, 176, 180-
    188, 204, 242
  diarrhea and, 156-159, 176, 182-
    184, 242, 335
  milk allergies and, 176, 204
  mucosal enzyme assay and, 158,
    184-186, 203, 206, 335
  primary, 180-188
  tests for, 158, 184-186, 203, 206
Lactic acid dehydrogenase, 78
Lactinex, 260
Lactose
  absorption test, 158, 184-186, 206
  feces test and, 158, 183, 184, 206
  intolerance to
    tests for, 158, 184-186, 206
Lactose-free diet, 156-159, 186, 204,
    243
Lactose-free formula, 156-159, 186,
    204, 243
Lactulose, 504
Lamina propria
  celiac disease and, 203
  diarrhea and, 155
Lavage, gastric, 490
LDH. See Lactic acid dehydrogenase
LE prep. See Lupus erythematosus
LES pressures. See Lower esophageal
    sphincter pressures
Leukemia, 471, 472
Leukocytes, 449
Levamisole, 450
Levator and muscle complex, 312,
    322, 323
Ligament of Treitz, 203
Linton tube, 489, 492
Lipase, 538, 540
  duodenal contents and, 538, 540
  fat digestion and, 538, 540

Picornaviruses, 153, 154
Pilocarpine iontophoresis test. See
  Sweat test
Pinworms, 383-388
Piperazine, 388
Pi system. See Protease inhibitor
  system
Pitressin. See Vasopressin
Pneumonia
  achalasia and. See Achalasia
  aspiration. See Reflux, gastro-
    esophageal
Polyposis. See Polyps
Polyps
  adenomatous polyposis of colon and,
    303, 304
  generalized juvenile polyposis and,
    302, 303
  intussusception and, 302
  juvenile polyposis coli and, 301-
    304
  lymphoid polyposis in, 267-272
  rectal bleeding and, 302
Porphyria, 508-516
Portacaval anastomoses. See Anas-
    tomoses, portacaval
Portal hypertension
  abdominal distention and, 489
  biliary atresia and, 77
  cirrhosis and, 421, 427, 429
  extrahepatic
    clinical features of, 487, 489
    etiology of, 490, 491
    laboratory studies of, 489-493
    medical management of, 492
  gastrointestinal bleeding and, 487,
    489-491
  hematemesis and, 487
  hemorrhoids and, 491
  hepatitis and
    chronic active, 448, 450
    neonatal, 421
  intrahepatic, 448, 450
    biliary hypoplasia and, 483
  Wilson's disease and, 462, 464
Portal vein
  obstruction of
    rectal bleeding and, 491
    portal hypertension and. See Portal
      hypertension
Portal-systemic shunting, 492, 493
Portoenterostomy, hepatic, 77
Postsinusoidal portal hypertension,
  491
Potassium
  ascites and, 449

chronic active hepatitis and, 449
Prednisone. See also Steroids
  and azathioprine
  in celiac crisis, 205
  in Crohn's disease, 244
  esophageal burns and, 94, 95
  hepatitis and
    chronic, 449, 450
    chronic active, 449, 450
  ulcerative colitis and, 292
Pregestimil
  in biliary atresia, 77
  in cirrhosis, 421, 429
  in contaminated small bowel syn-
    drome, 27
  diarrhea and, 159
  fats in. See Medium-chain trigly-
    cerides
  gavage feedings and, 159
  intrahepatic biliary hypoplasia and,
    482
  milk allergy and, 176
  short bowel syndrome, 27
Pregnane-3alpha-20beta-diol, 78
Prematurity. See Neonate
Primperan. See Metoclopramide
Pro-Banthine. See Propantheline
  bromide
Procarboxypeptidase, 547
Proctitis, 291
Proctologic disorders, 316-328
Prolapse of rectum. See Proctologic
  disorders
Propantheline bromide, 293
Prostaglandins, 138
Prostigmine, 233
Protease inhibitor system, 428-430
Protein electrophoresis
  serum. See Liver function tests
Protein homeostasis, tests of, 215-
  217
Protein-losing enteropathy
  albumin metabolism in, 215-217
  chylothorax in, 214
  chylous ascites in, 214, 400
  clinical findings in, 214
  differential diagnosis in, 214
  eosinophilic gastroenteritis in, 214
  immune homeostasis and, 215, 216
  intestinal lymphangiectasis in, 214-
    217
  milk allergy in, 214
  pathogenesis of, 216, 217
  tests for, 215-217
Proteins
  allergy to, diarrhea and, 174-175

of fat absorption and metabolism,
206
gastric acid, 124-126, 135, 144
glucose tolerance. See Glucose;
Lactose; Sucrose
lactose absorption, 158, 184-186,
206
of liver function. See Liver function tests
maltose absorption, 158, 186
for occult blood in stool. See Bleeding
pancreatic function. See Pancreatic
function tests
of protein homeostasis and enteric
protein loss, 213-215
red cell peroxide hemolysis. See
Vitamins, E
Schilling, 206
sucrose absorption, 158, 186, 192,
193
for sugars in feces, 158, 186, 192,
206
sweat. See Sweat test
Tetany
celiac disease and, 202
short bowel syndrome and. See
specific condition
Tetracycline
in contaminated small bowel syndrome, 232, 233
in Crohn's disease, 244
in Yersinia infections, 225
Thalassemia, 78
Thiamine. See Vitamins
Thorazine. See Chlorpromazine
Thrombocytopenia
cirrhosis and, 448
hematemesis and, 489, 490
Shwachman's syndrome and, 538
Thrombus
of inferior vena cava, 492
of protal vein, 491
Tocopherol
obstructive jaundice and, 75, 76
Tonometry, anorectal. See Hirschsprung's disease
Total parenteral alimentation. See
Parenteral alimentation
Toxic megacolon, 293, 294
Toxin-induced hepatitis, 471-474
Toxins
diarrhea and, 166
jaundice and, 471-474
Toxoplasmosis
jaundice and, 421

neonatal hepatitis and, 421
TPA. See Total parenteral alimenta-
tion
TPN. See Triphosphopyridine nucleo-
tide
Transaminases, serum hepatitis. See
Hepatitis, acute viral and chron-
ic active
Transcobalamin. See Anemia, perni-
cious
Transferrin. See Iron
Transfusion
esophageal varices and, 492
hepatic coma and, 504
Reye's syndrome and, 504
Transit time, intestinal, 263
Transplantation
liver. See Liver, transplantation of
Trasylol. See Chymotrypsin inhibitor
Trauma to gastrointestinal tract
pancreatitis and, 546
Triglycerides
medium-chain. See Medium-chain
triglycerides
Trisomy 21. See Down's syndrome
Tri-Vi-Sol, 539
Trypsin
duodenal contents and, 538, 540
pancreatitis and, 546-549
Trypsinogen
deficiency of, 538-540
pancreatitis and, 546-549
Tube feedings, 159
Tuberculosis, 239, 242
Tumors
adenocarcinoma and, 281
carcinoid, 159
carcinoma and. See Carcinomas
hemangioma and. See Hemangiomas
hematemesis and. See Bleeding
hepatic. See Hepatic tumors
jaundice and, 519
lymphosarcoma of small inteetine
and. See Lymphosarcoma
pancreatic. See Pancreas, tumors
of
polyps, 301-304
Tween 80. See Polysorbate 80
Tylenol. See Acetaminophen
Typhoid fever, 168

UDPG dehydrogenase. See Uridine
diphosphate glucuronyltransferase
UDPG-T. See Uridine diphosphate
glucuronyltransferase